The Veterinarian's Encyclopedia of Animal Behavior

The Veterinarian's

Encyclopedia
of Animal
Behavior

BONNIE V. BEAVER
BS, MS, DVM, Diplomate ACVB

IOWA STATE UNIVERSITY PRESS / AMES

BONNIE V. BEAVER, BS, MS, DVM, Diplomate ACVB, is Professor and Chief of Medicine, College of Veterinary Medicine, Texas A&M University, College Station.

© 1994 Iowa State University Press, Ames, Iowa 50014

∞ Printed on acid-free paper in the United States of America

First edition, 1994

Library of Congress Cataloging-in-Publication Data

Beaver, B. V. G.

    The veterinarian's encyclopedia of animal behavior / Bonnie V. Beaver.–1st ed.
      p.   cm.
    Includes bibliographical references (p.   ) and index.
    ISBN 0-8138-2114-2
    1. Domestic animals—Behavior—Encyclopedias.   2. Veterinary medicine—Encyclopedias.   3. Animal behavior—Encyclopedias.
    I. Title.
    SF756.7.B43   1994
    599´.051´03—dc20   94-27257

The charter diplomates of the American College of Veterinary Behaviorists are internationally recognized experts who have joined their talents and resources to accomplish the difficult task of getting such a specialty organization off to a firm beginning. It is to the other seven ACVB charter diplomates that I dedicate this book—Robert K. Anderson, Sharon Crowell-Davis, Benjamin Hart, Katherine Houpt, Elizabeth Shull, Victoria Voith, and Tom Wolfle.

Contents

Preface

VETERINARY BEHAVIOR is unique to veterinary medicine because the growth of this discipline is based on the demand from outside the profession, rather than from within. Animal owners want to know how to raise "good citizens"; the public is demanding psychological well-being for laboratory animals; humane groups want to decrease needless euthanasia because of behavior problems; and livestock raisers want increased production with consideration of behavioral needs. Issues such as these require veterinarians to look at animal behavior as a service to their clients. The development of veterinary behavior actually draws from several closely related disciplines, including animal science, dermatology, ethology, internal medicine, neurology, neuroanatomy, neuropathology, neuropharmacology, neurophysiology, psychology, wildlife science, and zoology. While this diverse relationship helps to define the uniqueness of veterinary behavior, it also complicates the understanding of the discipline and the complexity of the language.

Because animal behavior is relatively new to the profession and not extensively taught in the curricula of colleges of veterinary medicine, veterinarians are having to learn what they can after graduation. Behavioral seminars are always popular at continuing education programs, but there is only so much a person can retain after one of those programs. Journal articles are widely scattered and only a few textbooks are available that are directed to the special needs of the practicing veterinarian. A bridge is still necessary between the common problems that most behavior seminars cover, the information in the literature, and those everyday questions that arise. This is the role of an encyclopedia—introductory knowledge about a lot of varied topics.

Much thought went into the format of this encyclopedia. It is not intended to read like a textbook, but rather to function like a reference for specific items. It should allow the reader to find specific subjects and learn something about them, find terms that are similar to or opposites of others, learn about the complexities of certain topics, and to compare behaviors between species. For me, one of the joys of having an encyclopedia or library around is to browse through various topics, learning about subjects I would never look up otherwise. Responses from others who have read the manuscript indicate this has been a plus for them as well. Because terms come from a variety of disciplines, one of the earliest problems a student of behavior encounters is finding a definition for a given word or concept. While there are at least three published dictionaries of ethology, none is complete relative to veterinary behavior. Nor do any discuss the diagnosis or treatment of the various problems practitioners see on a daily basis in the variety of animals served by the profession.

The terms in *The Veterinarian's Encyclopedia of Animal Behavior* are arranged in alphabetical order. Following the discussion of each term is a list of cross-references to other related topics for the reader. The cross-reference that is itself simply a synonym under which the information is actually found is introduced by "SEE"; all other cross-references are introduced by "ALSO SEE." Where appropriate, therapies are mentioned in the text of the discussion, and the reader is referred to a more in-depth discussion of the implementation under another section. For example, in the discussion of suggested treatments for lick granulomas, exercise and control of the dog's daily schedule are part of a long-term management protocol. Specifics on how each can be part of a behavioral modification program are found under "exercise" and "schedule." Complicated behaviors are broken down into more specific parts where possible. The topic of aggression is discussed in very broad terms and then the reader is directed to the various types of aggression, such as "fear-induced aggression," "hypothyroid aggression," or "play aggression."

Three appendixes are included for the convenience of the reader. The first (A) is a sample behavior problem history form, to assist in getting answers from an owner. While every behaviorist uses a different system, the one included here incorporates many of the features discussed under the history-taking section. The second appendix (B) includes general species information for quick reference. Veterinary psychopharmacology is changing rapidly, and a number of human drugs are currently being tried for animal behavior problems. While any list can never be complete, the third appendix (C) lists several drugs currently being tried in animals, with indications and doses cited from a variety of references.

Improvements can always be made in any project. In this encyclopedia, the reader might find a term forgotten, an incomplete discussion, or disagreement about a definition or a suggested treatment. But the project represents an important first step, a basis for discussion. New things will be learned, new drugs used, another technique refined to replace an old one.

Acknowledgments

IT TAKES A LOT OF PEOPLE to successfully complete a project like this, and I owe a big thanks to them all. In the very beginning, there were those who pioneered the field of animal behavior in its broadest definition. Some like Ivan Pavlov, B. F. Skinner, Paul Leyhausen, Konrad Lorenz, Nico Tinbergen, Karl von Frisch, Erich von Holst, Fritz Walther, John Alcock, Irenäus Eibl-Eibesfeldt, Edward Wilson, Jane Goodall, and Dian Fossey come to mind. Certainly, there were many others who were perhaps less well known by the general public. The formal relationship of animal behavior to veterinary medicine is much newer, but it has already benefited from work by other pioneers, including William Campbell, Michael Fox, Andrew Fraser, E.S.E. Hafez, Ron Kilgore, Hal Markowitz, John Scott, and John Fuller. From these and many other colleagues, I have been able to gather the benefits of their work and pass on some of the knowledge to the next generation of veterinary behaviorists.

There are always improvements that can be made in any project. In this encyclopedia the reader might find a term forgotten, an incomplete discussion, or disagreement about a definition or a suggested treatment. But the project represents an important first step, a basis for discussion. New things will be learned, new drugs used, another technique refined to replace an old one.

For me, the most important support for this project came from home, because much time sitting in front of the computer is taken away from other aspects of family life. Thanks Larry. It also took the support of my department head, Dr. John August; college dean, Dr. John Shadduck; and departmental colleagues. I am indebted to a host of talented people for all kinds of help with the technical aspects of this project, including Dr. Margaret Fischer, Dr. Kelly Helmick, Dr. Kelly Chaffin, Jay Morrow, Tricia Dicky, Debbie Choate, Kirsten Hamilton, Beverly Pedulla, Krista May, and those who reviewed the rough draft manuscript for Iowa State University Press. A special thanks goes to Gretchen Van Houten for her enthusiasm and drive to see this idea come to completion.

The Veterinarian's Encyclopedia of Animal Behavior

Abnormal Behavior

Any behavior that varies from the norm expected for a species can be called abnormal. This variation can relate to the style or timing of the act, represent a normal behavior used in an inappropriate place or time, or be a behavior not typically used by a species.

ALSO SEE: *Genetic Problems, Improper Socialization, Medical Problems, Stereotyped Behaviors, Stress-related Behaviors*

Acral Lick Dermatitis

This is another name for lick granulomas.

SEE: *Lick Granulomas*

Action-specific Exhaustibility

This is another name for a refractory period.

SEE: *Refractory Period*

Active Submission

Active submission is a series of distance-reducing silent communication postures exhibited by an animal when approached by another individual. In dogs, these postures include diverted eyes, lowered ears, lowered head, lowered body, no movement when touched, lowered tail, a wagging tail, licking or tongue flicking, a raised forepaw, lying down, rolling over, and submissive urination, indicating a degree of submission to the approacher. Each posture can be seen individually or in combination. Be cautious when reading the lowered head and neck and the tail motion because in dogs these can also be aggressive postures.

ALSO SEE: *Ambivalent Postures, Distance-increasing Silent Communication, Distant-reducing Silent Communication, Passive Submission, Submissive Behavior, Submissive Urination*

Adaptation

Adaptation is the adjustment to change, usually over time, and is most often related to environmental changes. For individuals, adaptation may require learning to accept changes, or it may require a physiologic or sensory habituation to adjust to sensory input variations.

When adaptation occurs within a group of individuals and results in selection in favor of environmental changes, Darwin's principles of evolution are in effect. If humans influence the characteristics of this selection, domestication can occur.

ALSO SEE: *Domestication, Sociobiology*

Added Food Bowls (Feeding Spaces)

This is a treatment technique that can be useful for cats that are urinating or defecating in a house and for groups of animals when feeding space is controlled by a few individuals.

For housesoiling cats, additional food bowls can be placed on particular spots where the cat is soiling. The principle behind this therapy is that a cat will not soil where it eats and will eventually go back to using the litter box. While it is an effective technique in some cases, most cats will simply move their elimination spot to a new location. A few cats will continue to soil in the same location, even though the food is soiled too. When only a few nonlitter box locations are used by the cat, added litter boxes are more successful. If a large number of spots are used, food bowls may be useful in combination with added litter boxes.

In some instances, a dominant individual in a herd or pack may control access to food, causing group members to either decrease their food intake or fight continuously with those controlling food access. The first situation, common in livestock species, limits growth and weight gains. The second decreases the group harmony in social species such as dogs. To prevent these situations, it may be necessary to provide added feeding bowls or spaces.

ALSO SEE: *Added Litter Boxes, Aggression—History Taking, Dominance Aggression, Housesoiling, Housesoiling—Defecation, Housesoiling—Urination, Material Protective Aggression, Social Behavior*

Added Litter Boxes

This is one technique that may be helpful for dealing with feline housesoiling, particularly in relation to urination or defecation outside of the litter box. The additional litter box, placed on the soiled spot, may be all that is required to correct the problem elimination. After a period of adjustment, the new box is gradually moved, approximately 1 inch/day, to a more acceptable location. For some cats, old plastic litter boxes apparently develop a disagreeable odor, and the addition of a new litter box causes the cat to use it exclusively.

ALSO SEE: *Housesoiling, Housesoiling—Defecation, Housesoiling—Urination*

Additional Pets

It is sometimes desirable to add another dog or cat to a household; however, the results are not always positive. A single dog would benefit from the addition of another dog if the owners are away for long periods, provided the single dog has been around other dogs in the past. Another dog might also work well for an owner who enjoys dogs. An added dog is not necessarily the answer when an existing pet begins showing destructive behaviors, and it could actually result in two dogs showing destructive tendencies.

Adding a cat to a household with pets frequently adds a problem. A resident dog that is not used to cats may spend its time chasing the cat. A resident cat may not appreciate the presence of a new pet. A new cat should be confined to a room by itself with food, water, a bed, and a litter box. This allows the resident cat time to get used to the smells and sounds of the newer pet, without having to encounter it. Confinement also allows the new cat time to develop a territory and learn some hiding places. After several days, the door can be opened to the room so the two can find each other, even though aggression between the two is likely to some degree.

ALSO SEE: *Asocial, Confinement, Feline Asocial Aggression, Pavlovian Conditioning, Social Behavior, Socialization*

Adipsia

The lack of thirst, adipsia, is an uncommon problem, but when it does occur, it is usually related to an animal being supplied with necessary liquids during fluid therapy. Cats on canned food or patients on gruel-type diets can approach their daily requirement for liquids and not seek supplemental sources. Outdoor animals may get water from puddles or at times when the owner does not see them drink, or they may be eating plants that contain large quantities of moisture. As a result, the owner may voice a concern that the animal is not drinking. Adipsia as a true problem would involve direct or biochemical depression of brain centers.

ALSO SEE: *Drinking*

Advertising Dress

Sexual selection of mates within a species is often based on physical differences between the sexes. Typically, but not exclusively, the males have a color pattern or physical feature that is used to advertise a territory or readiness to mate. This advertising dress may be a permanent feature of that animal or it may only be present during a particular season or hormonal state. The bright red of a male cardinal and the colored sex skin of the estrous female baboon are examples.

ALSO SEE: *Color Change, Sexual Selection*

Aerophagia

Aerophagia is another term for wind sucking in horses. The term is occasionally applied to cribbing as well.

SEE: *Cribbing, Wind Sucking*

Affective Aggression

This represents a broad category of aggression characterized by an intense, patterned, autonomic activation and includes interactions between the sympathetic nervous system and the adrenal glands. The animal would show species-specific signals of a distance-increasing silent communication. Affective aggression generally includes intrasexual, pain-induced, fear-induced, competitive, dominance, protective, learned, and redirected aggression.

ALSO SEE: *Competitive Aggression, Distance-increasing Silent Communication, Dominance Aggression, Fear-induced Aggression, Interfemale Aggression, Intermale Aggression, Intrasexual Aggression, Learned Aggression, Pain-induced Aggression, Protective Aggression, Reactive Distances*

Age Dimorphism

Age dimorphism refers to physical characteristics that vary between juvenile and adult animals. Proportional differences in juveniles such as rounded heads, larger eyes, and longer legs make age differences more obvious and help signal to adults which individuals do not represent a threat. In other cases, physical differences may help camouflage the young, as with the spots on fawns.

Three or more stages of age-related differences would be called age polymorphism.

ALSO SEE: *Child Schema, Dimorphism, Paedomorphosis, Polymorphism*

Aggregation

An aggregation is a grouping of animals, not dependent on social attraction or necessarily of the same species, that occurs when individuals seek to be in a particular location. Typically, an aggregation would occur near a watering hole or limited food resource.

ALSO SEE: *Animal Sociology, Social Behavior, Society*

Aggression

Aggression is a threat or harmful action directed toward one or more individuals. The diversity of actions range from verbal threats by humans to vocal communications that generally imply a distance-increasing message or tone, body postures and facial expressions that are used to communicate "go-away," inhibited attack, and actual physical attack.

Aggression can be subdivided into a number of different types based on external signs, intended victims, neurological control, and related problems. In veterinary medicine, a more specific diagnosis is needed to effectively work with problem animals. Aggression as a complaint is similar in its broad representation to the symptom of coughing. It describes a behavior but does not help to distinguish the cause — pneumonia, bronchitis, tracheitis, foreign body, allergies, or local laryngeal stimulation. Likewise, in behavior problems, causes of the aggression must be determined before any meaningful advice can be given or treatment prescribed. This is where an in-depth behavioral history becomes important. Since a good history is critical and takes time, appropriate scheduling allows the veterinarian to spend the time needed and charge for the time and expertise. Normal forms of aggression, such as predatory aggression, may require control of the environment. Medically related types can be helped with medication. "Shotgun" therapies are no more appropriate for behavior cases than for traditional medical problems, and castration, tranquilizers, and hormones are not panaceas.

As members of a profession charged with the protection of public health, veterinarians also have a responsibility to evaluate the potential danger to the public and family members. It is the author's opinion that human safety must have the highest priority. With the intense emotional attachment some owners have for the animal, it is at times necessary to direct their options toward those that ultimately protect the public, even though in another set of circumstances the same condition could be treated.

ALSO SEE: *Affective Aggression, Aggression—History Taking, Aggression and Doorbells, Aggression and Food, Aggression and Mail Carriers, Aggression and Telephones, Agonistic Behavior, Avoid Situations, Biting, Canine-Tooth Threat, Cannibalism, Death Shake, Defensive Behavior, Diet Change, Distance-increasing Silent Communication, Electroshock Therapy, Epileptic Aggression, Erythrocytosis, Euthanasia, Fear Biting, Fear-induced Aggression, Feline Asocial Aggression, Feline Dispersion Aggression, Feline Dispersion Aggression—Atypical, Feline Ischemic Encephalopathic Aggression, Filing Canine Teeth, Food Allergy, Frustration, Frustration-induced Aggression, Ground Pecking, History Taking, Hormonal Imbalance Aggression, Hydrocephalic Aggression, Hyperthyroidism, Hypothyroid Aggression, Hypoxia, Idiopathic Aggression, Improper Socialization Aggression, Ingestive Behavior, Inhibited Bite, Interfemale Aggression, Intermale Aggression, Intrasexual Aggression, Irritable Aggression, Jaw Chomping, Legal Concern, Material Protective Aggression, Maternal Aggression, Mental Lapse Aggression Syndrome, Mimic Grin, Mobile Aggression, Nape Bite, Nonaffective Aggression, Ovariectomy, Owner Protective Aggression, Pack Response Aggression, Pain-induced Aggression, Pariah Aggression, Play Aggression, Predation,*

*Predatory Aggression, Prefrontal Lobotomy, Protective Aggression, Puer-
peral Aggression, Rage Copulation, Rage Syndrome, Redirected Aggres-
sion, Ritualized Fighting, Self-Mutilation, Senile Aggression, Sex-related
Aggression, Solitary, Temper Tantrum, Territorial Protective Aggression,
Testosterone-induced Aggression in Mares, Threat Displays, Trained
Aggression, Unconsciously Learned Aggression, Warning Behavior,
Appendix A*

Aggression—History Taking

History taking for problems with aggression should contain some additional information beyond that obtained using a general behavior-taking form, such
as that in Appendix A.

Target. *Person*—It is necessary to determine if the aggression is directed
toward adults, children (what ages), owners, familiar people, or strangers. *Other
animals*—Aggression can be directed toward other animal species, such as dogs
chasing cats or horses biting cattle. It can also be directed toward members of the
same species. Here, the victim's sex becomes important. *Self-trauma*—If aggression is self-directed, the part being damaged can be diagnostic.

Associated actions. *Predictability*—Some forms of aggression can be predicted by the owner, either because of the type of situation that triggers aggression, or by a certain look that occurs before it happens. *After reactions*—Immediately after the aggression ends, some animals seek close contact with the victim, others want to be left alone, and the rest act as if nothing has occurred.

ALSO SEE: *Aggression, History Taking, Housesoiling—History Taking,
Appendix A*

Aggression and Doorbells

Some dogs attack doors or guests whenever the doorbell rings. This is usually a learned behavior, unconsciously encouraged by the owner's behavior. A
person may use words like "take it easy" or "that's all right," but the tone of voice
and physical encouragement actually reward the barking and escalate excitement. In other homes, children may run to answer a guest's arrival, which can
also excite the family dog. As a result, the dog quickly learns to associate the
ringing of the doorbell with excitement.

This behavior can be stopped in several ways. One way is habituation by
repeated ringing of the doorbell until the dog no longer reacts. The dog can also
be made to "heel" and "sit" by the door whenever the bell rings. The procedure
is repeated with corrections of "no" and "time-out" being used for inappropriate

responses. Initially, the door should not be opened, but as the dog learns the appropriate behavior, the door should be opened. Eventually the bell ringer should be allowed to enter and to interact with the dog. Because habituation learning or the substitution of an appropriate behavior takes time for the dog to learn, the owner should make an extended commitment to solve the problem.

ALSO SEE: *Avoid Excitement, Classical Conditioning, Desensitization, Habituation Learning, No, Substitute a Behavior, Sympathetic Induction of Mood, Time-Out*

Aggression and Food

Aggression over food can occur for a number of reasons. Competitive aggression occurs when a more dominant animal wants to take over access to food. In many cases, a simple threat is sufficient to get a subordinate to relinquish its position; however, a threat will often be followed by a more-intense act of aggression. If a dog considers itself dominant to a family member, especially a child, aggression will be directed toward that person if he or she tries to take away a food bowl or treat. Antiaggressive puppy training, relative to the food bowl, is helpful in preventing this type of aggression.

Material protective aggression is another reason animals show aggression over food. Some individuals will stand guard over food, as if protecting it from pack or herd mates, even though they have no interest in eating it. Dogs commonly show this behavior over bones or toys. While dogs are thought of as the primary animal showing this problem, it also occurs frequently in cats, horses, and other species. Horses often become aggressive toward people bringing their feed or hay, and they may show aggression toward any intruder, human or animal, while eating.

Horses that are hand fed treats, especially sugar, may show aggression when they expect the treat. Cats also may become very aggressive if an expected tidbit is not forthcoming. This type of food-related aggression should not be confused with accidental nipping that occurs when an animal gets a part of a hand while trying to reach a handout. Nipping is not true aggression.

The aggressive behavior toward humans may reach such an intolerable state that it may become dangerous to be around the animal. Since the behavior is being rewarded by food or by the departure of the person or animal, there is a good probability that aggressive behavior will continue. The most practical approach may be to feed the individual in a specific place and at a specific time, with no food treats given between meals. If additional treatment is needed, the animal should not be given any food until a friendly behavior is shown, and then given a small amount of food so the session can be repeated several times. Horses in particular may threaten the owner if approached while eating hay or grain, in much the same way they would react to a herd mate trying to claim the food.

Horses displaying this behavior may gradually develop a trust in the person if it is allowed to continue eating while the person approaches a little closer with each feeding. Each move is maintained until the distance-increasing signs are stopped. The animal will develop a trust in the person because it can continue eating. For the horse or dog that actively goes after someone who approaches, a mechanism can be rigged so that the food is pulled away when the threat is made and given back when the threat stops.

ALSO SEE: *Antiaggressive Puppy Training, Competitive Aggression, Distance-increasing Silent Communication, Dominance, Dominance Aggression, Material Protective Aggression*

Aggression and Mail Carriers

Canine aggression directed at mail carriers, meter readers, and other regular visitors is related to territorial invasion or is a learned response. Many dogs react with territorial defense to people approaching their home. People engaged in occupations in which they frequently encounter unfriendly dogs develop a protective reaction and may overreact to a dog's approach. The dog recognizes this increased threat and quickly learns to establish a more aggressive posture toward specific individuals.

The best overall response is to confine the animal away from the mail carrier or meter reader so that a negative situation cannot develop and so that the animal cannot demonstrate the extent of its territorial protectiveness. Friendly introductions using a food reward (bribe) given by the potential victim can also successfully manage the situation.

ALSO SEE: *Desensitization, Territorial Protective Aggression*

Aggression and Telephones

Some dogs develop the behavior of attacking the telephone whenever it rings. This usually occurs in a family with teenagers or others who race to answer the phone. The high level of excitement gets the dog excited as well. The pet learns to anticipate excitement with the ringing, and eventually the behavior is triggered by the phone even though no one may be at home. Once the behavior problem starts, owners often perpetuate it by trying to race the dog to the phone.

Several sessions of habituation to a ringing phone, which is placed out of the dog's reach and which no one answers, can extinguish the behavior. Substituting a behavior, such as "sit," places the dog in a conflicting situation; therefore, he must choose. Praise for following the command reinforces an acceptable behavior. Punishment can also effectively stop the attacks. "No," a collar jerk, time-out in social isolation, and a remote-triggered air blast are a few examples. It is also important to drastically lower the excitement levels associated with the phone, perhaps by providing additional phones to make answering easier.

ALSO SEE: *Desensitization, Extinction, Habituation Learning, No, Punish-*

ment, Remote Punishment, Substitute a Behavior

Aggressive Personality

Aggressive personalities are both made and born. This means that traits, such as those for guarding, as with the German shepherd, can be inherited. Training can also change a personality, but is most effective if used to accentuate an innate characteristic. The ease of aggressive training in the shepherds, Dobermans, and Rottweilers takes advantage of an inherited characteristic that has been selected over many generations. Individuals can have particularly aggressive personalities, with some very dominant and some just mean.

ALSO SEE: *Personality*

Aggressive Play

This is also called play aggression and represents distance-increasing behaviors shown in play.

SEE: *Distance-increasing Silent Communication, Play Aggression, Play Behaviors*

Agonistic Behavior

Agonistic behavior is that which does not promote group harmony or peaceful coexistence, implying a degree of combativeness or contesting. This term is applied to the broad group of behaviors usually associated with distance-increasing silent communication and fighting.

ALSO SEE: *Allelomimetic Behavior, Distance-increasing Silent Communication*

Allelomimetic Behavior

Allelomimetic behaviors are those that promote group harmony and the coexistence of members. For social animals, most behaviors are of this type, since without them, there would be no major reason to preserve the group. Social behaviors, including reproduction, group living, distance-reducing communications, mutual grooming, and cooperative hunting, reflect the allelomimetic nature of many species.

ALSO SEE: *Agonistic Behavior, Distance-reducing Silent Communication, Fear of People, Male Behaviors, Mutual Grooming, Social Behavior*

Allergy Workup

Food allergies are suspected when accidental or planned dietary changes result in calming hyper animals and relaxing irritable ones. Confirmation of a behavior change due to an allergy can be accomplished only by reintroducing specific dietary components to find the one causing the allergy. From a clinical viewpoint, owners are often so pleased with the initial behavior change that they are reluctant to try the appropriate food challenges.

ALSO SEE: *Diet Change, Food Allergy*

Allogrooming

Allogrooming is another name for mutual grooming.

SEE: *Mutual Grooming*

Allomother

This is a term applied to a foster mother.

SEE: *Fostering*

Altricial Animals

These are animal species, such as rodents and carnivores, that give birth to young that require quite a bit of additional development. Typically, the young are naked, blind, deaf, and unable to walk. The young of altricial birds are called nidicolous nestlings.

ALSO SEE: *Nidicolous Nestlings, Precocial Animal*

Altruism

Altruistic behavior by an individual benefits another member of its species without regard to the individual's own welfare. People who heroically save others are the best examples of this behavior. In animals, altruism is difficult to document and harder to explain. To some, parental behavior is considered altruistic; however, most do not include it within the definition.

Explanations for this behavior usually include a relatedness of the animals and the survivability of a certain gene pool, making altruism beneficial to the group as a whole.

ALSO SEE: *Hero, Kin Selection*

Ambivalent Postures

Animals in emotional conflict show mixed body postures, usually a combination of distance-increasing and distance-reducing signs. The fear biting dog is the classic example of ambivalence. The stare, piloerection on the shoulders, and/or bared teeth give a "go away" message, while the lowered body and tucked tail are submissive signs. A dog that stares and barks at an object as it shifts its weight or moves back is another example.

The only safe way to work with these animals is to read the "worst" end. If the dog is cornered or pressed to react, the aggressive reaction usually prevails.

ALSO SEE: *Conflict, Distance-increasing Silent Communication, Distance-reducing Silent Communication, Fear-induced Aggression, Fear Biting, Mixed Motivation* .

Ambush Predator

An ambush predator is one that waits for its prey rather than stalks it. Spiders are examples of this type of predator.

ALSO SEE: *Predation*

Anaclitic Depression

Anaclitic depression is the separation anxiety that occurs when the symbiotic dependence of an infant on its mother is broken. In animals, an example is the stress behaviors shown by a foal or calf when separated from the dam after the pair has been together for several days. Behaviors of weaning are also examples, but are usually less extreme in form.

ALSO SEE: *Deprivation Syndrome, Separation Anxiety, Separation Syndrome, Weaning*

Analgesic Tranquilizer

An analgesic is a drug used to relieve or minimize pain. Some problem behaviors can be controlled by controlling the underlying pain. Three of these drugs have been particularly useful with certain behavior problems. Oxymorphone can be used to incapacitate a particularly aggressive dog so that appropriate medical attention or anesthesia can be given. The combination product fentanyl citrate and droperidol will also incapacitate a dog, but it can have the opposite effect on some aggressive dogs, so should be used with caution. Detomidine hydrochloride is particularly useful in managing difficult horses during procedures when their cooperation is needed.

ALSO SEE: *Drug Therapy*

Analogy

An analogy consists of patterns or physical features that are similar between species because of convergent evolution rather than common ancestors (homology).

ALSO SEE: *Homology*

Anesthesia

In veterinary medicine, anesthesia is the loss of consciousness or the loss of sensations to part or all of the body. In certain behaviors, particularly aggression, anesthesia has been used as a therapy. In some situations it works successfully, but the reasons for the success may have to do with other factors.

Severe anorexia, particularly in cats, has been treated on rare occasions with general anesthesia. Food is made available as the cat recovers. This procedure is generally not recommended because of the possibility of aspiration pneumonia during recovery. Stress-related factors are the most likely cause of anorexia that responds to this type of treatment.

Fighting dogs have been treated by anesthetizing both individuals and allowing them to recover together. The cause of aggression has not been classified in cases where this type of therapy has been used; however, it is most likely competitive (dominance) aggression. If the dominant dog is removed from the home environment, the second-ranking dog assumes the number one position and is not willing to relinquish that position when the first dog returns. While anesthesia and simultaneous recovery might be useful in this situation, it is usually as effective to remove the number two dog for a day or so and then return it with the healthy dominant dog present.

Deep anesthesia for prolonged periods is known to result in personality changes. Aggressive animals have become nonthreatening; outgoing animals have become shy and reserved. Barbiturate anesthetics have lasted excessively long times—a common happening in cats—and the level of anesthesia has been very deep. Oxygen deprivation to the brain is the most likely cause of the behavior changes seen.

Another short-term anesthetic, ketamine hydrochloride, has also caused dramatic personality changes when used alone. Hallucinations during recovery are reported in humans and may occur in cats as well. Over time, the behavior changes back toward normal.

ALSO SEE: *Anorexia, Anorexia Nervosa, Competitive Aggression, Dominance Aggression, Drug Therapy, Hypoxia*

Animal Psychology

By strict definition, animal psychology would apply to the behavioral study that originated from human psychology. In general use, however, the term refers to comparative psychology and studies in learning. In the broadest sense, animal psychology refers to the behaviors of animals. While the terms animal psychology and animal psychologist are commonly used in the popular press and by animal trainers, these have generally been replaced by the terms ethology or animal behavior, and animal behaviorist.

ALSO SEE: *Ethology, Learning, Psychology*

Animal Rights

Animal rights is a moral, and often emotional, issue that has received a great deal of discussion over the last several years. Rights have to do with those concerns that are in accordance with moral law or some other standard of rightness. Animal rights may overlap the subject of animal welfare, but the two are not synonymous.

ALSO SEE: *Animal Welfare*

Animal Sociology

The establishment and maintenance of the various types of social structure are studies under the title of animal sociology.

ALSO SEE: *Aggregation, Social Behavior, Social Groups, Society*

Animal Welfare

Animal welfare has to do with the general well-being of an animal or group of animals. This subject is currently undergoing a great deal of research to learn more about specific needs to meet the physical and psychological well-being of the various species and individuals within the species. Included are a broad range of topics such as lighting, temperature, social spacing, social interactions, feeding schedules, exercise needs, environmental interactions, perception of stress, neurological reactions, and restraint and handling procedures. Behavior of and psychological changes in the animal are the major factors in assessing results from these studies.

ALSO SEE: *Animal Rights, Psychological Well-being*

Ankle Attacks

Cats commonly attack the ankles of their owners or of guests entering the home. If the animal is not allowed to express normal predation on rodents, insects, or toys, the threshold stimulus for the behavior decreases. Eventually, any motion can trigger the predatory behaviors. The easiest way to stop frequent ankle attacks is to encourage the cat to play with movable toys. These can be objects on a string, windup mice, or any other items that encourage the cat to stalk and pounce.

During history taking, it is important to record the age and environment of the cat. Feline dispersion aggression is common in pubertal cats and should be differentiated from this predatory behavior.

ALSO SEE: *Damming-up Theory, Feline Dispersion Aggression—Atypical, Predatory Aggression*

Annual Periodicity

Annual periodicity is a term applied to the annual or circannual rhythms of an animal. They may relate to yearly reproductive changes, hibernation, or migrations. External influences, such as the length of daylight, are often associated with these changes.

ALSO SEE: *Biological Rhythms, Circadian Rhythms*

Anomalous Milk Sucking

Anomalous milk sucking, or galactophagia, occurs when one animal sucks from another that is not its dam or foster mother. The behavior is most commonly a problem in adult cattle, which may even pair up and nurse one another. There is a suspected hereditary basis in cattle; however, husbandry practices, such as early weaning, are related. Aversive conditioning is most often used to prevent the behavior from becoming well ingrained. Devices that stick the animal's face or nose or administer an electric shock are most commonly used. While aversive condition is generally helpful, occasional individuals must be culled for this problem.

ALSO SEE: *Aversive Conditioning, Nursing*

Anonymous Group

An anonymous group is a social group of animals in which members do not recognize individuals. In open anonymous groups, individuals may come and go without apparent impact on the group. In closed anonymous groups, members are recognized by a particular group-specific trait, such as an odor. Insects typically are members of anonymous groups.

ALSO SEE: *Animal Sociology, Individualized Group*

Anorexia

Occasional anorexia (inappetence) is a normal occurrence in animals. It is generally short in duration and does not require treatment. It can result from unpalatable food, nausea, or individual variations in appetite. Long-term anorexia is more severe because of the degree of emaciation it produces. This problem can result from stress (anorexia nervosa), lesions in the hypothalamus, or medical problems that act on the gastrointestinal system or brain. To combat long-term anorexia, appropriate therapies should be instituted based on the cause. In some cases, frequent changes in food flavors or textures may be necessary, or the animal may eat enough of a high-quality food that the wasting may be slowed. Forced feeding orally or through a gastric tube may be necessary in a few cases, at least until the animal recovers enough to eat on its own.

ALSO SEE: *Anesthesia, Anorexia Nervosa*

Anorexia Nervosa

Various types of stress can stop an animal from eating. The problem is most common and the outcome potentially the most serious in the cat. For the house cat, stress can come from a number of sources—invasion of its territory, a new cat in the household, a visitor, a new family member, a move to a new home, hospitalization, or boarding. Since this behavior is stress related, it is generally responsive to therapy. In most cases, the cat will begin eating again in two to five days because it adapts to the situation. For cats that do not begin to eat after a week of gentle coaxing and for those that are obese and subject to the severe manifestations of fatty liver problems, removing the source of the stress should be enough to stop the anorexia. If, however, the problem has been long standing, extremely severe, or unavoidable, other approaches must be used. Confinement in a small area away from the stress is one approach. Providing a cardboard box or paper sack to hide in is very useful for cats taken outside their normal homes. Treatment with antianxiety tranquilizers, anabolic steroids, progestins, or anesthesia may be necessary.

Anorexia nervosa can occur in species other than cats. Fortunately, it tends to be less of a problem in those species. The most common cause of anorexia nervosa and decreased food consumption in social animals is the presence of a highly dominant group member near the food. The mere presence of such an individual can produce psychosomatic changes, such as decreased production of saliva.

ALSO SEE: *Anesthesia, Anorexia, Progestins, Stress-related Behaviors, Appendix C*

Anthropomorphism

Anthropomorphism is the assigning of human characteristics, values, or feelings to animals. This trait in animal owners can result in unrealistic expectations and thus in the expression by the animal of undesirable behaviors.

ALSO SEE: *Animal Rights, Zoomorphism*

Antiaggressive Puppy Training

Puppies will develop a social position within a human group as they would within a canine pack, but in the human group it is important that the puppy is subordinate to its owner. Since this relationship can be established before four months of age, early lessons are important while the puppy is still small enough to control.

Play biting is the first major problem encountered by most owners. This is a time when the dog learns jaw pressure. A littermate will yelp and stop playing when pain occurs; however, humans may tolerate the pain because it is "cute." Thus they teach the puppy that it takes a lot of pressure to cause pain. Instead, owners should discourage the puppy from biting people by diverting its attention or stopping play. Punishment is not appropriate because it is not understood relative to a normal behavior.

Toys, "stolen items," and food will occasionally need to be taken away from an adult dog, so this is a good lesson for a puppy to learn. The owners should remove the food bowl and note the puppy's reaction. If it growls, bites, or objects, the dish should not be returned for at least five minutes. If there is no reaction, the bowl can be returned immediately. Children should also practice this procedure, under adult supervision, before the puppy becomes large enough to cause harm. Occasionally, toys should be removed the same way, and "stolen" or guarded objects should be taken away without the use of a food bribe.

Chewing should be discouraged because it reinforces mouth-oriented behaviors that can become destructive chewing or aggression as the puppy matures. Games like "tug-of-war" should not be played. Only a few chew toys are desirable, and they should differ from common items in the environment. Old shoes cannot be differentiated from new shoes. Leather slippers are similar to leather purses or leather chairs. Old socks are no different to the puppy than new socks. The puppy should expend extra energy through appropriate exercise rather than chewing.

The owner's dominance can be established and reinforced by other lessons as well. An owner should repeat activities the puppy does not like and especially emphasize those things it may have to accept when older. Lay the puppy on its back and firmly hold it in place by its chest. If the puppy bites and struggles, continue to hold it down until the struggling stops. Firmly hold the muzzle and move the head around. Manipulate the ears, especially on floppy-eared dogs. Holding the feet, manipulating the toes, and trimming the toenails are valuable lessons for later. Let the puppy wear a collar and leash so it will accept them later. Baths and general grooming are important for good skin condition and parasite control, and puppyhood is the ideal time to start these lessons. These techniques help the dog become accustomed to its owner's control.

Obedience lessons are suggested as an important follow-up for antiaggressive puppy training.

ALSO SEE: *Destructive Chewing, Divert Attention, Dominance, Dominance Aggression, Obedience Class, Play Aggression, Punishment, Social Order*

Antisocial

This term describes the behavioral response of an individual or a species that actively discourages any interaction among individuals. An antisocial animal will be a loner at all times, except perhaps during mating season or when a female has young. The Indian tiger is an example.

ALSO SEE: *Asocial, Social Behavior*

Antler Rubbing

This is the rubbing or scraping of the antler covering against tree limbs. Animals probably show the behavior in response to the physiological changes in nerve and blood supply to the covering skin, and behaviorally it progresses into the aggressions associated with the mating season.

ALSO SEE: *Ground Rutting*

Anxiety

Anxiety is the anticipation of dangers. Some people distinguish anxiety from fear by defining anxiety as the anticipation of dangers from unknown or imagined origins that results in physiological reactions within an animal. This is distinct from fear, where the response is caused by a consciously recognized external threat. Anxious states can occur in animals when they are sensitized to a noxious stimuli and then generalize the lesson to other situations.

ALSO SEE: *Fear, Hysteria, Phobia,*

Appeasement Behavior

Patterns of behavior that inhibit attacks by others of the same species are called appeasement behaviors. In general, these behaviors do not involve intimidation, but rather are the opposite of the expected action. As a threat occurs, behaviors such as a mating posture, a juvenile play display, or an extremely submissive signal would seem inappropriate. It is this degree of inappropriateness that probably defuses a tense situation.

Some behaviorists separate submissive behavior from appeasement behavior. Submission is the presentation of signals that communicate the opposite of aggression. Appeasement activates tendencies incompatible with aggression. In general usage, submission is a variation of appeasement.

ALSO SEE: *Automimicry, Cut Off, Distance-reducing Silent Communication, Infantile Behavior, Inhibition, Passive Submission, Social Inhibition, Submissive Behavior*

Appetitive Behavior

In the broadest sense, appetitive behavior represents the first phase of a behavioral series that leads to the actual behavior, or consummatory phase, and then the refractory period.

In the narrower definition, appetitive behavior is the goal-seeking, investigative phase of ingestive behavior that normally precedes the actual act of eating or drinking. In animals that depend on humans for food, this behavior is often abbreviated. The hunting behavior of the outdoor cat changes to the meowing demand with the whirring of the can opener. Components of appetitive behavior also can be seen as stereotyped behavior.

ALSO SEE: *Consummatory Phase, Ingestive Behavior, Refractory Period, Stereotyped Behaviors*

Approach Distance

An animal may approach an intruder by walking forward a short distance. This short distance is the approach distance, and it represents one of the social (reactive) distances.

ALSO SEE: *Reactive Distances, Social Distance*

Asocial

Asocial describes the behavioral response of an individual or species that avoids, but does not necessarily discourage, interaction among individuals. While an asocial animal would be alone a great deal of the time, it would interact to some degree with other members of its own species. The domestic cat is an example.

ALSO SEE: *Antisocial, Feline Asocial Aggression, Feline Dispersion Aggression, Hiding, Social Behavior, Solitary*

Associated Movements

Basic postures or movements of a specific behavior are accompanied by other postures or movements that can vary somewhat. These accompanying postures are called associated movements. While a horse grazes, the associated body posture is usually that of a slow walk; however, under certain conditions the horse may actually be laying down. Defecation is usually accompanied by a standing position with the head upright, but the animal could use a second associated head-down movement to graze, too.

Association

In behavior, association refers to animals of the same or different species living together. In learning, association refers to the connection between a stimulus and a response.

ALSO SEE: *Animal Sociology*

Attachment

The attraction of an animal to a place, an object, or another animal (including humans) is described as an attachment. The attachment to a social creature is also described as a bond.

ALSO SEE: *Bond*

Attention-Deficit Hyperactivity Disorder

This is a condition diagnosed in humans where there are inappropriate degrees of inattention, impulsiveness, and hyperactivity. Novel environments and strict controls minimize the expression of the condition. Certain neurological conditions or chaotic environments are thought to be predisposing factors. The relationship of this disorder to hyperactivity and/or hyperkinesis in animals has not been studied.

ALSO SEE: *Hyperactivity, Hyperkinesis*

Attention Seeking

Animals seek the attention of humans or conspecifics in a number of ways and for a variety of reasons. Social species tend to want acceptance by group members, and use mutual grooming (or petting) to meet this need. Animals can solicit attention—cats by rubbing against a person, dogs by leaning against your side, horses by pushing with their nose. Other livestock species and individuals within species learn unique ways to get the message across.

When attention does not come on a regular basis or if it is withheld, the attention-seeking behaviors become more abnormal. Housesoiling, licking, digging, vocalizing, psychogenic expressions, and other behaviors can be attention seeking. Negative attention, even as punishment, can be perceived as better than no attention at all.

Owners need to schedule attention time and reward specific positive behaviors. They must also be sure not to reinforce the unacceptable behavior. Attention should not be given to the wrong behavior, or the behavior should be punished but quickly followed by a rewardable command.

ALSO SEE: *Digging—Indoors, Excessive Grooming, Excessive Vocalization, Extinction, Frustration, Licking of Objects, Mutual Grooming, No Attention to Behaviors, Psychogenic Problems, Schedule, Sympathetic Lameness*

Atypical Narcolepsy

This is an unusual behavior that owners mention in a casual manner. It is more of a curiosity than a serious problem. The typical history is that of a dog, purebred or mixed, that barks at its food bowl each time food is presented. The duration of the barking period varies with individuals, but it is followed by the dog eating its meal.

The author theorizes that these individuals are mild narcoleptics and have learned that excitement before eating will keep them awake through the meal. One dog barked, ate part of his meal, and barked again before finishing eating. In another case the dog was presented for aural hematomas caused by it shaking its head instead of barking. A stockinette was placed over the ears before meals to control the problem.

Specific treatment is not recommended unless secondary complications warrant such measures, and then treatment is selected on an individual basis.

ALSO SEE: *Narcolepsy*

Atypical Sexual Behavior

Any unusual variation from a species' typical sexual behavior can be called atypical. There are many such behaviors, including inappropriate mounting, masturbation, hypersexuality, and the buller steer syndrome. It is important to understand that these are uncommon variations of normal and not truly abnormal behavior.

ALSO SEE: *Buller Steer Syndrome, Female Behaviors, Hypersexuality, Inappropriate Mounting, Male Behaviors, Masturbation*

Automimicry

Automimicry describes the behavior of imitating another sex or age in vocal or body posture communication. Usually automimicry is used as an appeasement. A tomcat will mount other male cats within its territory, and these intruders respond with a crouched posture similar to that used by a female during mating.

ALSO SEE: *Appeasement Behavior, Female Behaviors*

Autoshaping

Autoshaping is a type of classical conditioning that occurs simply because of repeated exposure to certain stimulus contingencies. Dogs and cats may quickly associate the noise of a can opener with presentation of food so that they come running and start drooling with the sound alone. This same set of relations can be used to teach a dog or cat to show "guilt" with housesoiling. The combination of urine or feces odor plus the presence of the owner becomes associated with the owner's body language of threat and eventual punishment. This pairing of stimuli eventually results in the submissive postures shown by the animal when the owner comes home.

ALSO SEE: *Classical Conditioning, Guilt*

Aversion-induced Aggression

This is another name for pain-induced aggression or redirected aggression.

SEE: *Pain-induced Aggression, Redirected Aggression*

Aversive Conditioning

Aversive conditioning is a type of learning that leads to the avoidance of a place or object by association with an aversive experience. The aversion can be any type of negative experience such as pain, nausea, or fright, and can involve one or more of the senses. The avoidance can take the form of staying away from a location or object, refusing to come near the object, or actually fleeing from it.

In a more specific sense, aversive conditioning is used to describe the development of food aversions owing to a delayed toxic response.

Aversive conditioning is a useful technique for controlling certain problem behaviors, particularly those that are mouth-related.

ALSO SEE: *Smell Aversion, Taste Aversion*

Avoidance Conditioning

This is another term for aversive conditioning.

SEE: *Aversive Conditioning*

Avoidance Disorder

While relationships with owners and familiar persons are considered normal, a dog or cat may show excessive withdrawal from unfamiliar people. This may be related to poor socialization, desocialization, or extremely shy personalities. Other influences may affect this behavior in animals much as it does in humans.

ALSO SEE: *Deprivation Syndrome, Socialization, Timid Personality*

Avoid Excitement

A number of behavior problems are related to a high degree of excitement. These include redirected aggression, irritable aggression, barking, digging, climbing, submissive urination, and destruction when an owner is not home. Efforts should be made to avoid the excitement. Owners should minimize their interactions with pet dogs and cats for at least 30 minutes before leaving and until they start a specific activity after they return. Keeping horses and dogs away from potential excitement also reduces the sympathetic induction of mood. This could mean, for example, fencing an area so the animal cannot directly interact with a neighboring animal that excitedly races back and forth along the property line. Exercise can be recommended to burn extra calories that might otherwise be used in the unacceptable behavior.

ALSO SEE: *Barking, Climbing, Destructive Behaviors, Digging, Emotional Come and Go, Excessive Vocalization—Barking, Exercise, Housesoiling—Submissive Urination, Irritable Aggression, Redirected Aggression, Separation Anxiety, Submissive Urination, Sympathetic Induction of Mood*

Avoid Situations

The occurrence of certain behavior problems can be predicted based on a thorough history. Some behavior problems can be related to specific events that seem to trigger their occurrence. Aggression may be directed toward one person or a specific group, such as small children. By identifying the stimuli, it may be possible to prevent the problem by confining a dog or cat when the situation is likely. Abrupt changes in social interactions or an animal's schedule should be avoided. Pastured animals abruptly confined can show a number of problems. Young horses taken for long trail rides alone commonly show problems such as rearing and running away. Gradual changes are much more desirable.

SEE: *Aggression, Frustration, Running Away, Self-Mutilation, Separation Anxiety*

B

Bachelor Groups

In some social species, young males are driven from the group soon after they become sexually mature, but while they are still too young to be lead males. These young males may band together in small bachelor groups, probably as a protection against predators. The social structure is typically a rigid dominance hierarchy to minimize the amount of intermale aggression and maximize the social benefits of group membership. Eventually, the bachelor groups split apart as individuals begin to put together their own female bands.

ALSO SEE: *Social Order*

Balking

Balking is the refusal to move, even with encouragement—a behavior typically associated with burros and donkeys. For animal species that evolved in mountainous areas, running away was not a viable reaction to possible danger, because the possibility of falling was a greater threat. Instead, waiting to evaluate a situation and then reacting was more conducive to preservation of the individual and the species. The flight distance for these individuals was very short.

ALSO SEE: *Flight Distance*

Barbering

Barbering is a behavior seen in group-housed laboratory animals when one individual rubs, pulls, or chews the hair of another, often around the face. The problem is most common in mice, where the dominant individual chews off the

whiskers and facial hair of others in the cage. A similar behavior has been reported in rats, guinea pigs, and rabbits. Hair loss can also occur on other parts of the
victim's body, and it can be self-induced and stress-related. The problem is eliminated when the dominant individual is removed or when the precipitating stress
is reduced.

ALSO SEE: *Psychogenic Dermatoses, Psychogenic Problems*

Bar Biting

Bar biting is an oral behavior problem of sows kept in crates. The behavior
is probably related to boredom, since environmental enrichment with things to
chew or root will generally control the problem.

Vacuous chewing is a related behavior of chewing movements without anything in the mouth.

ALSO SEE: *Boredom, Environmental Enrichment, Vacuous Chewing*

Bark Collars

Bark collars are specially designed collars used to control excessive barking by dogs. There is a great potential for abuse with the bark-activated shock
collars if they are inappropriately used and if the initiating cause of the problem
is not also addressed. A bark-activated sound-producing collar is relatively successful in controlling nuisance barking but much less so for barks of excitement
or anxiety. Serious barking is still punished, but not so severely as to prevent the
appropriate warning.

ALSO SEE: *Excessive Vocalization—Barking, Shock Collars*

Barking

Barking is a form of vocal communication used by canids to express a threat
or warning. Domestic dogs often bark more than their wild relatives, even to the
point that excessive barking may be considered a behavior problem. Pigs express
a barklike vocalization as a warning.

ALSO SEE: *Excessive Vocalization—Barking, Howling, Vocal Communication*

Behavioral Characteristics Favoring Domestication

There are at least five behavioral characteristics that are useful in changing
a wild population into a domestic one, although recent discussions suggest there
may be more. The process of domestication takes many generations, and the
selection criteria for breeding usually include certain physical, as well as behavioral, factors.

Human need is the primary reason for domestication. While wild species
may meet human needs in part, easy access and the ability to manage the animals

make domestication desirable. The decision to domesticate is usually not conscious, but based on accessibility of breeding animals. The five useful behavioral characteristics were described by E. B. Hale (in Hafez, 1969).

Group structure is a desirable trait in animals associated with humans. Animals that live in a group can be kept in larger numbers within a given space without major aggressive bouts causing harm to individual members. Castration also increases the numbers that can be kept together, by decreasing the tendency for intermale aggression.

Promiscuous sexual behavior allows humans to choose the mates for the perpetuation of selected traits. Color and physical traits of mates become less important for successful reproduction.

Recognition of their young by features other than color by parents, dams in particular, is another characteristic useful in domestication. When recognition is not dependent on the color of offspring, crossbreeding, artificial insemination, and embryo transfer can be used in modern production systems. Smell of the young is the sense for offspring identification in many domestic animals. This sense can be "fooled" by rubbing the smell of the adoptive mother onto a young animal that is to be fostered.

Tameability of a wild species is often a critical factor as to whether or not the species will eventually be changed enough to fit into a program leading to domestication.

Noncompetitiveness with humans for food or space is a desirable characteristic. Animals that can live on the by-products of human culture and that occupy little space will survive best. Dogs and cats tend to fit this category. Horses and cattle compete with humans for grain and space, and thus have to be very efficient in converting feed into meat or in satisfying a strong human need.

ALSO SEE: *Domestication, Intermale Aggression, Roles of Domesticated Animals*

Behavioral Ecology

This is a branch of science that deals with the relationships between a species' behavior and its physical environment.

ALSO SEE: *Sociobiology*

Behavioral Embryology

The branch of ethology that studies behavioral development from conception to birth is called behavioral embryology. It typically parallels the development of the nervous system, but examines more than just reflex development.

Behavioral Endocrinology

Behavioral endocrinology is the study of the relationship of hormones and behavior. It has also been called ethoendocrinology and is considered a part of behavioral physiology.

ALSO SEE: *Behavioral Physiology, Stool Eating—Another Species*

Behavioral Genetics

This is the study of the heritability of behavioral traits and the way genetics interacts with behavior. Genetics can affect normal behavior, and recent studies show frequent involvement in behavior problems as well.

ALSO SEE: *Genetic Problems*

Behavioral Mimicry

Behavioral mimicry involves the imitation of a species' behavior to gain protection or some other advantage. This mimicry may resemble a physical action or a vocalization. Also called ethomimicry, it is in contrast to morphological mimicry.

Behavioral Phylogeny

In studying evolutionary concepts, behavioral traits, as well as physical traits, can be compared. This branch of ethology is called behavioral phylogeny. The relative sameness of a behavior between species is often used in deciding the relatedness of the species. It has also been used to theorize how extinct species might have behaved.

Behavioral Physiology

This is the science that deals with the relatedness of physiology and ethology. It includes behavioral endocrinology and neuroethology.

ALSO SEE: *Behavioral Endocrinology, Neuroethology*

Behavioral Seizures

A seizure represents the sudden onset of an uncontrollable behavior, usually associated with the chronic condition called epilepsy. Behavioral seizures can be associated with distorted electroencephalographic activity manifested in several different ways, including aggression, tail chasing, fly snapping, and hyperesthesia.

ALSO SEE: *Seizures*

Behavior Modification

Behavior modification refers to any of several techniques used to modify or eliminate a particular behavior. The use of the techniques involves understanding the principles of learning.

ALSO SEE: *Conditioning, Counterconditioning, Desensitization, Extinction, Fear of Noise, Flooding, Learning, Phobia, Punishment, Reinforcement Schedules*

Bioacoustics

Bioacoustics is the study of sound production and reception in animals. Thus, it includes the study of the auditory organs and pathways, the areas of sound production, the sound characteristics, and the sound-environment relationships.

ALSO SEE: *Hearing*

Biological Rhythms

Biological rhythms are the cyclic phenomena of life. They can be daily (circadian), monthly, annual (annual periodicity), or other patterns, and they can influence everything from reproduction to effectiveness of medication. The terms biorhythm and biorhythmicity have also been used.

ALSO SEE: *Annual Periodicity, Circadian Rhythms, Lunar Periodicity, Time Synchronizer*

Biting

Biting is a behavior shown by most animals but will be discussed relative to dogs, cats, horses, and swine. For these animals, the teeth must be considered potential weapons. While pointed canine teeth (tusks in pigs) can do a great deal of damage, any of the teeth can cause serious injury. The severity depends on the type of aggression, the location of the injury, the accuracy of the attack, and the difference in size and strength between the animal and the victim.

Biting as a problem is common in puppies and young stallions, and occasionally in cats. If the victim is of the same species, it breaks social contact or returns the aggression. When the victims are people, they are often reluctant or too surprised to punish the behavior in an appropriate manner. Correction is necessary to teach which behaviors are acceptable and which are not. A muzzle may be necessary to protect the owner, especially in the case of the horse.

ALSO SEE: *Aggression, Antiaggressive Puppy Training, Distance-increasing Silent Communication, Filing Canine Teeth, Muzzle, Reactive Anomalies*

Bloodletting

Bloodletting was an early therapy for aggression that reportedly caused a dramatic improvement in the behavior of dogs and cats. This procedure is no longer advocated for several reasons. The specific type of aggression in which it was useful has not been defined. The mode of action may have been oxygen deprivation from the brain, similar to deep anesthesia, resulting in actual neurologic changes. The specific changes, if any, are unknown, and the part of the brain affected by hypoxia could not be controlled.

ALSO SEE: *Aggression, Anesthesia, Erythrocytosis, Hypoxia*

Body Language

Silent communication by posture, or body language, is the most important form of communication used by animals. The type of message is generally friendly (distance-reducing), threatening (distance-increasing), or confused (ambivalent).

ALSO SEE: *Active Submission, Ambivalent Postures, Distance-increasing Silent Communication, Distance-reducing Silent Communication, Hard-to-Read Postures, Mimic Grin, Nonverbal Communication, Pavlovian Conditioning, Play Behaviors*

Body Pecking

Body pecking is a cannibalistic behavior problem of poultry under intensive management. The problem bird will peck with a stabbing and plucking action and will eat the feathers and flesh it gets. Body pecking is usually directed toward wounds where feathers have been picked out; however, it can also be directed toward the toes, back, or vent.

Control is usually achieved by debeaking or using red lights, neither of which addresses the cause of the problem. The cause is often husbandry-related where there is not adequate space to allow escape.

ALSO SEE: *Cannibalism, Feather Picking*

Bolting

Bolting has two meanings as it relates to behavior. Animals that eat fast and gulp their food are said to be bolting their food. In the second meaning, animals, particularly horses, that suddenly start running are also bolting. The tendency to run is often a response of flight instincts to a potential danger. The animal may also learn to associate the behavior with successfully getting away from the rider or handler, so bolting can become a learned response for escape.

ALSO SEE: *Gulping Food, Running Away*

Bond

The social attachment between two or more individuals in which there is a mutual dependence is called a bond. This relationship can be between mated partners (pair bond), young and parent(s), group members, or animals and humans (human-animal bond). Determining whether a true bond exists can be difficult.

ALSO SEE: *Attachment, Human-Animal Bond, Pair Bonding*

Boredom

Boredom is a mental state of tiredness resulting from uninteresting, monotonous, or repetitive events. Whether the feeling of boredom can actually occur in animals is a topic for scientific debate; however, there are suggestions that it can be a contributing factor in an animal's problem behavior. When the environment is barren, social contacts are minimal, and meaningful amounts of exercise do not happen; thus, an animal starts showing problems. Stereotyped behaviors are the most common, but destruction, pica, and several others can also occur.

A successful outcome is more easily accomplished if causative factors can be identified. Recommendations usually include environmental enrichment (particularly helpful with laboratory animals and those in zoos) and increased exercise. If the behavior has developed into a habit, its elimination becomes more difficult.

ALSO SEE: *Bar Biting, Coprophagia, Cribbing, Destructive Chewing, Environmental Enrichment, Excessive Grooming, Excessive Vocalization—Barking, Excessive Vocalization—Howling, Exercise, Habit, Hair Pulling, Inappropriate Licking, Offensive Threat, Polydipsia, Stereotyped Behaviors, Stress-related Behaviors, Tongue Rolling, Vacuous Chewing, Wind Sucking, Wood Chewing*

Brain

The brain is the center of all behaviors. Cerebral areas are associated with learning, the senses, and motor activity. The limbic system is composed of deeper components that relate to the emotional response to incoming stimuli. The following are six major areas in the limbic system of the brain with the most significance to behavior.

The amygdala regulates some of the aggressive behaviors, primarily those associated with fear-induced aggression (fear biting), and has some regulatory control over the hypothalamic output.

The cingulate gyri help maintain a lack of aggression and probably help in the functional organization of certain behaviors.

Behaviors of a very broad context are usually associated with the hippocampus. These include personality, attention mechanisms, emotions, recent memory, and distance-reducing silent communication postures (submissive behavior).

The hypothalamus is part of the limbic system having a broad influence over behaviors. Physiologically, the hypothalamus controls metabolism, the autonomic nervous system, body temperature regulation, and water balance. It also contains the hunger center, the satiety center, and areas that control predation, sexual behavior, the sleep-wake cycle, and certain emotions such as fear, anger, aggression, and rage.

The primary functions of the septal nuclei are to integrate and moderate sensory stimuli for control of level of activity, emotional response, and water consumption. Additionally, the septal nuclei suppress aggression from the amygdala and hypothalamus.

The thalamus, also part of the reticular activating system, regulates the states of consciousness. It also has a regulatory function over the hypothalamus.

ALSO SEE: *Ingestive Behavior, Sleep*

Brain Disorders

Changes in behavior can be related directly to changes within the brain. With any type of problem behavior, brain disorders must be considered. There is still a great deal of research to be done to learn the full extent of the brain-behavior problem connection, as well as to understand how certain medical conditions exert a neurologic effect. Known disorders include epilepsy, narcolepsy, mental lapse aggression syndrome, hydrocephalus, polyphagia, psychogenic conditions, and stereotyped behavior.

ALSO SEE: *Hydrocephalus, Mental Lapse Aggression Syndrome, Narcolepsy, Polyphagia, Psychogenic Problems, Seizures, Stereotyped Behaviors*

Brontophobia

Brontophobia is the fear of thunder.

SEE: *Fear of Thunder*

Broodiness

Broodiness is the part of maternal behavior directed specifically to the hatchlings, most commonly associated with poultry hens. The maternal behaviors directed to the young include calling, protecting, and covering of chicks. The behavior is probably associated with prolactin, and there may be a genetic component as well (Guhl and Fischer in Hafez, 1969). Since egg production decreases as broodiness increases, the behavior is selected against in the modern poultry industry.

ALSO SEE: *Brooding, Maternal Behavior*

Brooding

Brooding is the normal behavior of birds (either male or female) involving the covering of the brood of chicks to protect them or provide warmth. This is in contrast to incubation, which covers the unhatched eggs.

ALSO SEE: *Broodiness, Maternal Behavior*

Brood Parasitism

A few species leave their eggs or young for another species to raise. This form of parasitism is best associated with the cuckoo, but occurs in other species as well.

Bruce Effect

Named after the person who noticed it, the Bruce effect describes the abortion that can occur in some pregnant mice when exposed to the odor of a male other than the one that sired the fetuses.

Buller Steer Syndrome

Steers that are closely confined, as commonly happens in feedlots, may develop some unusual behaviors. According to A. J. Edwards (1988), as many as 4% of the steers in a feedlot become "bullers," depending on the time of the year and the length of time in the feedlot. They stand for mounting by other steers called "riders." If the behavior continues, it can reduce weight gains of individuals being ridden or result in injuries or exhaustion. These bullers are usually separated into a pen with others showing the same behavior. Stress from intense social interactions probably plays a role in this syndrome, and the more recent increase in frequency is related to hormone implantation.

ALSO SEE: *Atypical Sexual Behavior, Bachelor Groups, Inappropriate Mounting*

Burying Food

Domestic carnivores commonly bury food. Dogs probably bury bones and food as a remnant behavior for protecting occasional excess from scavengers. Because the behavior has no survival value to the domesticated dog, it has gradually been extinguished from the ingestive behavior patterns of dogs in general. In fact, most dogs do not seem to remember where they buried something.

Cats bury food for another reason. This behavior is usually shown toward a new type of food, often less palatable. The animal smells the food and then begins covering it for the same reason cats cover feces. The odor triggers the response to cover.

ALSO SEE: *Earth Raking, Elimination Behavior, Ingestive Behavior*

Butting

Butting is a distance-increasing behavior shown by many ungulates as they aggressively strike with the head. Horns can make the animal more dangerous if sharp points can contact the intended victim. If people tease animals that tend to play by butting with their heads, the animals may increase their aggressiveness, becoming dangerous to be around.

ALSO SEE: *Distance-increasing Silent Communication, Reactive Anomalies*

C

Canine Cognitive Dysfunction Syndrome

The canine cognitive dysfunction syndrome was first defined by W. W. Ruehl (1993) in his work studies of *l*-deprenyl in geriatric dogs. The syndrome is characterized by one or more clinical signs that suggest a decrease in the dog's interest in, or ability to interact with, its environment. In humans, cognitive dysfunction is usually associated with a neuronal degenerative process such as Alzheimer's disease or hypoxia. Clinical, physiological, and pathological components have not been well studied in dogs.

ALSO SEE: *Senile Aggression*

Canine-Tooth Threat

This is a threat display most common in the deer family in which the upper lips are elevated to expose the canine teeth. At the same time, the eyes are rotated so that only the white sclera is seen by the threatened animal.

ALSO SEE: *Threat Displays*

Cannibalism

Cannibalism refers to the eating of another animal of the same species. This behavior is usually associated with carnivores and omnivores—dogs, cats, and pigs of the domesticated species.

Dogs in geriatric beagle colonies are known to cannibalize others under certain circumstances. The cause is speculative and may relate to single or pack response aggression. Bitches can cannibalize puppies. An obvious runt in a litter may be killed and partially eaten. This behavior may be a response to the instinct to keep the nest area clean so as not to attract predators.

Queens and sows have also been known to eat their dead or stillborn young.

Females may chew through the umbilical cord while cleaning up a neonate and actually chew into the abdomen. Inexperience and/or inadequate hormone levels may account for the behavior, since it is most often associated with the first litter. This is generally not regarded as true cannibalism. When on an extremely deficient diet, queens have been observed to kill and eat kittens.

Feather picking by birds can progress to the killing of flock members and then to cannibalism if allowed to continue.

ALSO SEE: *Body Pecking, Cronism, Feather Eating, Feather Picking, Fratricide, Infanticide, Pack Response Aggression, Senile Aggression, Tail Chewing*

Car Chasing

Car chasing is a variation of prey chasing (predatory aggression) in which a dog chases a car that is moving away from it. Other variations include bicycle or jogger chasing, as well as livestock chasing. The behavior can be learned from another dog or it can possibly result from boredom, not enough exercise, and access to cars.

Elimination of the problem is particularly difficult because the behavior is internally rewarding. At best, success can be achieved in no more than 50% of car-chasing dogs, even in dogs injured by a car. The only sure cure is confinement in a house, in a fenced yard, or on a chain. Other methods depend on the ingenuity and determination of the owner.

Because any successful chase will be a reward, each attempt must be punished. Confinement must be employed when the owner cannot punish the chasing behavior. The owner should plan for quick punishment at the start of the behavior. It tends to be more effective if there is an element of surprise involved (for example, if it is arranged that the target car suddenly stops). The dog can be hit with a water balloon or squirt-gun spray, or the owner can jump from the passenger side and run yelling and arm-waving at the dog. The animal could also be allowed to drag a long rope that may be grabbed and the animal hauled in while being told "No" all the way. Eventually, the owner may have to remain concealed and use different cars to tempt the dog into action for punishment. Remote controlled shock collars have also been used. This problem behavior usually requires long-term therapy, since it is often well established by the time the owner seeks help.

ALSO SEE: *Internal Reward, Livestock Chasing, Predatory Aggression, Prevent Access, Reinforcement Schedules, Shock Collars*

Car Phobia

The fear of riding in a car, car phobia, is often the result of a poor introduction to the vehicle. Dogs and cats are usually taken for relatively long trips, often associated with an unpleasant event such as vaccinations, rather than taken on short, quick, enjoyable outings.

Teaching a dog or cat to ride in a car is best accomplished by a gradual introduction to the experience, with rewards for appropriate behavior. This is true for problem animals as well as the youngsters. The pet is asked to come to the owner and is rewarded with food or praise, as appropriate. Each successive time the owner moves closer to the car. Eventually the dog approaches the open back seat door but is not asked inside. At the next approach, the dog is asked to come inside for its reward. Then it is asked inside, and the door is closed and opened; then the door is shut for a longer period of time. Next, the engine is turned on and off. The sequence then progresses from moving a few feet to moving several feet, to moving to the end of a driveway, to driving around a short block. Eventually short trips with enjoyable outcomes are taken. These gradually are lengthened and then varied in length. Another important aspect of the program is to vary the purpose of the car rides. If all the trips end at a boarding kennel or veterinary office, the dog quickly learns to dread the ride.

Illness in a dog, and occasionally in a cat, is commonly induced by the motion of a car. It typically occurs in puppies and in dogs that have developed a fear of riding in a car. The problem can be prevented or resolved by an owner who is willing to take a little time to work with his or her pet before the inevitable long trip.

ALSO SEE: *Skinnerian Shaping of Behavior*

Carrying In

This is the behavior of carrying objects or young to a nest area. The phrase describes the behaviors of birds or fish bringing in nesting materials, and of carnivores and rodents that carry their young to new dens, burrows, or nests. Some species such as cats move their young every several days. Others move their young only if a nest site is perceived to be unsafe. The behavior continues until all young have been relocated and the female has returned for one trip more than the number of young. Carrying in also describes the retrieval of young that have wandered from the nest.

ALSO SEE: *Maternal Behavior, Transport of Young*

Caste

Caste describes a group of individuals within an insect society that are specialized by morphology and behavior to carry out a specific duty. Typically castes include workers, soldiers, and a queen.

ALSO SEE: *Division of Labor*

Castration

Castration is the surgical, chemical, or psychological removal of the testicles or their influence. This procedure has been used to alter the behavior of animals, originating with livestock kept in herds or flocks. In this way, males could be kept in large numbers in confinement without expressing intermale aggression or showing the tendency to collect female groups. It has allowed better meat production and more dependable service animals.

Castration is successful only at eliminating behaviors that are dependent on testosterone—urine/feces marking, roaming, intermale aggression, and male reproductive behaviors. In some animals, notably dogs, there is a learning component to the male sexually dimorphic behaviors. Thus, castration or the use of progestins to reduce serum testosterone levels is less successful in older animals that have had the opportunity to use specific behaviors.

Castration rates vary considerably between the dog and cat populations. Approximately 15% of male dogs in the United States have been castrated, while the castration rate is 40% to 60% for cats (Manning and Rowan, 1992; Wilbur, 1976). This difference may be attributable to two major factors. Feline spraying behavior generally is considered unacceptable in a house cat and thus more likely to be controlled with castration. On the other hand, the dog more often is regarded as a child substitute, making castration less acceptable.

ALSO SEE: *Intermale Aggression, Intrasexual Aggression, Male Behaviors, Masturbation, Progestins, Sexually Dimorphic Behaviors*

Catatonic Reaction

A catatonic reaction is characterized by stupor and marked muscular rigidity. Cats may not be able to escape an environment where they undergo severe emotional stress, resulting in a catatonic reaction. The animals are aware that things are going on around them and will slowly turn to follow movement, but there is little change in the general body position. They may be frozen in this position for several hours. This reaction is not as extreme as psychogenic shock.

ALSO SEE: *Hypotonia, Psychogenic Shock, Stress-related Behaviors, Thanatosis*

Caterwauling

This is the vocalization used by cats, particularly intact tomcats, to advertise their territory to potential mates and to warn intruders away. It is most common to hear this noise during the mating season. Since cats are usually separated by space, vocal communication is a necessary first step for cats to find potential mates. Only after caterwauling and the heat cries have attracted attention and brought the cats close can physical behaviors be used in sexual behavior.

ALSO SEE: *Male Behaviors, Vocal Communication*

Catnip

Catnip (*Nepeta cataria*, catmint) is one of several plants known to affect the

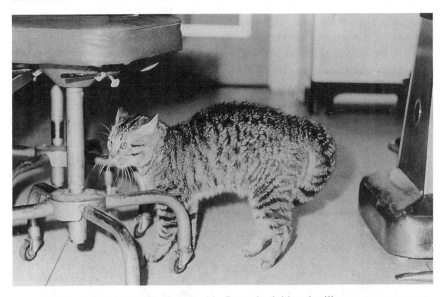

Catatonic Reaction. The cat in this figure is rigid and will not move except to slowly follow with its head a person's motion around the room. After 2 hours, his normal responses returned.

behavior of cats that smell them. The reaction is thought to be hallucinogenic. The reaction of a cat is variable, but usually consists of smelling the catnip, perhaps licking or chewing it, staring, salivating, twitching the skin of the back, and rolling. The response generally lasts a few minutes, but can continue for up to 15 minutes, followed by a refractory period of approximately one hour. Fifty to seventy percent of cats will react to catnip odors to some degree, and this is controlled by an autosomal dominant gene (Hatch, 1972). Age and experience can modify the response.

Other plant odors that can cause behavior changes include those from cat thyme (*Teucrium manum*), Matatabi (*Actinidia polygama*, silvervine), and valerian (*Valeriana officinalis*).

ALSO SEE: *Refractory Period, Smell*

Cats

Fossil evidence for feline ancestors goes back to *Miacis*, a shared ancestor with the dog, which lived approximately 40-60 million years ago. *Miacis* gave rise to *Cynodictis* (which became the dog), the bear-dog group (which became the bear), *Hoplophoneus* (which gave rise to the saber-toothed tiger), and *Dinictis*. The African wild cat, *Felis lybica*, is the probable immediate ancestor of the modern cat, *Felis catus*. The European wild cat, *Felis silvestris,* may have played a role in the development of the modern cat, although this theory is not universally accepted.

Cats first associated with humans in ancient Egypt around 1600 BC, because of the large granaries. The Egyptians incorporated cats into their religion, as Bastet and other part-cat figures, and mourned the animal's death. Cats spread to Europe with merchant traders and were initially held in high regard. At some time, however, the cat became associated with the moon goddess Diana, which eventually led to an association with witchcraft. After the Crusaders returned to Europe with the rat, which brought with it the plague, cats were again tolerated as the principal method of rodent control (Beaver, 1992).

Throughout its association with humans, the cat has undergone little selective breeding. Even today, the homogeneity of physical size, the relatively small number of pedigreed cats, and the asocial behavior of the species indicates the relative lack of human influence on the species.

ALSO SEE: *Domestication, Appendix B*

Cattle

Modern European breeds of cattle, *Bos taurus*, are generally accepted to have come from the *Bos primigenius primigenius*, also known as aurochs or extinct giant ox (Clutton-Brock, 1981). The last aurochs died in Poland in 1627. *Bos primigenius namadicus* is the probable ancestor of the humped zebu cattle of India, *Bos indicus*. Recent analysis of cattle DNA samples by D. Bradley and P. Cunningham indicates the European and Asian lines diverged approximately 200,000 years ago (Two Eves for Daisy? 1994). Lesser known cattle species may have other ancestors. Bovine remains have been found with human sites dating back to 6400 BC. Early associations between species were probably more for religious, ceremonial, or barter purposes. Later they were used for draft, then food, shelter, and clothing.

ALSO SEE: *Domestication, Appendix B*

Central Filters

When an animal's senses respond to an environmental stimulus, the information is received in the brain for processing. Central filters are those areas in the brain and central nervous system that determine if the information is received and how it is interpreted. A severed spinal cord or damaged area in the brain can mean the input passes a peripheral filter, but is not received. Inappropriate early experiences can also result in a varied filter. Experimentally, it has been shown that a lack of vertical lines during a kitten's early visual experience can result in a lack of their perception later (Ganz and Fitch, 1968).

Central filters can also result from the environment and the arousal state. An individual's mood can result in different responses to the same stimulus at different times.

ALSO SEE: *Filters, Mood, Peripheral Filters, Stimulus Filtering*

Central Hierarchy

In certain species of primates, a group of males can form an organization known as the central hierarchy. The individuals support each other in disputes so that the group strength allows them to dominate the troop and gain a status higher than that attainable by individual members. There is also an internal social rank within the group.

ALSO SEE: *Social Order*

Chasing Cars

Chasing cars is a form of predatory aggression that can be particularly dangerous for the dog. The internal reward of the chase makes elimination of the problem very difficult.

ALSO SEE: *Car Chasing, Internal Reward, Predatory Aggression*

Chasing Livestock

Dogs chase livestock as a form of predatory aggression. Since this behavior is self-rewarding, it becomes very difficult to stop except by preventing access to the livestock. Other techniques attempt to make the chase less rewarding. In desperation, some dog owners have hung the killed animal's body around the dog's neck or tied it in the dog's mouth. With aversive conditioning, the meat is treated to induce vomiting or nausea if eaten.

Breeds that work livestock, like border collies and Welsh corgis, were developed for their predatory tendencies. These were modified to a controllable, nonaggressive form through selective breeding. The chase is still in the breed, but the killer instinct has been minimized.

ALSO SEE: *Aversive Conditioning, Predatory Aggression*

Child Schema

Certain physical features tend to arouse care-giving tendencies in humans. The schema is characteristic of human infants—big head, round eyes, small chins—and is often characteristic of animal infants as well. Toy breeds of dogs, toys, and cartoon characteristics (like E.T.) often play on the child schema.

ALSO SEE: *Age Dimorphism, Paedomorphosis*

Choice Test

A choice, or preference, test is a form of behavior testing to determine preferences between various items or the ability to discriminate under very specific conditions. In a feeding trial, the animal chooses between two or more flavors or textures of food. Experimentally, livestock species have been given choices for "light" or "no light" and "on" or "off" radio.

ALSO SEE: *Preference Test*

Circadian Rhythms

Various systems within an individual maintain a cycle in a natural rhythm of approximately 24 to 28 hours. These physiologic and behavioral rhythms are generally tied to the earth's rotation. Air travel does not disrupt them, resulting in jet lag, and only time or light-dark shifts can reset the biologic clock. As scientists have come to understand more about circadian rhythm, they have been better able to adapt timing of medications to the body's natural rhythm.

ALSO SEE: *Annual Periodicity, Biological Rhythms*

Circannual Rhythms

This is a term used to refer to annual periodicity of animal behavior.

SEE: *Annual Periodicity*

Classical Conditioning

Classical conditioning is a type of learning popularized by Ivan Pavlov, thus its other name—Pavlovian conditioning. An unconditioned stimulus produces a response that is reflexlike, usually involving the contraction of smooth muscle or the secretion of a gland. A neutral (conditioned) stimulus is then paired with the unconditioned stimulus until the neutral stimulus alone can trigger the same response. In Pavlov's studies, food was the unconditioned stimulus that resulted in salivation as the response. He used a bell as a neutral stimulus and eventually was able to get the dogs to produce saliva simply by ringing the bell.

Classical conditioning is a form of learning that commonly occurs in animals, either through intentional use or by accident. Dogs and cats frequently begin drooling when their owner uses a can opener or opens a cupboard door. Dairy cows let down their milk when they enter a milking parlor.

ALSO SEE: *Autoshaping, Learning, Pavlovian Conditioning, Pseudoconditioning*

Claw Sharpening

Cats claw objects as a part of grooming, marking, and stretching. The behavior of extending foreclaws into soft wood or fabric helps remove fragments of claw that are being shed and keeps the claws sharp. Marking takes on two dimensions with clawing. There is an olfactory message left by sweat glands on the feet and a visual cue by the changes in the surface that occur over time. Since a number of the episodes occur soon after a cat wakes up, a stretching function may also exist.

Problem behaviors occur with indoor cats when owners fail to recognize the animal's need to express the clawing behavior. Kittens should be encouraged to climb and play on scratching posts, and the posts should be in accessible locations. Access to furniture and curtains should be limited, and the kitten disciplined immediately every time it tries to claw them.

ALSO SEE: *Claw Sharpening—Carpet, Claw Sharpening—Curtains, Declawing, Destructive Behaviors, Furniture Scratching, Marking, Punishment*

Claw Sharpening—Carpet

Many cats like to condition their foreclaws on horizontal objects rather than vertical objects. If outdoors, they use a board or tree root. Indoors, a carpet provides the alternative. While they tend to prefer certain areas for clawing, it may occur anywhere. Stopping claw sharpening on carpet is more difficult than on other surfaces. The first and easiest attempt is to put a horizontal scratching post on the spot of carpet used by the cat and then to put the cat on the post as an introduction to it. The scratching post should be soft or bark-covered wood or a unique-weave carpet. If the cat simply moves to a new location without using the new post, other methods should be tried. Ideally, the cat should be kept off the carpet and be offered a horizontal scratching post until it has learned to prefer the post to the carpet. This can be accomplished by confining the cat to a noncarpeted room that contains a scratching post. Carpet may have to be covered with a different textured material, such as plastic or newspaper.

ALSO SEE: *Claw Sharpening, Claw Sharpening—Curtains, Declawing, Destructive Behaviors, Furniture Scratching*

Claw Sharpening—Curtains

A few cats will reach up and use a curtain as a scratching post. This is apt to happen on full-length drapes of a heavy, loose-weave fabric. Once the problem develops, it takes some time to get it stopped. A scratching post should be put at the curtain location. It is best to replace the curtain with an inexpensive substitute having a different weave and texture. Plastic drapes generally work well. Because a behavior must be unlearned and an alternative learned, it could take as long to get the cat to use the scratching post as it did to develop the original problem.

ALSO SEE: *Claw Sharpening, Claw Sharpening—Carpet, Climbing Curtains, Declawing, Destructive Behaviors, Furniture Scratching*

Claw Sharpening—Furniture

This behavior is generally called furniture scratching.
SEE: *Destructive Behaviors, Furniture Scratching*

Cleaning Symbiosis

This is a mutually beneficial relationship between individuals of two species. One gets the benefit of ectoparasite removal, the other gets food. Birds often congregate on ungulates and other large mammals or on reptiles. Cleaner fish also are groomers.
ALSO SEE: *Commensalism, Grooming Behavior, Mutual Grooming*

Climbing

Problems with climbing can take a number of forms, depending on the species involved. Cats climb curtains in play and to get to higher places for rest or escape. Since climbing down is often viewed as more difficult for the cat, the owner may feel it is necessary to help the cat that is "stuck" in a tree.

Dogs show climbing problems differently. A few can climb certain trees if they get a running start. Most commonly, however, dogs climb out of their yard by going over fences or kennel runs. Owners may take elaborate precautions to keep their pets from digging out of a yard, only to find them climbing over the top instead. A number of control methods have been used. The tops of fences have been electrified using an electric fence wire made for livestock, or they have been designed to point inward, or made to completely cover the kennel top. While these efforts might prevent the dog from climbing over the fence, they do not address the cause of the problem, and many dogs develop another problem. The climbing dog becomes the digging dog. When this is stopped, barking may become the new outlet. For dogs, climbing and digging out of an enclosure are signs that the animal may be seeking social attention or that it is not expending enough energy. The pet confined to the backyard may get enough attention initially, but as the novelty wears off, owners spend less time with it. Attempts at social interaction with people on the front sidewalk or down the block cause the dog to escape. Excess energy will also cause the dog to seek routes to get rid of this, and escaping to run alone or with other dogs will meet the need. Scheduling attention and adequate exercise can prevent or correct the problem. The solution involves a commitment by the owner. If external sources of excitement precipitate the climbing, efforts should be taken to minimize them.

Goats are another domestic animal in which climbing is a problem. Kids challenge each other in their own version of "king of the hill," where the hill is anything taller than the surroundings—feeders, wagons, and cars. As goats get older, they climb net wire fences and become hard to contain.
ALSO SEE: *Avoid Excitement, Climbing Curtains, Digging, Excessive Vocal-*

ization—Barking, Exercise, Locomotion, Running Away, Schedule, Stress-related Behaviors

Climbing Curtains

Cats climb because they like to position themselves in high places. Kittens often scurry up objects in play, and older cats frequently rest or sleep in high spots. Most complaints are about the climbing behavior of kittens, but occasionally older cats use the behavior to get to a shelf or other favorite resting place. If the problem occurs frequently, remote punishment with limited access to the area may offer the best solution. It may also be necessary to change the curtains to blinds or plastic to discourage the behavior.

ALSO SEE: *Claw Sharpening—Curtains, Climbing, Remote Punishment*

Clinch

Fighting cows can use a clinch as a rest period during battle. One cow will allow her opponent to slip past her head and gain a flank approach with the poll of her head, but at the same time she will gain a flank approach to her opponent. Neither animal can gain a successful position because when one moves, the other maintains body contact. After a period of time, both back away and the fighting continues.

ALSO SEE: *Distance-increasing Silent Communication*

Clinging Young

In many mammalian species, including primates, the young reflexively cling to the mother for several weeks. This behavior ensures the young will have access to food until it is able to travel with the mother on its own.

ALSO SEE: *Nursing*

Cloth with Odor ("Security Blanket")

Animals can be reassured or frightened by odors in their environment because for most the sense of smell is more acute than in humans. If there is a significant odor of the owner, many stressed pets will develop a calmer nature. One method to provide the odor is to have the owner handle a handkerchief or small cloth and then let the animal have access to the cloth when the owner is away. A specific odor, like a perfume or aftershave, wintergreen extract, or a kitchen spice can be used in the same way if that odor has been used when the owner is around. The odor is thus associated with nonstressful situations and serves as an olfactory reminder of less stressful times.

ALSO SEE: *Fear of Thunder, Separation Anxiety, Smell*

Cognition

Cognition applies to an individual's mental functions, including the ability to learn, remember, and think. While the term is generally applied to human abilities, it may have limited use in ethology, especially relative to primates.

ALSO SEE: *Intelligence, Learning*

Coital Misalignment

A sexually aroused, experienced bull or billy may show interest in an estrous female but not align itself properly to mount and make no attempt to mount. Although juveniles often show a misalignment as they develop their behavioral patterns, this early behavior generally is not included under the heading of coital misalignment.

ALSO SEE: *Male Behaviors, Mounting*

Colony

Colony is a term used for a group of individuals of the same species without any implication as to the nature of the group.

ALSO SEE: *Animal Sociology*

Color Change

As the term implies, certain animals have the ability to change part or all of their body color. The change may occur instantaneously or seasonally and remain for seconds or months. This change may serve as camouflage in some species, such as snowshoe rabbits and ptarmigans, which turn white in winter and brownish in the summer. It can also communicate such things as aggression or reproductive states.

ALSO SEE: *Advertising Dress*

Color Vision

Because vision is especially important to humans, visual capabilities of animals, particularly color vision, have interested researchers. Many carefully designed projects have come up with differing results about color perception. Most domestic animal species can be found to react at least partially to certain colors. Functionally, most of these animals are physiologically capable of detecting a few colors; however, since color vision is not necessary for their survival, behavioral color vision is not developed. This makes the animals behaviorally color blind. Movement, with its contrast in background, is more important where camouflage plays a role in survival.

Primates, insects, and birds are believed to use color vision behaviorally, although the ranges of colors perceived may vary from the red-to-blue range of human vision.

ALSO SEE: *Vision*

Comfort Behavior

The term comfort behavior is applied to those behaviors that are generally felt to provide some degree of comfort to an individual. Grooming behaviors and relieving behaviors (eliminating, stretching, yawning, and perhaps sleeping) are usually included.

ALSO SEE: *Grooming Behavior*

Commensalism

This is a type of relationship between individuals in which one benefits while the other neither gains nor loses.

ALSO SEE: *Cleaning Symbiosis*

Communal Courtship

Courtship where more than two individuals take part is called communal. Often there are several males interested in one or more estrous females. Following of estrous bitches by dogs and competition in bulls and birds are examples. In some species, the presence of more than one male may be necessary for successful reproduction.

ALSO SEE: *Courtship*

Communal Song

This is a vocalization where two or more individuals vocalize at the same time. The chorusing of canids and primates may help group cohesion and definition of territories. In some insects, reptiles, and birds, the behavior is primarily associated with attracting mates.

ALSO SEE: *Vocal Communication*

Communication Behaviors

Communication is the act of transmitting information between individuals. Animals communicate through vocal patterns, body language, and body odors. The vocal forms of communication are generally used to transmit emotional states rather than specific messages because the vocabularies are so limited. Silent communication, or body language, is well developed in animals, particularly for the types of messages most useful to a particular species. Distance-increasing silent communication postures indicate a "go away" message, while distance-reducing silent communication postures show "friendly" or submissive behavior.

ALSO SEE: *Distance-increasing Silent Communication, Distance-reducing Silent Communication, Interspecies Communication, Interspecific Releaser, Mechanical Communication, Pheromone, Song, Vocal Communication*

Competitive Aggression

Competitive aggression is a variation of dominance aggression where two animals compete for a favored food or location. When animals do not share equally, a solution to possession usually is decided by the dominant animal getting the prize of the competition.

ALSO SEE: *Dominance Aggression*

Concaveation

Concaveation is the expression of maternal behavior that occurs as the result of a female being exposed to the young of her own species for a long enough period of time.

ALSO SEE: *Maternal Behavior*

Concept Learning

This is the ability to understand a certain concept and apply it in new situations. Conceptualization implies a high form of intellectual achievement and is most commonly observed in primates. Sign language has been used to test for concept formation in chimpanzees and gorillas. Other species have been able to demonstrate the ability to learn same/different pattern recognition.

ALSO SEE: *Learning*

Conditioning

Conditioning is a process where an animal learns to respond in a certain way to a certain stimulus.

ALSO SEE: *Behavior Modification, Classical Conditioning, Counterconditioning, Operant Conditioning, Pseudoconditioning*

Confinement

Confinement is a treatment that is useful for a number of behavior problems. It can take several forms, and the appropriate choice depends on the specific problem. An animal can be confined to a small area such as a crate, chute, or stall. It can also be confined to areas of increasingly larger size, such as in a room or group of rooms or in a paddock or pasture. Confinement can also mean to be kept out of an area, such as preventing access to a particular room where a problem occurs. For many problem behaviors, confinement alone will not stop a recurrence.

Problems can also result from excessive confinement with minimal exposure to conspecifics, people, different environments, or adequate exercise. For the deprived individual, stereotyped behaviors are common. Other problems include improper socialization, digging, kennelosis, barking, climbing, cribbing, wind sucking, stall kicking, and self-mutilation.

ALSO SEE: *Climbing, Crate, Cribbing, Excessive Vocalization—Barking, Housetraining, Kennelosis, Self-Mutilation, Socialization, Stall Kicking, Stereotyped Pacing, Stereotyped Weaving, Time-Out, Wind Sucking*

Conflict

Conflict applies to the aggressive interactions, or contest, between two or more individuals. It also applies to an individual's internal dispute when opposite tendencies are aroused simultaneously. Ambivalent behaviors, displacement activities, stereotyped behaviors, and redirected aggressions are the external manifestations of these internal conflicts.

ALSO SEE: *Aggression, Ambivalent Postures, Displacement Activity, Mixed Motivation, Redirected Aggression, Stereotyped Behaviors*

Consort Pair

In some species, such as primates, a male and female may temporarily pair during a female's estrous period and minimize their interactions with other group members.

Consummatory Phase

In a series of actions that together constitute a specific behavior, the action that completes the series is called the consummatory phase, or end act. For cat hunting behavior, the consummatory phase is the eating of the prey. The series consists of stalking, catching, killing, carrying to a secluded location, and eating. Copulation would typically be the consummatory phase of sexual behavior. The successful completion of this phase may be related to the onset of a refractory period.

ALSO SEE: *Appetitive Behavior, Ingestive Behavior, Refractory Period*

Contact Animals

Many animal species tend to maintain body contact with conspecifics when resting. Examples include pigs, primates, certain fish, and some birds.

ALSO SEE: *Contact Behavior, Density-Tolerant Animals*

Contact Behavior

This is another name for huddling behavior and involves close physical contact between individuals. It is a common behavior with contact animals, in species with clinging young, and between individuals as protection against the cold or wet.

In a broader sense, contact behavior includes vocalizations and other messages that keep animals apprised of each other's whereabouts.

ALSO SEE: *Clinging Young, Contact Animals, Contact Greeting, Density-Intolerant Animals, Huddling*

Contact Greeting

A contact greeting is any form of greeting behavior that involves touching. It is as common as the handshake, or rubbing against an individual, as cats commonly do.

ALSO SEE: *Greeting Behaviors*

Coolidge Effect

After mating with a female several times, a male's refractory time between matings increases until mating no longer occurs. If a new female is introduced, it can stimulate the male to resume copulation. This effect of stimulus novelty is called the Coolidge effect, or action-specific exhaustibility.

ALSO SEE: *Male Behaviors, Refractory Period*

Coprophagia

Coprophagia is a form of pica where the animal eats feces. This behavior is common in the young of most species and is seen as a problem in several others.

As young animals begin the transition between nursing and adult forms of ingestive behavior, many go through a stage of eating the feces of their own species, especially that of their dam. While the exact cause is not known, certain theories have been proposed (Crowell-Davis & Houpt, 1985). The first is that the young use their mouths to explore their environments; coprophagy may be one expression of that exploration. A second theory explains the behavior as useful in helping the youngster establish an intestinal microflora. This theory has not held true, at least in rats. A third theory says the behavior is used to compensate for a nutritional deficiency. Deoxycholic acid, present in feces, may promote myelinization and intestinal immunocompetence.

Maternal behaviors often include licking the anogenital areas of neonates. With puppies and kittens, this behavior is necessary to stimulate the anogenital reflex, which is the only way to promote urination and defecation. Also, by swallowing the excreta, the female can help reduce the odors that could attract predators to the area. Cows and mares will also lick the young and may elicit elimination as well as consume some of the feces or urine.

Dogs are the animals most commonly presented with coprophagia as a complaint. These complaints fall into one of four groups: the dog is eating its own feces, another dog's feces, cat feces, or horse/cow feces. The dog that is eating its own stool needs to be evaluated for possible metabolic problems, including pancreatic deficiencies. Hydrocephalic dogs, dogs with heavy internal parasite loads, and dogs that are apparently bored have also been known to eat their own feces. The second type of canine coprophagy, when a dog eats the stool of other dogs, is most frequently done by puppies and by dogs that have few other outlets for activity. The eating of cat feces occurs because of the apparent olfactory attractiveness. Since canine aesthetic values differ from those of humans, the odor attracts the dog to another source of protein. The feces of horses or cattle represents a source of predigested vegetable matter and are eaten for many of the same reasons that dogs eat grass.

In the nonmedical cases, preventing dogs from eating feces is difficult because the behavior is self-rewarding, and in some cases, a habit. The only certain prevention is to deny access to the feces. Taste aversion can be used, but owners must be persistent at keeping the aversive taste strong enough for a long enough time for it to become discouraging. Substances added to the food to pass through with the feces generally are not strong enough to discourage the problem dog, although they may work on the beginner. If lack of activity is suspected as a contributing factor, exercise and scheduled interactions may become important.

Coprophagia is seldom a problem for cats. Even young kittens usually leave feces alone. They can be seen eating litter or dirt within a few days of beginning to eliminate on their own, but the behavior does not include feces-eating.

Foals, calves, and piglets do show moderate degrees of coprophagia. While foals have been shown to investigate feces in general, they only eat the dam's feces.

Laboratory-held primates commonly develop coprophagia, possibly because of a lack of adequate environmental stimulation. A trend toward enrichment of the environment should help prevent the development of this behavior.

Eating feces from other species is normal behavior for a number of animals. Birds pick out seeds and grains. Pigs may also get nutrients from bovine fecal matter.

ALSO SEE: *Boredom, Eliminative Behavior, Fefection, Grass Eating, Habit, Litter (Bedding) Eating, Pica, Stool Eating—Another Species, Taste Aversion, Transitional Phase*

Counterconditioning

Counterconditioning is a learning process aimed at establishing a new response to a stimulus as a replacement for an undesirable behavior. For example, if a dog that is food motivated is fearful of a gunshot, it should be fed immediately after the gun is fired. It may gradually replace the fearful behavior with anticipatory excitement. This technique is often coupled with desensitization, which in this example would also simultaneously lessen the fear reaction to the loud noise.

Counterconditioning is the opposite of conditioning.

ALSO SEE: *Aggression and Doorbells, Aggression and Mail Carriers, Aggression and Telephones, Behavior Modification, Classical Conditioning, Conditioning, Desensitization, Operant Conditioning, Trailer Problems*

Counterphobic Behavior

Counterphobic behavior is the expression of a behavior because of a fear. For example, in humans, a person who is afraid of heights might go mountain climbing. While this behavior is difficult to demonstrate in animals, occasional feats suggest that it may be possible.

Courtship

The first stage of reproduction is courtship, or the pre-mating phase. It can involve males or females, although it is most commonly associated with males. Courtship typically involves the male showing interest in the female, often following her. The duration of this phase varies depending on the recent number of breedings the male has made and the number of estrous females available. The actual determination of the female's readiness to mate is determined by her odors and/or her behaviors. These behaviors include standing to be mounted, returning pressure from chin resting, standing for a foreleg-kick, male soliciting, rolling, vocalizing, neck-biting, mounting, and others.

Species differences do occur. In cats, the sex call by the male advertises a territory to an estrous female while warning other toms. Since cats are asocial, the vocalizations by both male and female are important for locating individuals ready to mate. Neck-biting is a well developed behavior in the tom.

For stallions, the courtship phase is very important because it takes considerable time for a vascular penis to become engorged with blood, especially when compared with a fibroelastic penis. The interactions of the stallion and the mare and other environmental stimuli during courtship are all important to complete the erection.

Bulls show chin resting as a courtship behavior. They put their chins on the rump of a cow, exerting a slight forward pressure as they do. Anestrous cows respond by moving away, while cows in heat do not move or will push back.

During courtship, boars show teeth grinding, with resulting foaming saliva. A similar behavior also is seen in aggressive interactions.

ALSO SEE: *Communal Courtship, Consort Pair, Epigamic Display, Estrous*

Behavior, Female Behaviors, Flehmen, Foreleg-Kick, Infantile Behavior, Male Behaviors, Mating March, Reproductive Behavior, Soliciting Behavior

Crate

The crate is a small area of confinement useful for transporting animals, housing pets, and treating certain behavior problems of dogs and cats. Owners frequently express concern about keeping a dog or cat in such a small space, but most pets spend a large portion of their day sleeping in one location, and a crate works well for that. Crating should not be used as punishment or for isolation only. Pets can be fed in them and have their beds in them to develop a feeling of security there. Gradual introduction, associated with food or play, increases acceptance of the confinement.

ALSO SEE: *Confinement*

Crawling under and through Fences

Dogs and livestock species contain individuals that learn to escape from a pen or pasture by crawling under or through a fence. Most commonly they do this to get to feed on the other side, but occasionally they do it to escape to reach a conspecific. These animals can become very proficient in the technique, and prevention can be a real challenge if correcting the initiating factor does not work. Yoke-like neck pieces made of wire are commonly used in cattle, but care must be exercised with horses because of the species' tendency to struggle after being caught in the fence. Alternative fencing types, including electric fences, can successfully contain most of the problem animals; however, many owners choose confinement or sale of the animal as a low-cost alternative. Twisted wire stays between strands of barbed wire, a strand of barbed wire at the bottom of hog fencing, and burying the lower fence are other alternatives.

ALSO SEE: *Climbing, Escape Behaviors, Fence Jumping*

Cribbing

Cribbing is a behavior problem in horses that involves biting and holding onto fences, stall walls, mangers, trees, and other objects. It is most likely associated with lack of activity, particularly when the horse is not getting enough exercise. Excessive chewing of an object may precede the development of this behavior. Cribbing is self-rewarding to a certain degree, so it becomes more difficult to control as time continues. Young horses that are stalled for prolonged periods are most likely to develop the problem. Pastured horses spend most of their time grazing and are less likely to develop the problem.

Treatment is most effective if it has several phases. Taste aversion is effective at getting the horse to stop chewing on certain objects. At the same time, it is important to address the cause of the inactivity. Since horses would normally spend the major portion of a day grazing, they need to be exercised to remove the excess energy, fed several times a day instead of just once or twice, and provided with things to do. Running in a pasture at least part of the day may be adequate. Muzzles can be used, but if the initial inactivity is not addressed, other problems will develop. Without treatment, some horses will develop into wind suckers.

ALSO SEE: *Internal Reward, Muzzle, Psychogenic Diarrhea, Taste Aversion, Wind Sucking, Wood Chewing*

Crib-Whetting

Crib-whetting is another expression for the behavior problem of excessive licking.

SEE: *Licking*

Critical Distance

This is the social (reactive) distance associated with the approach of an intruder. When the intruder approaches an animal, the animal normally would flee as the intruder reaches the flight distance. If the animal is not aware of the intruder's approach or if it cannot flee, it will attack as the intruder reaches the critical distance. The difference in spacing between the flight distance and critical distance varies with species. For bears, for example, the gap is quite narrow so that a fast-moving, unobserved intruder could pass the flight distance and reach the critical distance before the bear had a chance to escape. An attack would result.

ALSO SEE: *Flight Distance, Reactive Distances, Social Distance*

Critical Periods

During an individual's development, there are specific time periods when important things must happen. When the period ends, the specific opportunity is lost. Critical periods include those for species identification, socialization, and maternal and infant imprinting. The specific times for each vary with the species.

ALSO SEE: *Imprint Learning, Sensitive Period, Socialization*

Cronism

Cronism refers to a type of cannibalism in which the parents eat their young. This is most frequently seen as a stress-related behavior in domestic animals, particularly pigs. Infanticide, which is the killing but not the eating of the young, is usually included within the broad definition of cronism.

ALSO SEE: *Cannibalism, Infanticide, Ingestive Behavior, Stress-related Behaviors*

Cross-Sucking

This behavior is another name for prolonged sucking.

SEE: *Prolonged Sucking*

Curiosity

An intense interest in a novel object or area is called curiosity. This term is usually referred to as investigative behavior.

ALSO SEE: *Exploratory Behavior, Investigative Behavior*

Cut Off

This is a behavior used to reduce the degree of stress between two individuals that would otherwise result in aggression. The shifting of weight away from an approacher or the diversion of eye contact are cut-off behaviors.

ALSO SEE: *Appeasement Behavior, Submissive Behavior*

D

Damming-up Theory

An animal will show a certain series of behaviors when the stimulus for that series reaches a threshold level. As the behavior is performed, the threshold will increase, and the amount of stimulus needed will be greater. If the animal does not express the behavior over time, the threshold will decrease. If the stimulus does not occur, the action-specific energy to perform the behavior continues to accumulate, as if dammed up behind an invisible barrier. When a slight stimulus does occur, the resulting behavior is often exaggerated.

If the stimulus does not occur or is not obvious, the behavior may eventually appear anyway. It would then be termed a vacuum activity.

ALSO SEE: *Masturbation, Vacuum Activity*

Dashing through Doors

Animals use dashing through doors as a method of escape. Horses use it to escape from a stall. Dogs and cats can use the behavior to either get out of a house or into a house, perhaps at a time when the owner does not want this to happen. To decrease the extent of the problem, increase the amount of exercise the animal gets, correct deficiencies in social interactions, or make the animal show a conflicting behavior. A dog that bursts into the house can leave muddy paw prints across the floor. A reward for obeying the "sit" command gives the owner time to wipe the mud off.

ALSO SEE: *Bolting, Escape Behaviors, Substitute a Behavior*

Death Shake

Canids often shake their prey after catching it. They may then toss it aside and attack it again. The combination of bite and shake is useful in killing the prey. Cats use the nape bite and directly penetrate the spinal cord instead of using a death shake.

ALSO SEE: *Nape Bite, Predation*

Deception

Deception is the use of a behavior or physical feature to create a misleading impression. The angler fish has an anatomic "worm" to attract prey. Some flowers attract insects by looking or smelling like a female insect. Many ground birds act as if they have a broken wing to distract predators from a nest.

ALSO SEE: *Display*

Declawing

Declawing is the surgical removal of the ungual process or the distal phalanges for the purpose of removing the claw. The procedure is most commonly done in the forelimbs of cats, although owners may request it for the rear limbs of cats, the forelimbs of digging dogs, and the limbs of certain exotic pets such as lions. There is no evidence of long-term problems as the result of the procedure (Bennett, Houpt, and Erb, 1988); however, it is elective surgery, and there remains moral controversy about that. There are times, however, when the animal would be euthanized if the procedure was not done.

ALSO SEE: *Claw Sharpening, Claw Sharpening—Carpet, Claw Sharpening—Curtains, Digging, Digging—Indoors, Digging—Outdoors, Furniture Scratching* .

Decrease Body Threat

For an animal that is showing an extremely submissive behavior to a person, the extremeness of the posture may be reduced if the person decreases the degree of his or her body threat posture. This problem is usually shown by the very timid or fear-biting dog. The human threat can be decreased by avoiding direct eye contact with the dog and by diverting the face. The body should be turned laterally with stooping or kneeling down useful to reduce the appearance of size. These postures minimize the vision of a huge "thing" towering over the dog. The person, instead, can encourage the dog's approach with a friendly, high-pitched voice. Reaching out and grabbing the dog is contraindicated. A few cats show the pariah threat to their owners. For those, an increased threat is counterproductive. Minimizing contact is actually the most effective.

ALSO SEE: *Fear-induced Aggression, Fear Biting, Housesoiling—Submissive Urination, Pariah Threat, Passive Submission, Submissive Urination, Timid Personality*

Decreased Sexual Behavior

Sexual behaviors, particularly mounting, are most frequent about the time of puberty and decrease somewhat with age and with opportunity. When there are multiple estrous females, the degree of interest and courtship by the male decreases so that mating may be the only behavior shown. The more often breeding occurs, the longer the refractory period between mating bouts. Castration (physical, psychological, or chemical) and pregnancy are the most common causes for the perception of decreased sexual behavior.

ALSO SEE: *Female Behaviors, Male Behaviors, Refractory Period, Sexually Dimorphic Behaviors*

Defecation

Defecation involves the removal of the waste by-products from the intestinal tract. This process involves a number of behaviors that are quite similar to those associated with urination.

Neonatal animals, particularly puppies and kittens in domesticated species, need stimulation of the perineal area from the dam's licking in order to defecate. This anogenital reflex is useful in minimizing odors that might attract predators.

Adult dogs do not differ greatly from prepubertal puppies in the defecation posture. The rear limbs are spread apart and the back is markedly arched, bringing the perineum relatively close to the ground. Dogs may posture and defecate multiple times during a single defecation period, walking a short distance between each defecation. An occasional dog will back up to a tree or onto a tree as if in a handstand, and push the feces onto it. This may serve as an olfactory marking behavior. Defecation normally occurs two or three times daily.

Cats use a defecation pattern similar to that of normal urination. They dig a hole in soft dirt or litter, assume a slight squat over the hole, defecate, turn and smell the feces, then earth rake, usually covering the feces. The earth raking is instinctive, triggered by the odor. Covering is learned; older cats can be encouraged to cover if the owner moves the cat's paws to help the covering act. The covering of nonexcrement, such as food, is related to the cat's perception of its smell. Defecation normally occurs one or two times each day.

Horses defecate 5 to 12 times during a 24-hour period. The posture includes a slightly arched back and rear limbs abducted slightly from normal standing. Stallions are particularly interested in the odors of fecal piles. They will smell them and may defecate (or occasionally urinate) on top and then re-smell. This can occur several times before the horse moves on. Horses also have a strong tendency to defecate in specific locations.

Defecation postures are minimal for cattle. There is a slight arching of the back and abducting of the rear limbs, but the animal may continue to walk or graze. There is some question as to how much control the animal actually has over when or where it defecates. There is no apparent social significance of feces to cattle and defecation is not restricted to specific locations.

Swine can be trained to eliminate in specific areas, a trait that has allowed pet pigs to use a litter box. In confinement, swine tend to eliminate near their water source. There is no obvious posturing associated with defecation.

ALSO SEE: *Elimination Behavior, Housetraining, Marking, Urination*

Defensive Behavior

Any behavior taken to avoid predation is a defensive behavior. Primary defenses are those that occur at all times. These can include camouflage, burrows, and other constants. Secondary defenses are behaviors that are in response to an immediate danger. These range from mobbing attacks on a predator by a group to an individual playing dead.

Defensive Threat

This is a distance-increasing silent communication threat posture shown by a cat until it has an opportunity to escape. Typically it is a lateral, arched-back stance with piloerection, a stare, flattened ears, and a downwardly arched tail. The teeth may be showing and a hiss is often used. The ultimate defensive posture involves the cat laying on its back with all the claws and teeth showing. This posture is reserved for intense confrontations when defense becomes necessary.

ALSO SEE: *Distance-increasing Silent Communication, Lateral Threat, Offensive Threat, Pariah Threat*

Demanding Personality

Certain individuals show a behavior that is almost continuously demanding of the owner. The tendency is encouraged by rewarding the behavior. Some cats always want to be petted, for example, and the act of petting rewards the demand and increases the likelihood of it being repeated. There is a fine distinction, and not always an obvious one, between a demanding personality and a learned behavior.

ALSO SEE: *Trial and Error Learning*

Density-Intolerant Animals

These are species that respond to crowding with a decreased reproductive rate. They are also called distance animals.

ALSO SEE: *Density-Tolerant Animals, Distance Animals*

Density-Tolerant Animals

These are species that are tolerant of crowding and able to maintain their reproductive rate until the crowding reaches a certain level. Generally these are contact animals.

ALSO SEE: *Contact Animals, Contact Behavior, Density-Intolerant Animals*

Depraved Appetite

Animals can eat a number of nonfood items as well as unusual food. This behavior is commonly called pica.

SEE: *Pica*

Depression

Clinical depression is difficult to document in animals and probably does not occur often. In order to be considered as a diagnosis, the depression should have a major, long-term effect on an animal's behavior, making that animal less responsive or interested in its surroundings for prolonged periods. Recovery is also gradual. Causes of depression are related to prolonged exposure to severely depressed, nonresponsive people or to an environmental change that drastically changes the animal's lifestyle.

Treatment for clinical depression is based on minimizing the cause. Owners should encourage activities that the animal enjoys and incorporate them at least daily. It may be necessary to work with human health-care givers if the depression is owner-related. Drug therapy with medications such as fluoxetine may be useful in severe or prolonged canine cases.

ALSO SEE: *Drug Therapy, Frustration, Appendix C*

Deprivation Syndrome

This is the general name applied to changes in behavioral development that result from social isolation in early life. This can be the result of premature breaking of the bond between the infant and its mother (separation syndrome), as has been well studied in primates. It also can result from minimal contact with a varied environment or with humans (isolated syndrome).

ALSO SEE: *Isolated Syndrome, Separation Syndrome*

Desensitization

Desensitization is the process of making an animal less behaviorally sensitive or reactive. This procedure often involves habituation. Desensitization works well on fears, phobias, and learned reactions, such as attacking ringing telephones.

The stimulus for a specific behavior can be repeated so often that it becomes meaningless. For example, when a dog attacks a ringing phone or doorbell, allow the ringing to continue without any reaction by the family until it no longer triggers the barking attack. After a rest, start the ringing again until the reaction stops. Gradually, the repetitive bouts become shorter, and finally the undesirable behavior stops altogether. Under some conditions, such as fear of thunder or gunshots, the initial stimulus must be minimized so that it is mute enough not to cause the reaction. Distance from the noise or decreased volume is useful. Gradually the volume is raised, giving the animal a chance to become accustomed to the sound and to learn that there is no danger. Antianxiety tranquilizers may be necessary initially. During desensitization, counterconditioning is often used to change the type of response as well.

ALSO SEE: *Aggression and Doorbells, Aggression and Mail Carriers, Aggression and Telephones, Behavior Modification, Cloth with Odor, Counterconditioning, Fear of Environment, Fear of Gunshots, Fear of Loud Noise, Fear of Noise, Fear of Thunder, Habituation Learning, Phobia, Trailer Problems*

Destructive Behaviors

In stressful situations, animals can respond with destructive behaviors. These generally include actions directed toward inanimate objects in the environment. The behavior may occur as an attempt to escape or as an action to relieve the stress. Behaviors included in this category are destructive chewing, digging, plant eating, cribbing, excessive licking, claw sharpening, prolonged sucking, and vocalizing.

Stresses that precipitate destructive behaviors often have to do with social isolation, excitement, emotional coming or going of the owner, lack of exercise, or a poor schedule. It is important to identify the stressor and eliminate it to cure the problem.

ALSO SEE: *Avoid Excitement, Cribbing, Destructive Chewing, Digging—*

D

Indoors, Digging—Outdoors, Emotional Come and Go, Exercise, Frustration, Licking of Objects, Plant Eating, Prolonged Sucking Syndrome, Schedule, Stress-related Behaviors

Destructive Chewing

In domestic animals the problem of destructive chewing occurs in three species—dogs, cats, and horses. In dogs there are three major causes of destructive chewing. Stress from changes in schedules or the lack of routine can result in chewing objects in the environment and in self-mutilation, including flank sucking and lick granulomas. Emotional coming or leaving related to owner activities and disruptions in the owner's life are other stresses that can be expressed as destructive chewing. The second major cause of this problem is the lack of adequate exercise, so chewing becomes an outlet for built-up energy. The third cause, fear of thunder, can result in some extreme cases of destructive chewing. Since puppies commonly chew, the behavior can be minimized by diverting the puppy's attention and decreasing the level of excitement. The puppy should not be allowed to chew on hands, in order to minimize the intensity of a bite in the future.

Chewing problems in cats are usually related to the prolonged sucking syndrome. In horses, protein, salt, and roughage deficiencies have resulted in destructive chewing or pica. Pent-up energy and/or the lack of environmental stimuli can also be associated with problem chewing in horses.

It is important to identify and eliminate the cause. This can mean using a strict schedule, increasing exercise, providing environmental stimulation, preventing access to favorite target items, and minimizing stress. Taste aversion or smell aversion may also be needed, particularly if the problem has developed over a long period of time. If fear of thunder is involved, habituation may also be useful.

ALSO SEE: *Antiaggressive Puppy Training, Avoid Excitement, Boredom, Destructive Behaviors, Divert Attention, Emotional Come and Go, Exercise, Fear of Thunder, Habituation Learning, Ingestive Behavior, Pica, Prevent Access, Prolonged Sucking Syndrome, Schedule, Self-Mutilation, Separation Anxiety, Smell Aversion, Spite, Taste Aversion*

Diary

Some behavior problems do not occur on a regular basis or do not seem to have an obvious stimulus. It may be impossible to determine critical factors that precipitate the problem on the basis of the initial history. For housesoiling, epilepsy, and stress-induced problems, appropriate diagnosis may require that the owner keep a diary of the frequency of the problem and the events that preceded the behavior for up to 24 hours.

ALSO SEE: *Epilepsy, Housesoiling, Stress-related Behaviors*

Diet Change

Animal diets may need to be changed for several reasons. Medical conditions such as food allergies and portosystemic shunts, which cause behavior changes, necessitate dietary changes. In dogs, other behavior problems can also have diet-related causes. Hyper or aggressive behaviors should be approached by changing to a good-quality regular commercial diet, if the animals are on a high protein diet or one with a large amount of additives or carbohydrates. In extreme cases, a restrictive allergy diet or a therapeutic diet used in specific conditions is appropriate.

To prevent kittens and puppies from becoming finicky eaters, dietary flavors and textures of food should be changed frequently. Food preferences are learned before six months in most animal species, so an early introduction to some variety is good preventive medicine.

ALSO SEE: *Allergy Workup, Finicky Eaters, Food Allergy*

Digging

There are a number of components to digging behavior. In dogs and some cats it is considered normal. It can become a problem if the animal owner does not appreciate the behavior or if it occurs to excess, in an abnormal location, or is combined with escape. A detailed history including location of the activity, simultaneous events, and events related to the area of digging is important in determining the cause and treatment approach. Declawing is rarely an appropriate solution. In each case it is important to evaluate social contact, external stimuli, amount of exercise, and environmental temperatures. Approaches to digging problems inside a home are different than those in a yard.

ALSO SEE: *Avoid Excitement, Declawing, Digging—Indoors, Digging— Outdoors, Digging Box, Escape Behaviors, Separation Anxiety, Stool Eating—Another Species, Appendix A*

Digging—Indoors

Occasionally, dogs dig indoors, usually on a carpet. In some cases this represents an effort to get out of a confined area in order to be with the family members. For that dog, attention means success, so the behavior must be extinguished with remote punishment and the cause of the problem evaluated. Schedule, exercise, and human attention should be adequate so that the dog is not just "deposited" someplace when its novelty wears off.

Geriatric dogs may also start digging in a carpet during the heat of summer or the coldest part of winter. When they lose some of their ability for thermoregulation, temperatures and drafts that had not been a problem begin to cause discomfort. This becomes noticeable when people try to save money on heating and air conditioning bills by adjusting their thermostats. Correction of this type of indoor digging can be accomplished by providing additional heat or cooling as appropriate. This can be done centrally or by adding a fan for summer cooling or wrapping the pet in a blanket during the winter.

Declawing would be a drastic last effort to control the problem.

ALSO SEE: *Attention Seeking, Declawing, Destructive Behaviors, Digging, Exercise, Hypothermia, Remote Punishment, Schedule*

Digging—Outdoors

Digging at various outdoor sites is a common behavior problem in dogs. It is important to understand that certain breeds are more apt to dig because of genetic tendencies to do so; however, digging can be a problem in most breeds under certain environmental conditions. History plays an important part in determining the cause of the problem, and that in turn is important in finding an appropriate approach to problem solving. Owners can go to extreme measures to stop the digging, such as filling the hole, filling the hole with water and holding the dog's head under the water, peppering the hole, declawing, and electric fencing. These methods are generally unsuccessful for the long term because the dog might avoid the one spot and move to another. Successful treatment is dependent on addressing the cause of the problem.

Holes dug randomly around the yard usually indicate the dog is getting rid of extra energy. It might be following small rodents or just digging for the "enjoyment" of the exercise. For this type of dog, exercise becomes an important part of its schedule.

Dogs that dig along a fence usually are pointing toward the source of the problem, whether or not they actually escape from the yard. The activity of a neighbor dog, cat, or child is the most common cause. Ideally, if the owner can stop the nearby activity, excitement, or exposure to that activity, the digging will stop. In some cases this can be done by timing trips so that the dog is out when the nearby activity is least likely to happen. In other cases, a kennel or fenced area away from the digging site will solve the problem. Additional exercise is usually helpful in these cases, too.

Destruction of flower beds, gardens, or other shady areas with moist dirt is common in the heat of summer as the dog seeks alternative methods for keeping cool. This behavior can be eliminated by correcting the overheating. Suggestions include keeping the dog indoors during the heat of the day, providing a fan to keep air moving in a certain area, putting a wading pool near the area, or landscaping a cool, shady area into a digging box.

Dogs that dig near gates, doors, or other areas where people tend to be are indicating another problem. Even those that actually dig out seldom go much beyond the front yard or the closest area with people. Dogs kept in the backyard tend to get less human contact over time. Instead of the playmate, they become the chore that must be fed once a day. When deprived of social contacts, dogs start seeking them out by escaping from the yard. The solution must incorporate human attention on a daily scheduled basis. This is best accomplished through three or four periods of 30 minute activities, such as grooming, playing ball, going for walks, and interacting in positive ways.

ALSO SEE: *Avoid Excitement, Declawing, Destructive Behaviors, Digging Box, Exercise, Running Away, Schedule*

Digging Box

For the outdoor dog, digging to cool off is always possible until the hot summer temperature changes. The usual presenting complaint is that a flower bed or a spot in the yard is being destroyed. In this case, the owners should choose an area that is shady in the afternoon, preferably in an area where the dog has been digging already. This area can be worked into the backyard landscape using timbers or railings. It should be kept slightly moist, and dirt should be replaced as necessary. It might also be necessary to fence off the unacceptable locations once a digging box has been built, to teach the dog where digging is tolerated. A digging area provides the dog with a spot to cool off and the owners with an acceptable alternative to total flower bed destruction.

ALSO SEE: *Digging—Outdoors*

Dimorphism

Dimorphism distinguishes two or more differences that occur in an individual, based on time or sex. Changes in body proportions occur with age and sex differences.

ALSO SEE: *Age Dimorphism, Sexual Dimorphism, Sexually Dimorphic Behaviors*

Direct Punishment

Direct punishment is the application of punishment by the owner, trainer, or the environment. This type of punishment is most effective when the problem directly involves the person or depends on the presence of or interaction with the owner. It can vary from a "No," to a jerk on a halter or collar, to the neck shake for a dog, to striking the animal with a hand or whip. As with any form of correction used for learning, the choice of punishment type and immediate timing of its application are critical. In addition to punishment applied directly by an owner, it can also appear to come directly from an environment. Cats and dogs can be kept off furniture by books, boxes, or chairs making the area uncomfortable. Horses, cattle, and swine learn to respect fences if an electric fence is used. Taste and smell aversion are other techniques that employ direct punishment.

ALSO SEE: *Competitive Aggression, Dog Collars, Motivation, No, Punishment, Remote Punishment, Smell Aversion, Taste Aversion*

Displacement Activity

A displacement activity is a normal behavior shown at an inappropriate time, appearing out of context for the occasion. An example would be when a cat that has been sleeping on its owner's lap, suddenly bites the person, and then jumps down. Immediately after landing it begins the displacement activity of self-licking. Pawing, barking, redirected aggression, self-mutilation, digging, and other forms of stress-induced behaviors may also be displacement activities if they occur out of context.

ALSO SEE: *Conflict, Digging, Excessive Vocalization—Barking, Habit Preening, Inappropriate Licking, Inhibition, Pawing, Redirected Aggression, Self-Mutilation, Stool Eating—Another Species*

Display

Behavior patterns that have a specific message or signal are called displays. They are typically used to communicate threat, submission, courtship, and other species-specific patterns. Occasionally, displays are used for deception or distraction of predator species, as with the "broken-wing" behavior of some birds.

ALSO SEE: *Body Language, Deception, Distance-increasing Silent Communication, Distance-reducing Silent Communication, Distraction Display*

Dissociation

Dissociation is the breaking or dissolving of a pair bond or other sexual pairing.

ALSO SEE: *Pair Bonding, Sexual Selection*

Distance Animals

Animal species that avoid close contact between conspecifics when possible and individuals that maintain some distance from each other are called distance animals. This behavior is typical for most ungulates, including horses, cattle, sheep, and goats. It also occurs in many types of fish and birds.

ALSO SEE: *Density-Intolerant Animals, Individual Distance, Social Distance*

Distance-increasing Silent Communication

Distance-increasing body language is displayed as a threat or warning to give a "go away" message. The general postural tendency is to show an increase in size, and that impression may occur suddenly to support the illusion of a rapid increase in danger.

Dogs. Dogs have certain behaviors that are generally associated with aggression, but more subtle ones can be recognized. The behaviors with distance-increasing messages tend to occur with increasing intensity, but they can occur in any order. In most dog-to-dog confrontations, direct eye contact by the dominant animal causes the subordinate to divert its eyes, and the matter is settled. Humans, especially children, often fail to recognize that they have made and maintained eye contact much longer than necessary. In another posture, the lips are lifted to show the teeth. The dog stands stiff-legged for maximum height, and the head, neck, and ears are held high. A word of caution is needed here because as an attack becomes more immediate, the head, neck, and ears are lowered for protection from injury, although the eyes maintain the stare. This lowering should not be confused with the similar posture of passive submission. The tail becomes more vertical and even can extend over the animal's back; there can be a flagging, high-frequency motion, not to be confused with wagging. Piloerection on the shoulders and rump may not be impressive on short-haired dogs, but it can rapidly add inches to a long-haired animal. Biting and fighting are the extremes of distance-increasing behavior, and ultimate victory is control of the throat.

Cats. Distance-increasing postures are well defined in cats. The first obvious sign is the twitching tail tip, an intense back and forth, almost rhythmic movement. Three types of well-defined threat postures could then follow. Offensive threat postures are based on a straight-on approach with a visual stare and bared teeth. The defensive threat postures are those of the classic Halloween cat—an arched back, piloerection, stare, and lateral position. The pariah threat is a crouched posture with teeth showing and ears flattened, usually directed toward the cat that controls the territory.

Horses. The usual distance-increasing silent communication posture of horses begins with the ears. They are pinned tightly back against the back of the head. Other head, tail, and limb signs are also used. For a stallion being approached, the first tendency is to raise the head, neck, and tail. The nose and lips are tensed, and the head may be shaken. Nostrils are flared. As the threat becomes more intense, the head becomes more parallel to the ground so that it can be rotated. The teeth are bared, and biting may follow. The tail is held tightly against the body and lashed back and forth. The feet, as well as the teeth, are weapons. The horse can paw, strike, or rear using the forelimbs as weapons. The rear quarters can be quickly turned toward an animal and a rear limb raised as a warning. Kicking with one or both rear limbs is useful for fighting.

Cattle. Before direct confrontations take place, tension may be released by pawing or rubbing the head, neck, and horns on the ground. The lateral, broadside position is a threat, often overlooked as insignificant. Little cues might help distinguish the lateral threat, such as the intensity that stops tail motion or a slight shifting of weight in front toward the person or animal being threatened. As an attack becomes more likely, the head is lowered so that the forehead is perpendicular to the ground to position the poll and horns, and the orientation shifts from broadside to straight on. Fighting in cattle is ritualized and occurs head to head. These bouts last until one animal submits or becomes exhausted. In the head-to-head battles, the animal tries to slip past the opponent's head and get a horn into its flank. Thus, great care is taken to prevent a flank approach from being successful. Equally matched opponents can fight for up to 10 minutes before one gives in. Cows have a type of rest period, called a clinch, that may occur during a long fight.

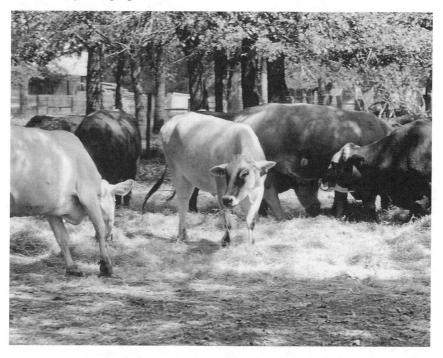

Distance-increasing Silent Communication. The cow on the left has just increased the intensity of her lateral threat by shifting her weight toward the cow on the right. As a result, the cow on the right is starting to move away.

Swine. Because of the general inflexibility of swine, signs associated with distance-increasing postures are minimal. The animals will grind their teeth and chomp their jaws, causing the saliva to foam. For boars, the odors in such saliva can incite aggressive behaviors. Piloerection is more obvious on some pigs than others, and pawing may occur. Teeth are the primary weapons, so sows try to bite, and boars use their tusks. Fights usually consist of tusk or teeth raking to the shoulder area as the aggressors stand facing each other. Pigs will also bite ears, the neck, or front limbs. Equally matched opponents may fight 30 to 60 minutes, but two or three quick attacks can end a mismatch.

ALSO SEE: *Ambivalent Postures, Butting, Clinch, Defensive Threat, Distance-reducing Silent Communication, Establish Dominance, Hard-to-Read Postures, Intention Movement, Kicking, Lateral Threat, Neck Shake, Nonverbal Communication, Offensive Threat, Passive Submission, Pawing, Piloerection, Rearing, Striking, Tail Switching, Threat Displays, Vocal Communication, Warning Behavior*

Distance-reducing Silent Communication

Distance-reducing silent communication is the type of body language that has a friendly or submissive message. Throughout the animal world, distance-reducing messages generally tend to decrease body size. This can vary from dropping eye contact, to lowering the head, to crouching. Specifics vary with species, their social structure, and the mobility of body parts.

Dogs. Canids have well-defined distance-reducing signals. They can be subdivided into three categories. Passive submission includes avoiding eye contact, lowering the head, neck, ears, tail or body, licking, mimic grinning, raising a paw, rolling over, and/or showing submissive urination. Active submission combines an active approach with one or more signs of passive submission. Play has several purposes in the young; in adult dogs, the classic play posture is the front-end-down, rear-end-up position.

Cats. Because cats do not have a great need to relay friendly messages, distance-reducing postures are not well defined. Felids will show an active approach to certain people and occasionally to other cats. As the cat gets close to the owner or a kitten to its queen, the tail goes up vertically into the air. Rubbing against nearby objects or legs with the side of their face or body may also represent a form of marking behavior. Rolling over to expose the abdomen has a distance-reducing or trusting message since this body area does not have skeletal protection. Play behaviors are generally reserved for kittens and shown only occasionally by adults.

Horses. Distance-reducing body postures of horses are expressed primarily by the head. Forward pointing ears indicate forward attention and may be accompanied by an active approach. The neck can be arched when the animal shows some apprehension or lowered with the nose out so the lip can make contact first. Ears to the side or partially back indicate where the horse's attention is or that it is not paying particular attention to anything. Nostrils generally flare when there is excitement, and eyelids open farther. The mobile upper lip may be extended forward with excitement or during mutual grooming. A raised lip, as in the horse laugh (flehmen), relates to the sense of smell. Young horses show jaw chomping, in which the mouth is partially open and moved up and down. The tail can also show distance-reducing postures. It can be carried away from the body and elevated during excitement or fall naturally in general activity.

Cattle. Distance-reducing silent communication is not well defined in cattle. Forward directed ears indicate where the animal's attention is. In the appeasement posture, the animal lowers its head and extends the head and neck until the forehead is almost parallel to the ground. When cattle submit to a threat, they usually divert their head first and then shift their weight caudally and away.

Swine. Body parts of pigs are not mobile, so distance-reducing postures are not well developed. An active approach and forward pointed ears are the main signals.

ALSO SEE: *Active Submission, Ambivalent Postures, Appeasement Behavior, Distance-increasing Silent Communication, Flehmen, Hard-to-Read Postures, Jaw Chomping, Marking, Mimic Grin, Nonverbal Communication, Passive Submission, Play Behaviors, Tail Wagging, Vocal Communication*

Distraction Display

This is a type of display used to distract a predator from the young. A bird may act as if it has a broken wing to lead an intruder away. Deer may rush past a predator to attempt to draw it away from a new fawn.

Distress Call (Distress Vocalization)

When frightened, infants of most species utter a unique call that brings a parent or sibling. Maternal aggression toward the intruder may result. The distress call is not associated with a specific infant, since any nearby female at about the same stage reproductively can show a high degree of arousal from it. This vocalization is well developed in domestic as well as wild animals.

ALSO SEE: *Maternal Aggression, Vocal Communication*

Divert Attention

Young animals in particular try a number of behaviors that are considered unacceptable. In many cases, however, they actually are showing normal behaviors, although excessive from an owner's perspective. Many puppies are chewers, a normal exploratory and learning behavior. Punishment does not work well for normal behaviors, so stopping the behavior is best accomplished by diverting the animal's attention to another activity.

Some owners have tried diverting their animal's attention, only to find that the behavior becomes worse, and the animal uses it to control the situation. A dog that is on the sofa may accept nothing less than a food bribe to get down. In time the dog may even learn to jump down to get the reward and race back up on the sofa before the owner can sit down. Horses may run at the stall door with teeth bared so the owner will give them some grain to get into the stall. In these cases, diversion of the animal's attention with a bribe should not be done. Appropriate correction of the behavior with punishment, shaping, obedience, or "No" should be used instead.

ALSO SEE: *Antiaggressive Puppy Training, Destructive Chewing, Masturbation, Shaping*

Division of Labor

A division of labor is a specialization in the types of jobs an individual would perform based on its body type (as in insects), sex (as in maternal behavior), or age.

ALSO SEE: *Caste*

Dog Collars

Dog collars serve a number of purposes and come in a number of styles. The standard round leather or web collar holds vaccination and name tags, as well as provides a place to attach a leash or chain.

Choke collars allow the collar to tighten around the neck when one ring is pulled. These typically come as fine metal chains, but some are made of soft cord. Choke collars are used in most obedience classes and help exert neck control, a lesson in authority not requiring excessive force.

German training (prong) collars are also controlled by increasing the amount of pull exerted on the free end. Pulling causes an inward rotation of paired prongs on each of the large links. This modified version of a choke collar is most commonly used on dogs with a heavy coat and those that are resistant to traditional collars.

Halters like the Promise™ (Gentle Leader™) and Halti™ are a newer concept in "collars." One piece goes around the neck and a second piece over the top of the nose. Pressure is applied to the back of the neck and to the nose by attaching the leash to the ring on the ventral nosepiece. This is thought by the developers to simulate the pressure a dominant animal puts on the back of a young dog's neck and the muzzle pressure used by a pack leader when it puts its mouth over that of the young dog. The Promise™ has an adjustable nosepiece, allowing it to be fitted for continuous wear.

The dog harness is a series of interconnected straps that encircle the neck and thorax. There is a ring on the dorsal part to connect to a leash. The harness serves much the same purpose as the rigid leather or web collars but offers greater resistance to escape.

Doggie Bag™ is a fabric harness that supports the thorax and abdomen. It can be used with a leash or as a handle to pick up and carry small dogs. Shock collars and bark collars are also available.

ALSO SEE: *Bark Collars, Obedience Class, Shock Collars*

Dog-Sitting

Occasionally, livestock animals are seen sitting in a position like that used by dogs and cats. It is most commonly seen in restrained breeding sows and to a lesser extent in veal calves. Bulls and horses have also been observed using this as a resting posture.

Dogs

Miacis, a small civetlike animal that lived 40 to 60 million years ago, is the oldest known common ancestor of dogs and cats. *Miacis* gave rise to *Dinictis* (which gave rise to cats), the bear-dog group (which gave rise to bears), *Hoplophoneus* (which gave rise to saber-toothed tigers), and *Cynodictis.* From *Cynodictis* came the hunting dogs of India and Africa and *Cynodesmus,* which gave rise to *Tomarctus,* and it to modern carnivores, including foxes, coyotes, and wolves. The wolf, *Canis lupus,* is generally regarded as the immediate ancestor of the dog, *Canis familiaris.*

The human/wolf-dog relationship may extend back as much as 30,000 years and was probably formed because they hunted the same prey. Initially the wolf could lead the human to prey, and eventually the scraps of the successful hunt could nourish the wolf-dog. The animals' highly social nature permitted easy taming and acceptance of humans as equals to pack members. The long relationship has permitted a great deal of selective breeding for characteristics, first of tameability, then of hunting skills, and eventually of size and appearance.

ALSO SEE: *Cats, Domestication, Appendix B*

Domestication

Domestication is the process of selectively breeding a group of originally wild animals over hundreds of generations in order to accentuate traits desired by humans. The process of domestication involves a change in morphology, physiology, and/or behavioral traits (Hafez, 1969). Decreasing reactivity to the environment is usually one of the changes that will occur, providing an interesting contrast between a tame wild animal and a tame domesticated animal.

Several factors are important for domestication to occur, and frequently more than one is present within the group undergoing change. The most critical factor is a human need. Without that, little attention would be paid to the species initially. The ability to subsist on food or in areas that are not in direct competition with humans is also desirable. Social animals have two advantages; many of them can be kept in a relatively small area without a great deal of agonistic inter-actions, and they are generally more willing to be tamed and handled by humans. Sexual behaviors that are promiscuous for breeding and nonselective for mater-nal care-giving are also favorable for domestication.

ALSO SEE: *Adaptation, Behavioral Characteristics Favoring Domestica-tion, Epigamic Traits, Feral Animal, Roles of Domesticated Animals, Selective Breeding, Tame Animal, Wild Animal*

Dominance

Social interactions among group animals are based on the ranking of indi-viduals. The top member (the alpha, or number 1) of the group exerts the major influence over the actions of other members, with lower ranking individuals exerting less influence, relative to their position. The highest rank is held by the animal that can threaten all the others without receiving a threat in return. Dom-inance is not related to the amount of aggression shown, just by who wins. The position an animal assumes is generally size-related. Smaller, younger females tend to have the lowest positions, although in each species other factors influence this generalization. For cattle and some wild species, the mother's rank or the mate's rank can also influence an individual's position.

Controlled access to food has been used to test the dominance relationship between two individuals, with the animal that can get or keep control of the food being judged dominant. While it is a generally useful indicator, dominance over food does not always relate to social dominance. For a complete picture of dom-inance, it is important to evaluate which animal grooms which, which animal will move away when approached, and which individuals spend time in closer proximity.

When new animals are introduced into a group, there will be restlessness, usually accompanied by some aggressive encounters. Once the new member's social rank has been decided, peace returns. One of the advantages of dominance is that a rigid social order can be established and confrontation between members reduced to gentle threats by the more dominant member.

For dogs, dominant-subordinate relationships can be established as early as 4 months of age. If puppies are around older dogs, they generally enter at the lowest rank and retain that position until removed from the group. The estab-lishment of a firm position is very important for a dog. There are individuals who change a dominance position as they get older, with confrontations most com-mon around 1.5 years of age. The typical situation involves a large male dog kept with its dam or a small female, or a dog with a dominant personality, trying to take control. Human dominance over pack members is typical although aggres-sion can occur when dogs consider themselves higher ranking.

Horses have complicated dominance patterns, although the older, larger stallions tend to be the highest ranking members of a herd. In the wild, each harem group has a dominant stallion, followed by the mares, and then the young. In managed situations, the dominance patterns are even more complicated because of the absence of stallions and the presence of geldings. Food dominance and social dominance can be different, since some subordinate horses become very aggressive in defense of hay or grain. So although food trials between individuals will give a general dominant-subordinate pattern, actual pasture observation is necessary to confirm regular social rankings. Human dominance is related to the ability to psychologically convince the horse that it is under the person's control. This is done by restricting the horse's ability to flee, first by a halter and strong rope and then by teaching it to trust the human as a guide.

Cattle herds of bulls, cows, and young stock have adult males dominant over all others, and cows dominant over juveniles. Young bulls change from the lowest group to the highest at between 1.5 and 2.5 years of age (Hafez, 1969), so a high number of aggressive encounters occur during the year. In addition to size-related factors, dominance is also influenced by strength, agility, and horns, but not by milk production. Identical twins share a position, while calves raised isolated from others tend to be less dominant. An estrous cow often disregards dominance and can disrupt a herd by ignoring the etiquette of interacting socially only within a few dominance rankings of its own position. Human dominance can be exerted by nose control. Since cattle need to lower their heads for a charge, lifting it prevents the threat.

Although barrows are generally dominant over gilts, dominance and weight gains in swine are influenced by their sucking order as piglets. The teat order established by a litter has a bearing on how fast and how large an individual pig will grow, and this influences which pigs will have the size and weight to control dominance orders.

Cats do not have dominance orders in the literal sense. All interactions are relative to a territory. Typically a tomcat is the dominant cat in a certain area. There will be a few very low ranking individuals (pariahs), with all others sharing a position under the tomcat and above the pariahs. If Tomcat A is the territorial owner, he may mount other cats, such as Tomcat B, within the territory. If Tomcat A enters Tomcat B's territory, A will be mounted. Dominance is less significant in cats because of the relatively asocial nature of the species.

ALSO SEE: *Asocial, Competitive Aggression, Distance-increasing Silent Communication, Dominance Aggression, Dominant Personality, Establish Dominance, Pariah, Social Order, Teat Order*

Dominance Aggression

Dominance aggression, an affective aggression, is the most common aggression problem presented to behavior specialists. The most common situation presented is when the dog considers itself dominant to one or more members of the family. The aggression might first present itself when a small child tries to take something away from the pet. It can also be seen when the dog is raised permissively and then is asked to behave in a certain way. A dog that sleeps on the bed may suddenly refuse to let one of its owners in bed, so nighttime becomes a game of seeing whether the owner can bribe the dog off the bed long enough to dive in before the snack is gone. A dog that guards tissues or toys may also control the owner's actions. A dominant personality may actually make owners fear the pet to the point that they are unable to take a collar off, brush the dog, or give it a bath.

The concept for changing dominance aggression is to change the dog's impression of the social order. When the owners have been permissive and the dog is regarded as a child substitute, the change is sometimes easier to make. First, the importance to the dog of social orders and dominance is explained to the owner. Once they understand that most dogs actually do better as a pack member, not as a leader, the owner is taught how to give a "No" response with a quick firm jerk on the collar. The Promise™ (collar) halter can be particularly useful on dogs showing dominance to an owner. Obedience class, where the owners work their dog, is recommended to help the people learn how to give commands and the dog can learn to obey. Since trouble is usually restricted to certain things, the environment can also be controlled. The dog can drag a leash around the house and then be allowed access to the bed, the guarded toy, the piece of tissue, or other objects. When the dog threatens the owners, they can grab the leash and give an appropriate jerk and "No."

Changing the dominance relationship between a dog and a person who is physically or psychologically unable to force the issue is difficult. Certain instructions can help owners who really want to try. They should be taught how to give a "No" and give a firm jerk on the collar if the dog does not become aggressive or frantic to that response. Obedience classes, where the owner works the dog, are often helpful. Submissive behaviors such as "shake hands," "roll over," and "down" can be practiced several times each day to reinforce the emerging relationship. Since neck control is the ultimate victory in a dog fight, this is a message that a dog can understand without incurring physical pain, and is the principle for most training collars. If the dog is physically small enough, the neck shake can be used to enforce dominance. The skin and hair on the neck is grabbed, and the dog is shaken. The technique can be used via a collar, with a tree limb, fence, or railing helping to give the person holding the leash (a parent should assist a child in this) a mechanical advantage to enforce a jerk correction. While slow and subtle games that teach submissive behaviors for food rewards will occasionally work, many cases of dominance aggression come to a physical confrontation. Owners should be aware of this and never give a command on which they are not willing to follow through.

The young puppy presented for its first vaccinations may already be showing signs of a dominant personality by biting, growling, and being strong-willed. When held on its back, the puppy that does not quit biting and struggling needs help right away. Owners should be counseled at that time about returning the puppy to the breeder or using antiaggressive puppy training methods to ensure a controllable pet.

Since many of the dogs showing dominance aggression to their owners are male dogs and since personality traits can be inherited, castration should be recommended as part of a program. Castration alone is not very successful, but when combined with retraining, the results improve.

A second type of dominance aggression—that between two dogs—usually involves dogs that get along when the owners are not present. At first the history indicates that these dogs fight all the time, but further questioning reveals that they stay together when the owners are gone, without bloody results. What usually happens is that the #1 dog subtly threatens the #2 dog with a stare to move away from the owner so that the #1 dog can receive the attention. The first time #2 fails to respond fast enough, #1 will increase the threat to a growl, at which point the owner yells at #1. The #2 dog quickly learns that it can get its way as long as people are around, and the #1 dog tries harder to enforce its social (dominance) ranking. This interaction can go on so long that it becomes difficult in a history to determine how the dogs actually rank, and favoritism by owners can compound the interaction even more. The highest ranking dog should be identified, or if a position is shared, the owners should decide which dog should be the highest ranking. From then on the owners should side with the #1 dog. If it growls at #2, the owners should reinforce that by making the #2 dog show a submissive posture (down, roll over) or go away. It is difficult for humans to do this because of the tendency to side with the underdog, but with appropriate measures, this type of dominance aggression can be quickly controlled. An alternative behavior by the owner would be to immediately walk away from both dogs, so not to influence their relationship.

Dominance aggression in horses, cattle, and other species of livestock is limited mainly to aggressive threats given by an animal to a lower ranking individual. The meaning of the threat is well understood and respected, so serious aggressive confrontations over dominance rarely occur. A new animal introduced into a herd or flock is most likely to be involved in aggressive bouts while finding its appropriate level in the social order. Removal of an individual from a group for variable periods of time can cause others to close up that position, and the individual may be treated as a newcomer when it returns. Dogs that are hospitalized can have this problem, as can cattle and swine returning from the show circuit. For dogs, remove the problem dog for a few days to reestablish the #1 dog in its appropriate rank. Show pigs and cattle are often kept in small groups or individually until the show season is over to minimize the aggressive interactions.

Competitive aggression is a form of dominance aggression in which two animals fight over a specific item, such as a bone.

ALSO SEE: *Affective Aggression, Antiaggressive Puppy Training, Competi-*

tive Aggression, Dog Collar, Dominance, Dominant Personality, Establish Dominance, Fight it Out, Mental Lapse Aggression Syndrome, Neck Shake, No, Obedience Class, Reestablish Dominance, Ritualized Fighting, Separate, Sibling Rivalry, Social Order, Submissive Tricks

Dominant Personality

Individual personalities can range from very dominant to very submissive. In dealing with the dominant individual, it is important for one to remember the significance of social orders to the species. While the animal is young, humans can most easily establish themselves as the leader of the pack (dogs) or as an accepted leader in certain situations (horses and cattle primarily).

An animal with a dominant personality places itself in the leadership role and reacts aggressively to any challenge to that authority. Dog owners can use the lessons of antiaggressive puppy training to establish dominance early. With the extremely dominant dog, it may be necessary to reinforce constantly the owner's position, a role many owners find uncomfortable. Establishing owner dominance over an older dog can be difficult.

Lessons of appropriate control over dominant horses and cattle are more difficult because of size differences. The lessons are somewhat easier if taught during the first few months of the foal's or calf's life.

ALSO SEE: *Antiaggressive Puppy Training, Dominance Aggression, Genetic Problems, Personality, Reestablish Dominance*

Drinking

Drinking is the ingestive behavior of taking in water or other appropriate liquids. The method of intake varies among the animal species. Dogs and cats turn their tongue's tip backward to form a ladle and lift the water into the mouth. Livestock tend to put their muzzles into the water and will use negative pressure to pull it into the mouth. While horses touch only their mouths to the water, cattle are more apt to submerge their noses. Birds usually scoop water in their lower bill and raise their heads up, allowing gravity to pull the water into the esophagus. Primates can drink from their hands, using them as a cup. Some animals, including cats, may stick a foot in the water and suck the moisture off it.

The amount an animal drinks is regulated by the hypothalamus and is dependent on several factors. These include the degree of current body hydration, body temperature, environmental temperatures and humidity, rapidity of body fluid loss, water content of food, availability of water, and salt intake. There are a few species of animals that can meet their requirements for water from their food, making drinking unnecessary.

ALSO SEE: *Adipsia, Ingestive Behavior, Polydipsia, Urine Drinking*

Drive

Drive is a term commonly used to describe the desire or motivation to accomplish a particular goal. There is a single focus of activity.

ALSO SEE: *Motivation, Motivational State*

Drug Therapy

Historically, treatments for behavior problems have progressively added therapies—euthanasia, castration, tranquilizers, progestins. In recent years, veterinary behaviorists have been adding research information about a number of the human drugs and their effectiveness in animal behavior problems. Appropriate drug therapy can be a very useful adjunct for treating certain behavior problems. When a medical workup reveals a specific medical problem, appropriate treatment is indicated. Some drugs have a more general use. These include anesthetics, anabolic steroids, progestins, and tranquilizers. Psychopharmacology is an ever-expanding field in veterinary medicine and should make tremendous progress in the next several years. Since this area is changing so rapidly, dosage recommendations given in Appendix C are expected to be refined over time.

ALSO SEE: *Medical Problems, Medical Workup, Psychopharmacological Drugs, Appendix C*

Dysphagia

Dysphagia is difficulty in swallowing. Causes vary from a physical origin, as in neuromuscular dysfunction, to an infectious origin, as with rabies. Psychological origin is felt to be relatively rare in veterinary medicine.

ALSO SEE: *Ingestive Behavior*

Early Ontogenetic Adaptation

Behaviors, reflexes, or instincts of neonates that help infants survive are called early ontogenetic adaptations. Rooting into warm objects by newborn puppies and kittens ensures warmth and helps locate the teats. The open-mouth gape of baby birds solicits feeding. Crawling from vulva to pouch by immature marsupial young takes them to a protected environment and food. Early ontogenetic adaptations disappear as the animal ages.

ALSO SEE: *Infantile Behavior*

Earth Raking

Earth raking is the movement made by a cat to move dirt or litter to make a hole to eliminate in or to cover the excreta. The behavior is instinctive and is triggered by the need to eliminate and by the smell of urine or feces. Earth-raking motions may be performed if the stimulus is present even though there is no dirt or litter to move. The number of paw raking movements is partially governed by inherited patterns. The actual covering of urine or feces is a behavior usually learned from the queen.

ALSO SEE: *Burying Food, Eliminative Behavior*

Eating Behavior

Eating behavior is another term for ingestive behavior, the broad category that includes nursing, eating, and drinking.

SEE: *Ingestive Behavior*

Egg Eating

When small flocks of chickens are kept in pens, an individual hen may start pecking at an egg until it breaks. She will then eat some of the contents. Once this behavior starts, it is important to identify and cull the individual quickly so that the behavior is not picked up by others. Grit should be available so that a deficiency will not precipitate the egg-eating behavior.

Electroshock Therapy

Electroshock therapy has been advocated for certain cases of aggression, although the specific type of aggression was not defined (Redding and Walker, 1976). While there may be certain cases where this treatment is appropriate, the parameters are not currently defined. In veterinary medicine, electroshock therapy has not been accepted as a major treatment for aggressive animals.

ALSO SEE: *Aggression*

Eliminative Behavior

Eliminative behaviors include those of urination, defecation, and anal sac expulsion. Since urine can be used in marking behaviors, the context in which urine expulsion occurs must be known to fully understand what type of behavior is occurring.

Individuals can develop a desire to eliminate on specific types of surfaces, even to the exclusion of all others. This behavior is most evident in our domestic carnivores. Dogs learn to eliminate on grass (which is occasionally translated into shag carpet), paper, concrete, asphalt, or other surface types and can be resistant to not using the favorite. Cats also learn this preference. Outdoor cats may not differentiate soil from dirt in potted plants. Abrupt changes in litter types will result in 50% of cats stopping litter box usage. One half of those will restart within several days; the remaining cats go to another location.

Horses have a strong tendency to eliminate in specific areas. In a pasture, these areas are easily spotted because of their rough appearance. Patterns of elimination also differ by sex. A stallion will walk into the rough area so that he reaches the far side. His feces are deposited in the center of the area. Mares and geldings walk to the area so that their feces are deposited at the outside edge, and the area continues to get larger. Stalled horses often choose one corner in which to eliminate, making stall cleaning relatively easy.

Cattle show no patterns as to where they eliminate, resulting in no easily distinguishable grazing or elimination areas. Swine tend to eliminate in group areas. There is a learning component to the elimination patterns where piglets are influenced by the sow.

ALSO SEE: *Coprophagia, Defecation, Housesoiling, House Training, Marking, Urination*

Emotional Come and Go

The interaction of an owner and dog can make a big difference in how the pet behaves while the owner is gone. If the dog is very attached to the owner, it may show some type of separation anxiety in the owner's absence. Owners can unconsciously contribute to this problem by leaving and/or returning in inappropriate ways. If the behavior problem occurs only when the owners are gone, it may occur immediately after they leave, during the entire period of absence, or after they have been gone for a long period. For those cases in which the problem occurs whether the owner steps out briefly or is gone all day, the emotional interactions between the owner and dog in the morning and evening must be examined. Owners often excite the dog unnecessarily before leaving in the morning. Since the animal needs time to calm down, the pet may redirect its excitement toward something in the house. Owners who make a show when coming home in the evening can inadvertently train the dog to anticipate the excitement. As the regular return time approaches and the animal becomes emotionally worked up, the excitement can be redirected as destruction.

In destructive behavior problems that occur while owners are away, the emotion of coming and leaving needs to be minimized. The last major interaction with the dog should take place at least 30 minutes before leaving, with a simple "Good-bye" given when the owner actually departs. When returning home, owners should say "Hi" and then start a specific behavior such as changing clothes. The second behavior, not the clock, should be the signal for the interaction.

ALSO SEE: *Avoid Excitement, Destructive Behaviors, Destructive Chewing, Hydrocephalus, Separation Anxiety, Star Gazing*

Encopresis

The defecation associated with extreme excitement or fear is called encopresis.

ALSO SEE: *Defecation*

End Act

This is another term for the consummatory phase.

SEE: *Consummatory Phase*

Engram

An engram represents the physical basis for learning and involves an actual change in cells along the pathway of the memory.

Enuresis

Enuresis is the urination that occurs at night during sleep or during emotional excitement. Dogs, for example, show this behavior during submission or in extreme fear.

ALSO SEE: *Submissive Urination, Urination*

Environmental Enrichment

Environmental enrichment is the term used to describe additions to an animal's environment that are psychologically stimulating and positively affect the animal's quality of life. There are five basic approaches to enrichment. The first creates an environment that mimics the wild habitat. The second, for social animals, provides access to peers to minimize abnormal behavior development. The third involves artificial appliances that allow animals to manipulate items, encouraging activity. A fourth approach, food gathering, can be as simple as finding hidden food scattered in bedding or as complex as working mechanical devices to earn food rewards. The last enrichment technique gives the animal some control over its environment; mechanical devices allow the animal to turn on or off lights or music.

ALSO SEE: *Frustration, Psychological Well-being*

Epigamic Display

An epigamic display is a courtship behavior in which secondary sexual characteristics (epigamic traits) are used to attract potential mates. The behaviors of showing colored feathers, presenting estrous skin patches, or spreading a particular odor are included. This type of display is associated with competition among those of the same sex to gain the interest of a member of the opposite sex.

ALSO SEE: *Courtship, Epigamic Traits, Presentation*

Epigamic Traits

Epigamic traits are those secondary sexual characteristics that evolve as a response to mate selection. Examples include bright color patterns, chemicals or odors associated with estrus, behavioral displays, and changing physical features.

ALSO SEE: *Epigamic Display, Female Behaviors, Male Behaviors*

Epileptic Aggression

Epileptic aggression is a form of nonaffective aggression due to a medical disorder resulting in a seizure. For these animals, the history is that of a Dr. Jekyll–Mr. Hyde personality. Most of the time the animal is normal in all respects, except there is a brief aggressive attack, which, to the owner, may seem longer. The history may indicate a pre-seizural period during which the owner notices the animal acting strangely or getting a "funny look in its eyes." If this stage is present, owners might say they can always tell when one of these bouts will occur. The actual seizure is the aggressive bout. Another abrupt change is the post-seizural phase in which the animal appears perfectly normal as if nothing had happened (which is difficult for owners to understand), and tries to get very close to the owner or goes off to be by itself.

Epileptic aggression has been diagnosed in dogs, cats, and horses, and probably occurs in other species as well. In dogs, it is a common medical cause of aggression (Beaver, 1993) and typically follows a history consistent with idiopathic epilepsy. Epileptic aggressive seizures start around 1.5 years of age and gradually increase in frequency and duration. If the bouts are frequent enough to be able to evaluate their response to therapy, epileptic aggression may be controllable with medications used for the more classical forms of seizure.

ALSO SEE: *Nonaffective Aggression, Seizures*

Epimeletic

Epimeletic refers to the care-giving behavior of a female toward her offspring. It includes allowing the young to nurse, protecting them, moving them, and searching for them if separated.

ALSO SEE: *Et-epimeletic, Maternal Behavior*

Erroneous Imprinting

Erroneous imprinting is the imprinting to a species other than that to which the animal belongs. Ducklings and chicks may imprint on the first large object moving by. In birds, song dialects can also be imprinted erroneously.

ALSO SEE: *Imprint Learning*

Erythrocytosis

Aggression has not been proven to be associated with excessive production of red blood cells or with high packed cell volumes. This is a speculative diagnosis based on the response to an old therapy of removing blood from aggressive animals. A specific diagnosis was never established before the blood was removed.

ALSO SEE: *Bloodletting*

Escape Behaviors

Escape behaviors are a series of actions that animals use to get out of an area or an environment. Behaviors include digging, climbing, opening stall doors, dashing through opened doors, jumping fences, crawling under or through fences, and running away. Other behaviors, such as rearing, may be included under certain conditions.

ALSO SEE: *Climbing, Crawling Under and Through Fences, Dashing Through Doors, Digging, Fence Jumping, Gate Crashing, Protean Behavior, Pulling Back, Rearing, Running Away*

Establish Dominance

A great deal of enjoyment can be shared with an animal when it respects the person as the dominant pack or herd member. Each species has certain behaviors associated with the social order that are useful in developing that respect. The lessons are most easily established when animals are young, because that is their normal time to learn how they relate to a social group. Later the lesson is more difficult.

Puppies usually enter at the bottom of a pack's social order, a place learned by interaction with older dogs. Human owners who never show dominance over the dog, letting it do as it pleases, may be surprised the first time they need to show authority. Dominance can easily be established in young puppies through the antiaggressive puppy training techniques, but older dogs may need to be confronted in a more serious manner. Obedience classes, where the owner works the dog, teach the owner how to give commands and the dog how to obey them. Commands such as "sit" and "down," as well as tricks such as "roll over" and "shake hands," ask the dog to show a submissive behavior. As soon as the dog knows how to do them, the owner should have the dog perform the behaviors multiple times each day. Another technique that can help an owner establish dominance over the dog is a jerk on a collar or leash along with a firm "No!" when the behavior is inappropriate.

When the dog has a very dominant personality, it may resist the more gentle attempts of the owner to gain control. Firm neck control with a Promise™ halter or a choke chain collar, or grabbing the skin at the neck and shaking, may be necessary. If aggressively resisted, the owners must be ready to reinforce their commands. The neck shake has two advantages in establishing dominance. It is understood by the dog, since throat control is the ultimate victory in a fight, and it does not inflict pain, which is itself a cause of aggression. There are owners who cannot exert the authority necessary to become dominant to their pet and are content to let the dog run their lives. For others, removing the dog from the environment may be the only practical solution.

Several techniques may be applied carefully to a strange dog to determine how dominant it is. The stare, direct eye contact, can be maintained until the dog looks away. A word of caution is necessary because extremely dominant dogs do not break eye contact and will grow irritable to the point of showing aggression if eye contact is not broken by the person. The "Captain-may-I" approach consists of taking a cautious step forward to test the dog's reaction to an approach. If the dog shifts its weight forward, it is increasing its threat. If, however, it shifts its weight back or diverts its eyes, there is a possibility of submission. Then another small, cautious step is indicated. The neck shake is a third technique useful for controlling some situations. At times, no gentle persuasion may work, and forced or chemical restraint may be necessary.

Since cats do not have well-defined social orders, it is not possible to establish dominance over them. It becomes a matter of getting them to accept human control. This is most easily accomplished by teaching a kitten to accept whatever restraint the owner uses. Some older cats may be controlled with direct eye contact or by picking them up by the dorsum of the neck. Forced and chemical restraint are needed more often for cats than for dogs.

Horses are controlled physically by the head. Each animal learns that a human can prevent its escape and can control the speed and direction of its movement by having control of its head. Usually this lesson in human dominance is learned with a halter and rope and reinforced with a bridle. Occasionally, it is learned with the bridle alone. Other devices can be used to control a horse. One-leg hobbles limit the horse's ability to flee, and most horses quickly associate the person who puts on the strap with the individual in control. Self-locking pliers, incompletely closed, can be used to pinch the skin to distract a horse while other things are being done. Chains on lead shanks can be placed between the upper lip and teeth. Tightening the chain when the horse acts up and releasing the pressure as soon as it stops is a quick way to teach an appropriate behavior. From the animal's perspective, it may be punishing itself because the handler is not reacting aggressively as would typically be expected.

Cattle are also controlled by the head. With particularly powerful animals, it may be necessary to use the sensitivity of the nose to assure complete control.

Swine respond to control of the nose. This form of control results in immobilization rather than true dominance over the individual.

ALSO SEE: *Antiaggressive Puppy Training, Competitive Aggression, Dog Collar, Dominance, Dominance Aggression, Dominant Personality, No, Obedience Class, Pain-induced Aggression, Social Order, Submissive Tricks*

Estrous Behavior

The behaviors of estrus vary among species, from elaborate courtship displays in birds to death of the male after mating in insects. Domestic animals are much less dynamic. In most domestic animals, an estrous female will allow breeding by any male of her species; however, mate selection or rejection can occur. If the female is actually in estrus, rejection is probably most often associated with an unacceptable style or odor.

There are three characteristics of estrus associated with all domestic animals to some degree. The female will flag her tail to one side, exposing her genitalia. She will lower her pelvis, tipping the perineum so intromission is more easily achieved, and she will stand to be mounted. By not moving, she indicates a readiness to breed. Specific information about the age of puberty, length of the estrous period, and length of the estrous cycle is included in Appendix B.

Bitches show a few variations from the other species in proestrus, including vulvar enlargement and a bloody discharge. The long proestrus (7-10 days) helps ensure that mating will occur by attracting a number of males. The estrous period is also long. Young female dogs may show an abbreviated or incomplete first estrus, followed by a complete, normal period in approximately one month.

Cats are unique in female estrous behavior. As solitary animals, their reproductive success is dependent on the estrous female and a male finding each other. The "heat-cry" is vocal advertising for surrounding males. Once in the female's general location, the male is then attracted by the obvious behaviors of rolling and rubbing. The queen assumes a crouched posture for copulation, tilting the pelvis upward. She is an induced ovulator, a physiological event evolved to ensure the best timing for fertilization. The penile spines of the male point caudally within the vagina so withdrawal produces a tactile stimulation that eventually results in ovulation. External evidence of this stimulation is a loud "copulatory cry" and an aggressive turning on the male.

Mares are undergoing a gradual change in breeding cycles as a result of human pressures to have foals born shortly after January 1. Evolutionarily, the mare is monestrous, with a seasonal receptivity of late spring and early summer. The pressure for early foals encourages the selection of mares with a true polyestrous cycle, ovulating year round. Currently there is a large group of mares considered as transitory polyestrous. These mares are sexually receptive year round but only ovulate on a seasonal cycle. Two behaviors are unique to the estrous mare—vulvar winking and increased frequency of urination.

In proestrus, a cow becomes restless and is apt to upset herd mates by violating social orders. The estrous cow will not only mount other cows, as an anestrous cow might, but she will also solicit and stand for mounts by other cows.

Sows in estrus actively search for boars and follow almost anything that moves. A herd can also be synchronized relatively easily by making an abrupt change in management, with estrus following in 4-6 days.

ALSO SEE: *Behavioral Characteristics Favoring Domestication, Female Behaviors, Male Behaviors, Silent Heat, Appendix B*

Et-epimeletic

Et-epimeletic refers to care-soliciting behavior by the young. It is primarily related to their distress vocalizations and requests for food.

ALSO SEE: *Epimeletic, Maternal Behavior*

Ethoendocrinology

This is another name for behavioral endocrinology.

SEE: *Behavioral Endocrinology*

Ethogram

To study a species, a catalog of all their behaviors is used in comparison with other species. This catalog, or inventory of behaviors, is called an ethogram.

Ethological Need

There has been a great deal of discussion recently as to whether or not animals have certain behavioral needs in addition to their nutritional needs. Proponents argue that there are cases in which the performance of the behavior can have significant consequences that are not necessarily related to functional requirements (Hughes and Duncan, 1988). The correct definition of what specific behavioral needs an animal has, if any, is still to be determined.

Ethology

Ethology is the scientific study of entire behavioral patterns in natural surroundings. Traditionally this has represented field study of wild animals, although more recently it has come to include behaviors of domestic animals in what has become their typical locations.

ALSO SEE: *Animal Psychology*

Ethomimicry

This is another term for behavioral mimicry.

SEE: *Behavioral Mimicry*

Ethostasis

Ethostasis is the adaptive use of various behaviors to establish and maintain physiological homeostasis and overall well-being. In Fox (1986), ethostasis is not equated with normalcy. Stereotyped behaviors might result in a physiological adaptation, but would have to be regarded as behavioral indices of abnormality.

ALSO SEE: *Stereotyped Behaviors*

Eusocial

Eusocial species describes an animal group where members of two or more generations coexist. This relationship between helper and helped is true in species such as termites, ants, naked mole rats, and some primates.

The term semisocial has been used where all members are of the same generation.

ALSO SEE: *Semisocial*

Euthanasia

This is the causing of a painless, humane death, especially to end suffering. Euthanasia may be the procedure of choice in a few behavior problems, especially when there is a strong possibility of people being injured by an aggressive animal. Generally, however, it is a choice made by the owner who is not willing or able to make the effort to change a problem.

Excessive Food Intake

Excessive intake of food tends to occur in situations where there is some competition among closely ranked individuals, where the food is extremely palatable, or when an individual has not had access to food for abnormally long periods of time. The behavior is common in individuals that had been abandoned for a period earlier in their life. Many of the commercial diets are extremely palatable, and if access is not limited, excessive caloric intake can result in obesity. Excessive food intake is a common problem in dogs because they evolved under a "feast-or-famine" pattern. Limiting access to food, using less-palatable foods, and using lower-calorie foods are approaches to working with this problem.

In certain medical conditions, such as hyperthyroidism, excessive food intake may be necessary to sustain the animal.

ALSO SEE: *Feast or Famine, Feeding Schedule Change, Hyperthyroidism, Ingestive Behavior, Obesity*

Excessive Grooming

Grooming is a normal maintenance behavior in animals that involves biting (combing), licking, scratching, rubbing, and rolling. Any of these behaviors can be carried to excess, even to the point of causing self-induced lesions. Excessive grooming behaviors can be the result of a medical problem (such as fleas), lack of other stimuli, excessive stimulation (stress), stereotypies, attempts to gain attention, or lack of ability to perform other behaviors. Problems associated with excessive grooming in animals include hot spots, lick granulomas, psychogenic dermatoses, and excessive licking.

After medically related factors have been controlled, the environment must be addressed, since it is important to minimize the stress or boredom. Increased exercise, rigid schedules, and environmental enrichment may be appropriate. It is important that the owners not reinforce the undesirable behavior through rewards or attention. Taste aversion, antianxiety tranquilizers, or narcotic antagonists can be used initially to break the pattern and may be helpful if environmental factors are addressed at the same time.

ALSO SEE: *Attention Seeking, Boredom, Environmental Enrichment, Excessive Licking, Exercise, Feather Picking, Frustration, Grooming Behavior, Hot Spots, Lick Granulomas, Over-Grooming, Psychogenic Dermatoses, Schedule, Self-Mutilation, Stress-related Behaviors, Taste Aversion, Appendix C*

Excessive Licking

Licking is a normal grooming behavior for most animals. Occasionally it is excessive, to the point of causing hair loss or skin problems. In many animals this behavior is a response to stress, and over time it may actually become a stereotyped behavior. Lick granulomas in dogs and self-induced hair loss in cats are examples of the extremes. Excessive licking can also be directed toward others, including owners, or toward inanimate objects such as floors, bricks, or salt blocks. The trait of licking inanimate objects can be associated with feline leukemia infections in cats, although the pathology is not understood.

Taste aversion may be useful for excessive licking problems caught early. Preventing access to the area is generally more successful in helping the animal break more thoroughly established patterns.

ALSO SEE: *Excessive Grooming, Inappropriate Licking, Lick Granulomas, Over-Grooming, Psychogenic Dermatoses, Self-Licking, Self-Mutilation, Sterotyped Behaviors, Stress-related Behaviors, Taste Aversion*

Excessive Sexual Behavior

Individuals may show an excessive amount of sexual behavior when compared to normal behaviors of the species. Around the time of puberty, males of most species show sexual behaviors more frequently. As the result of the increased testosterone production in the internal testis, males with retained testicles tend to show excessive degrees of sexual behavior. It was thought that this high degree of sex drive, or libido, was related to fertility, but it is now recognized that there is no correlation.

For males, castration is the method of choice to control excessive sexual behavior. Progestins can be used for short-term control because they reduce testosterone levels, but they can have serious long-term side effects. Increased amounts of exercise also help reduce available energy, which otherwise might be used inappropriately.

ALSO SEE: *Drug Therapy, Exercise, Masturbation, Monosexual Syndrome, Mounting, Sexually Dimorphic Behaviors*

Excessive Vocalization

A common complaint of some pet owners is excessive vocalization. Other owners live with vocal animals without any problem, recognizing it as a normal part of a breed's behavior. Excessive vocalization usually does not become a problem until it keeps the owners awake or bothers the neighbors. There can be individual, breed, and environmental influences that affect the amount of noise an animal makes. The behavior may even be rewarded by the receipt of food or attention. Specific types of complaints are discussed separately.

ALSO SEE: *Excessive Vocalization—Barking, Excessive Vocalization—Howling, Excessive Vocalization—Meowing, Excessive Vocalization—Whining, Separation Anxiety, Trial and Error Learning*

Excessive Vocalization—Barking

Barking tends to become a problem if it occurs at night and keeps the owners awake or if it occurs during the day and bothers the neighbors. Barking can also be a problem if the dog barks at everyone who passes by a house or apartment. Methods of control and owner motivation to affect a change vary in the three situations.

For the dog that barks at night, the owners are highly motivated to change the behavior because they are being bothered. Often the owners contributed to the severity of the problem without realizing it. The dog may have first barked because it heard a sound or another dog barking. The owners were awakened and yelled at the dog for quiet, which was a reward from the animal's perspective. Through trial and error, the dog begins to use barking to get attention at night. The owners unknowingly comply by yelling more or by letting the dog into the house. This problem dog can be managed in several ways. If the dog continues the behavior, remote punishment will extinguish it. Bark or shock collars can help some cases. More ingenious techniques can also be used, from water pistols or blasts of water from a spray nozzle, to water hose blasts, loud bangs from balloons breaking overhead, or the loud rattling of a soft drink can containing a few pebbles. Remote punishment works well on barking for attention and to negate the internal reward of "boredom" barking. In the latter situation, exercise and alternate activities must be added. Ignoring the behavior can lead to its decrease if the dog is barking for attention. For the dog that barks too much when the owners are home, another technique is useful. Instead of letting the dog in the house or giving it attention, the owners should reward silence. Initially the duration of that silence required before letting the dog in should only be a few seconds, but the length can then be increased gradually and eventually randomized.

The dog that barks when the owner is away may bother the neighbors. In theory, antibarking laws are helpful to give the neighbors some peace. The dog owner is often not motivated to control the problem unless there is accompanying destruction in the house or until the police start insisting, and then they want a quick, easy solution. Bark collars can be considered. Surgical removal or ligation of the vocal folds is a drastic alternative to the owner's lack of motivation. Some problems can be controlled simply by leaving the radio or television on for noise. In other cases, remote punishment can be useful, triggered by the owner hiding outside or by a noise-activated device. Behavior modification can be useful when the owner leaves for increasingly longer periods, returning during the quiet period before the barking starts again. Other therapies for separation anxiety can help associated barking.

Dogs that bark at everyone and everything passing by usually have become that way because the owners have rewarded the behavior or encouraged the associated excitement. Initially, they felt the behavior was protective and their actions and tone of voice were rewarding. Once the owners recognize the reward they are actually giving, extinction by habituation, direct punishment, or remote punishment is generally successful.

ALSO SEE: *Avoid Excitement, Bark Collars, Barking, Behavior Modification, Exercise, Habituation Learning, Remote Punishment, Separation Anxiety, Stress-related Behaviors, Trial and Error Learning*

Excessive Vocalization—Howling

Excessive howling occurs more easily in some dogs and is often associated with those times in which the animal is left alone. The behavior may then represent a domesticated version of that vocalized by the lone wolf. Scheduling of human interaction and exercise is often helpful. The dog learns when to expect attention and has less excess energy to spend on howling. If the behavior is associated with separation anxiety, more specific programs should be used. For the real problem dog, a nonshocking bark collar may be useful.

A few dogs howl when the telephone rings but is not answered. This may be a minor distraction to neighbors, and is usually just an interesting observation by an owner. Habituation to the ringing phone or use of an answering machine can stop the behavior if it is considered a problem.

ALSO SEE: *Bark Collars, Boredom, Exercise, Habituation Learning, Howling, Separation Anxiety*

Excessive Vocalization—Meowing

Cats occasionally vocalize in excess. While this is a common trait in Siamese, any cat can learn that meowing brings a desired reward. A few cats have a deeper pitched meow associated with distress, as when another household cat dies.

ALSO SEE: *Behavior Modification, Habituation Learning, Remote Punishment, Stress-related Behaviors, Trial and Error Learning,*

Excessive Vocalization—Whining

Whining vocalizations by dogs win sympathy from owners. Sympathy often results in the dog being picked up and spoken to in a reassuring tone of voice. In other words, the behavior is rewarded and likely to continue as an attention-seeking effort. The simplest correction is to stop rewarding the behavior. Initially, the dog may actually increase the frequency and/or intensity of the whining because the technique had been rewarded in the past. Eventually the behavior will stop. Because owners may have trouble ignoring this behavior, success is often difficult. They may be more willing to try if they realize that their pet is using this behavior to get attention on demand and that the owner no longer controls the relationship.

ALSO SEE: *Attention Seeking, Extinction*

Exercise

Excessive energy is a major component of numerous behavior problems. There are several reasons for this. 1) Most animals receive a good-quality diet but are not given appropriate exercise for their caloric intake or genetic makeup. 2) Dogs of many large breeds were developed to work for extended periods of time, not to lie around a house. 3) Cats, horses, cattle, and swine would normally spend a large portion of their day traveling to find food. Today we confine animals to houses, stalls, small paddocks, drylots, or feedlots for the management's convenience. As a result of these various situations, there is a need to get rid of built-up energy through increased exercise. Behavior problems that are usually responsive to some degree include digging, self-mutilation, stereotypies, escaping, excessive barking, destructive chewing, and pica.

ALSO SEE: *Ankle Attacks, Avoid Excitement, Climbing, Cribbing, Dashing through Doors, Destructive Behaviors, Destructive Chewing, Digging—Indoors, Digging—Outdoors, Excessive Grooming, Excessive Licking, Excessive Vocalization—Barking, Excessive Vocalization—Howling, Fence Jumping, Flank Sucking, Frustration, Habituation Learning, Hair Pulling, Hot Spots, Hyper Syndromes, Inappropriate Mounting, Masturbation, Psychogenic Problems, Self-Mutilation, Soil Eating, Stereotyped Behaviors, Stress-related Behaviors, Tail Chasing, Wind Sucking, Wood Chewing*

Experienced Female

As with many behaviors, the individual components of sexual behavior are instinctive. The proper sequencing and coordination are dependent on learning. Successful mating by a young male will take longer than for an experienced breeder. An inexperienced female can compound the problem of successful copulation, even to the point of complete intimidation. The use of an experienced female for the first few matings, especially with dogs, helps the male establish appropriate mating behaviors.

ALSO SEE: *Experienced Male, Fainting, Female Behaviors, Male Behaviors*

Experienced Male

In many species, females mating for the first few times may be behaviorally difficult. They tend to pull away or show aggression toward the male. An inexperienced male is also learning the sequencing of the mating behaviors and may still lack the appropriate advances for his species. Some are too timid, and some are too aggressive or rough. An experienced male will take less time to accomplish a successful copulation even with an inexperienced female, and she will learn those components of sexual behavior necessary to mate with most males of her species.

ALSO SEE: *Experienced Female, Fainting, Female Behaviors, Male Behaviors*

Exploratory Behavior

This is the behavior of curiosity. It allows an animal to explore a novel situation, location, or object even though there is no specific need to do so. Exploration is common in young mammals and may play a role in early latent learning. At first it allows them to socialize to other species. After the socialization period is over, the animal turns its attention to the environment. The degree of curiosity that remains into adulthood tends to be less, although there are probably species and individual differences.

ALSO SEE: *Curiosity, Investigative Behavior, Latent Learning, Socialization*

Extensor Dominance

As the central nervous system continues to develop after birth in certain species, external indications of the maturation can be evaluated. Extensor dominance is the overriding of vertebral flexor muscles by the extensors when the young is suspended by its neck. This gives the appearance of an arched back. Extensor dominance is consistent in puppies from day 5 through approximately day 18. In kittens, extensor dominance is not consistently present.

ALSO SEE: *Flexor Dominance, Nape Bite*

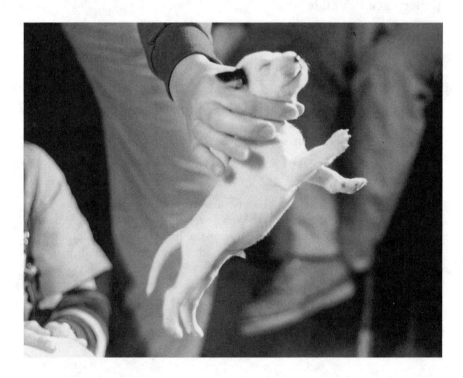

Extensor Dominance. This 2-week-old puppy is demonstrating the position of extensor dominance.

Extinction

Certain behavior problems can be stopped by withdrawing all of the reinforcement for the behavior. This technique works best on certain attention-seeking behaviors that are not rewarding in themselves, and it may be coupled with alternative behaviors that are acceptable.

Initially, when the reinforcement is withdrawn, the animal may try harder to get the results it anticipates, and so the frequency, duration, or intensity of the bout will increase. This phenomenon is known as the extinction burst. If no reinforcement comes, the animal quickly changes its behavior.

ALSO SEE: *Attention Seeking, Behavior Modification, Habituation Learning, Learning*

Facilitation

A behavior, mood, or environmental factor that enhances a behavior is said to be a facilitator of that behavior. An alert state can quicken the response of an animal to a potential predator over the response in a relaxed state. Also, the excitement of other herd members can alert the individual member to possible danger.

ALSO SEE: *Social Facilitation*

Fainting

Fainting is the temporary loss of consciousness resulting from an inadequate flow of blood to the brain. While it is most common in humans, fainting can occur in animals. Stallions servicing a mare for the first time may faint, frightening the owner. By the time the owner can call for veterinary attention, the stallion has usually regained consciousness and is completely normal within a few minutes. Fainting also occurs in certain goats, usually as the result of some type of excitement.

Fear

Fear is a feeling of apprehension resulting from the nearness of some situation or object. When the degree of fear is excessive, the feeling is called a phobia.

ALSO SEE: *Anxiety, Fear Biting, Fear-induced Aggression, Fear of Change, Fear of Environment, Fear of Falling, Fear of Gunshots, Fear of Loud Noise, Fear of Noise, Fear of People, Fear of Thunder, Phobia*

Fear Biting

When an animal is in a fearful situation, it may respond aggressively. This is called fear-induced aggression, or fear biting.

ALSO SEE: *Ambivalent Postures, Fear-induced Aggression, Fear of People*

Fear-induced Aggression

Aggression in response to a fearful situation is called fear-induced, and the severity can vary from an inhibited warning to a severe attack. When an animal cannot escape an approacher, it may strike out to warn the approacher that it is too close. Body postures may indicate distance-increasing signs, which warn of an attack, or they may be ambivalent, indicating the conflict of fear, submission, and aggression. The classic fear biter is a small dog, placed in a top cage, that crouches in the corner staring at the technician or veterinarian trying to get it out. Fear-induced aggression is also commonly shown by a cornered cat, horse, or cow. Animals that have had limited human contact or are away from familiar places (isolated syndrome) are more prone than others to show fear-induced aggression.

Working with these animals means decreasing the threat of the approach as much as possible or allowing controlled escape until they learn to accept the approacher. For fearful dogs, a decreased threat includes avoiding direct eye contact (not staring), a squatting posture, a sideways presentation, a friendly voice, and not reaching out for the animal. Backing into the fear biter's cage avoids direct facial presentation. Once held, the dog usually calms down.

Fearful cats sit in the back of a cage and often hiss and growl when someone approaches. A box or sack for the cat to hide in decreases stress and provides a container in which to capture the cat. Stress can be minimized in the cat being worked with if cupped hands are held over its nose and face. This works best if the owner's smell is on the hands, but any hands are helpful.

Horses can be worked in a round pen and the person gradually moves closer with gentle talking. It is important that the person does not leave until the lesson is accomplished and the horse touched or haltered. Cattle can be worked with by staying outside the critical distance until the animal accepts the person's presence.

Fear-induced aggression is one type of affective aggression.

ALSO SEE: *Affective Aggression, Ambivalent Postures, Critical Distance, Decreased Body Threat, Desensitization, Direct Punishment, Fear of People, Isolated Syndrome*

F

Fear of Change

Animals may show behaviors that indicate that they are afraid of changes within their environment. While most changes are obvious, some are subtle and require detective work to determine what they are. Cats started hiding under beds or stopped coming to the living areas of a home when a large plant was introduced or a toddler was visiting. Changes in an animal's schedule can be disturbing as well and difficult to single out in a behavioral history unless owners can identify changes in their schedules, too. Cats and dogs quickly learn to associate a suitcase with upcoming changes in feeding schedules and social interactions, or boxes with upcoming moves. Dramatic changes in behavior can follow, from soiling in the house to hiding.

ALSO SEE: *Fear of Environment, Negative Reinforcement, Schedule*

Fear of Environment

Animals that have been kept in a specific environment can develop sudden and extreme fears of that area. There may be no readily apparent cause for this onset of fear; however, investigation usually reveals the problem. Horses have suddenly become very destructive to a stall or have strongly resisted entering one. Careful inspection can show that the stall has accidentally become electrified, there was an unacceptable odor in it, or that stinging or biting insects were present. Bad experiences, as in a horse trailer, can also result in a specific fear. Dogs have suddenly become afraid of lawn sprinkler systems, the sun, or living room carpet, and the initiating factor could not be determined.

Gradual desensitization can eliminate the fear eventually if the problem fear is not continually reinforced by the environment.

ALSO SEE: *Desensitization, Negative Reinforcement*

Fear of Falling

Studies in a number of species, including cats, rats, dogs, sheep, and humans, indicate an age where the young begin to show a reluctance to cross a visual drop off. Very young animals will walk onto the glass continuation of a visual cliff. As vision develops, the infant can distinguish a drop off and will not continue past that point even though there is a glass continuation of the level.

ALSO SEE: *Vision*

Fear of Gunshots

The fear of gunshots is most frequently a complaint in hunting dogs and occasionally in horses that are used for the hunt. Although this phobia may be an inherited problem, it usually is acquired when an early exposure is too close and too loud.

Desensitization involves getting the animal accustomed to an increasing volume of gunshots. Dogs should know how to heel and sit. Gunshots can be muffled, and cap guns make effective alternative to a real gun. Begin with the dog as far from the gun as necessary, where it shows no reaction to a shot, and call that the start location. Have the dog heel to a position one yard closer to the gun and sit, then fire the gun. If the dog shows no reaction to the gun, give it praise or a food reward for the appropriate response of sit with no startle. Then return to the start position. Now heel the dog two yards closer to the gun, having it sit, and fire the gun. Reward appropriate behavior and return to the start position. Continue moving toward the sound source at one yard increments. If the dog shows any negative responses, such as quivering, leaning on the owner, or salivating, do not give the praise or food reward at the sit. Go back to the start and heel to the last position of acceptable behavior. Repeat the heel, sit, and fire procedure at this yardage several times before continuing forward again. The program can continue forward when the appropriate nonreaction is obtained at the former problem distance.

ALSO SEE: *Desensitization, Fear of Noise*

Fear of Loud Noise

Animals may show a reaction to a sudden, sharp, loud noise, and a single event can result in an extreme reaction to future occurrences of that noise. Typically, firecrackers and cars backfiring are associated with this fear; however, other events, such as a child hitting a pot near a dog or cat, can also precipitate the phobia.

If the fear-inducing events are limited and predictable, the animal may be confined away from the sharp noise, perhaps with a radio as background noise. If the problem occurs frequently enough and in random, single events, control involves desensitization through repetition with gradually increasing volumes.

ALSO SEE: *Desensitization, Fear of Noise*

Fear of Noise

Fear of noise can be related to several different noises, such as gunshots, thunder, firecrackers, and car backfiring. In the few cases where puppies show the fear, there may be a genetic component. More typically, dogs acquire the fear of noise as the result of a very negative experience or because the owner reinforced the behavior to a mild reaction. Horses and other animals that typically flee potential danger are somewhat more reactive. Even the relatively soft noises of a rattlesnake can be very upsetting to an animal that has been bitten before. Fear of noise can be restricted to a specific noise or generalized to a number of sounds.

Typically, the longer the fear of noise persists, the more difficult it is to eliminate, especially if other cues also trigger the phobia. For example, the fear of thunder is easier to control by itself than when it is coupled with fear of rain, ozone, or barometric changes. There are a number of ways to use counterconditioning to eliminate or minimize the fear. The basic concept is one of desensitization. The technique is to gradually accustom the animal to the sounds. Begin at a volume that is too soft to evoke a reaction and gradually increase it over several training sessions. This can be done by bringing the animal gradually closer to the source of the sound and reinforcing positive behaviors or by slowly increasing the volume of recorded sounds. Antianxiety tranquilizers may be useful in the early stages of desensitization. Owners should be told that this process requires time and effort on their part. It should not begin until external sources of the noise can be controlled.

Flooding—surrounding the animal with the specific noise until it no longer shows a reaction—can be used in carefully selected cases. It is generally inappropriate for noise phobias and can actually worsen the condition.

ALSO SEE: *Behavior Modification, Counterconditioning, Desensitization, Drug Therapy, Fear of Gunshots, Fear of Loud Noise, Fear of Thunder, Flooding, Generalization, Negative Reinforcement, Phobia, Appendix C*

Fear of People

Certain animals show an obvious and well-developed fear of people. The reaction can be directed toward an individual, a group of people, all but a few individuals, or all people. Fear of people often results from poor socialization or a negative experience that resulted in desocialization. Veterinarians frequently see animals that do not want to be handled by them, a behavior that may have resulted from some painful experience. Animals with timid personalities, especially dogs, can show a fear of people with dominant behaviors. The degree of expression can range from submissive postures to hiding to fear-induced aggression.

ALSO SEE: *Fear Biting, Fear-induced Aggression, Improper Socialization, Isolated Syndrome, Negative Reinforcement, Phobia, Socialization, Timid Personality*

Fear of Thunder

Fear of thunder (brontophobia, thunderphobia) is one of the most common noise-related fears in dogs. While a few dogs may have a genetic predisposition for this problem, most develop it gradually. In some dogs, the fear develops as a result of the owner's fear. Loud thunder scares the owner, who then strokes the dog for reassurance. Over time the dog learns to associate trembling at the sound of thunder with owner attention. Other dogs develop the fear suddenly because of a sharp noise at close range. A gun fired immediately overhead or an extremely loud thunder clap may start the fear, and continued exposure can then escalate the problem.

Owners generally do not worry about the problem while they are home to let the dog in, or if they live in a rural area. Only when the dog runs away or causes damage from its frantic digging, chewing, or tearing through doors, windows, and walls do owners seek help.

The destructive behaviors should not be punished. In many cases, the dogs are already bleeding from their feet or mouth from attempts to get inside. Conversely, the behaviors should not be rewarded by human reassurance. The owner should remain neutral.

The goal of treatment is to control the problem rather than to eliminate it completely, and it takes a committed owner. Initially, it may be necessary to tranquilize the dog until thunder season is over. While waiting, owners should record the sounds of thunderstorms. Commercial recordings of storms are another alternative. The dog then should go through a desensitization program using the recordings. It is helpful to use a specific location for training and a "security cloth," such as a handkerchief with the owner's scent on it. Eventually the location is viewed as a safe haven, and the cloth can be left with the animal as an olfactory reassurance during bad weather.

For indoor dogs, access to a closet or other dark quiet area, or the playing of a radio or TV may minimize the fear.

ALSO SEE: *Brontophobia, Cloth with Odor, Desensitization, Destructive Chewing, Drug Therapy, Fear of Loud Noise, Negative Reinforcement, Overshadowing, Phobia, Thunderphobia*

Feast or Famine

Predators that hunt as a group and those that kill large animals live with a feast-or-famine eating pattern. Their success at hunting depends on the skill of the group as a whole or the individual hunter's skill and also is dependent upon the availability of prey. Meals may occur daily or several days apart. These animals have developed a pattern of eating in which they consume as much as possible each time in order to survive until the next kill. Dogs have inherited this feast-or-famine background from their wolf ancestors, so it is difficult to keep most dogs at a reasonable weight with free-choice feeding. Some individuals can adjust to self-feeding, particularly if the food is not very palatable. Most dogs, however, do not adjust.

Predators that kill several small animals or supplement their diets with insects generally do not have the problem of overconsumption unless prepared meals are too palatable or fattening. For that reason, fat cats, foxes, and coyotes are uncommon unless humans interfere.

ALSO SEE: *Eating Behavior, Predation*

Feather Eating

The eating of feathers, which is closely related to feather picking and cannibalism, is a behavior problem of chickens. The feathers of the tail and pinions are preferred sites. It is generally believed that the problem is related to feeding, nutrition, or lack of appropriate environmental stimuli, since the problem usually decreases when bulk is added to the diet and when birds do more searching for favorite foods.

ALSO SEE: *Cannibalism, Feather Picking*

Feather Picking

Pet birds and poultry raised under intensive management systems can develop feather picking problems. In the pets, self-picking is most common, while group-housed birds are more apt to peck and pull each other's feathers. In flocks, the sight of blood will increase the severity of the behavior and increase the likelihood of its progression to body pecking and cannibalism. While the exact cause is not known, high stock rates and general stresses, including lack of environmental stimuli and crowding, are considered major factors.

Control of feather picking in commercial flocks has been achieved by beak trimming (removal of the rostral part of the upper beak), using red light (infrared lamps, red bulbs, red painted windows), and restricting a bird's vision with a type of blinder called "poly-peepers." Modifying the environment to address the pet bird's social needs and changing stocking rates of poultry should also be considered.

ALSO SEE: *Body Pecking, Cannibalism, Feather Eating, Stress-related Behaviors*

Feather Ruffling

Feather ruffling in birds is similar to piloerection in mammals. The usual function is to help prevent heat loss during cold weather. The behavior can also function as a display, particularly if a specific region is involved, such as a head crest or tail.

ALSO SEE: *Display, Piloerection*

Feces Eating

The eating of feces from an animal's own species or from an unrelated species is called coprophagy or fefection.

ALSO SEE: *Coprophagia, Fefection*

Feces Throwing

Caged primates often develop the behavior of throwing their feces at people passing by. This is most frequently done by animals kept in relatively barren environments and may be a learned technique that results in action, as people dodge the fecal material. The behavior in itself may have an internal reward.

Environmental enrichment, especially where social interactions can occur, minimizes this problem.

ALSO SEE: *Internal Reward*

Feeding Ceremony

This is the presentation of food as a greeting or to help establish a social relationship. In some animals, the food presentation protects the male from being eaten. In others, it is more of a gesture.

ALSO SEE: *Ingestive Behavior*

Feeding Schedule Change

Some dogs and cats have behavior problems associated with their feeding schedules. Since eating tends to stimulate defecation, dogs that defecate in the house at night might be able to stop the problem by eating earlier in the day.

Free-choice feeding may not be appropriate for certain individual dogs or cats, either because they eat any food present, the food available is too palatable, the food has too many calories for its bulk, or a combination of several factors. In these cases, a specific feeding schedule is recommended.

Feeding schedules should change as a puppy or kitten gets older. The specific frequency recommended will depend on the age, size, and caloric requirements of the individual. Very small dogs, young puppies and kittens, and lactating females need multiple feedings. Adult animals can usually get by on one to three.

ALSO SEE: *Excessive Food Intake, Housesoiling—Defecation*

Feeding Tradition

The young often learn food preferences from their dam. If a particular preference is localized to a region because of this learning it is called a feeding tradition. Food preference in humans from exposure to ethnic or regional flavors is one example.

ALSO SEE: *Food Preferences, Ingestive Behavior*

Fefection

The normal behavior of certain rodents and lagomorphs of eating their own feces is fefection. This is a natural behavior, unlike coprophagy in other species.

ALSO SEE: *Coprophagia*

Feline Asocial Aggression

Cats are generally considered to be an asocial species, although some individuals will act socially toward a few cats with which they are in frequent contact. When strange cats come around, the resident cat is usually aggressive toward them. While territorial and intermale aggressions may precipitate similar reactions, the feline asocial nature is generally responsible for triggering the aggressive behavior.

When one cat in a household dies or leaves, owners may get another cat to replace their loss. The older remaining resident cat is much less receptive to the new addition than is the owner. The new cat is often a kitten that tries to interact with the older cat. The resulting aggression is upsetting to the owners, although it is a common form of feline asocial aggression. Minimizing contact between the two cats until the younger cat gets older and less social tends to reduce the aggression. It is best to bring in a new cat that is at least a year old, for this cat will have gone through the personality change from social to asocial and thus seek less interaction with the resident cat.

ALSO SEE: *Asocial, Feline Dispersion Aggression, Feline Personality Change, Intermale (Interfemale) Aggression, Territorial Protective Aggression*

Feline Dispersion Aggression

Kittens live with their dam and littermates from their birth until about six months, plus or minus a few months. During this time they learn and perfect the behaviors that they will need to survive in a more solitary lifestyle. As the time approaches for dispersion from the maternal grouping, the behaviors among siblings gradually change, as do their individual personalities. The social play behaviors become rougher and end in aggressive bouts. Gradually, the play portion becomes shorter and the aggressive portion becomes more intense. The group eventually disperses when the level of aggression becomes greater than the need to remain together. Each cat is then on its own.

ALSO SEE: *Asocial, Feline Asocial Aggression, Feline Dispersion Aggression—Atypical, Feline Personality Change*

Feline Dispersion Aggression—Atypical

When a cat does not have its littermates to play with, it may direct the same behaviors at an owner. At first it may just pounce on the owner walking by, but by 8 to 10 months of age the more aggressive behaviors that would eventually dispel littermates become painful to the owner.

The behavior must be discouraged. The owner can carry a squirt gun or water sprayer, or use a soda pop can with rocks for a rattle. Physical punishment, while not recommended, has been used. Time will lessen the extremes of this behavior, provided the cat is not allowed to attack the owner. If the problem occurs at a certain time or location, it may be possible to restructure activities to decrease the aggression.

ALSO SEE: *Ankle Attacks, Damming-up Theory, Feline Dispersion Aggression*

Feline Hyperesthesia Syndrome

The feline hyperesthesia (rolling skin) syndrome is a relatively common condition in cats; however, the etiology is unclear and there may be multiple causes. An affected animal will show a sudden dilation of its pupils, a rippling of the skin over its back, and perhaps a sudden yowling vocalization, before it starts running. Severe chewing of the tail, even to the degree that amputation is required can also be part of this syndrome. No age, sex, or breed specificity has been defined. It is important to differentiate this behavior from normal play activities in kittens.

Some cats show a dermal sensitivity, usually to fleas, and appropriate control for the primary problem controls the hyperesthesia. Other cats develop this behavior as a result of environmental stresses, perhaps associated with a more nervous type of personality. Control of the environment by removing the stress is important in managing their problem. Short-term use of antianxiety tranquilizers or progestins may be useful initially as the environment is being stabilized. Some animals have been treated as epileptics, and the phenobarbital has controlled the rippling skin bouts. In other cases, owners may learn to accept occasional bouts of this syndrome if they know it is not particularly harmful to the animal.

ALSO SEE: *Drug Therapy, Remove the Stress, Seizures, Self-Mutilation, Stress-related Behaviors*

Feline Ischemic Encephalopathic Aggression

Neurologic and behavioral changes, including aggression, can result from cerebral infarcts in cats. Signs have an acute onset, and typically occur in one- to three-year-old cats. Most clinical chemistry tests are normal, although the cerebrospinal fluid and/or electroencephalogram may show changes. The prognosis depends on the location and degree of ischemia. Aggression and seizures are the most common residual problems.

ALSO SEE: *Aggression*

Feline Personality Change

In kittens, the need for staying in a group is strong. At first, the kitten needs the care of the queen. Eventually, it needs to learn and perfect the hunting behaviors that will sustain it as a solitary hunter. Kittens gradually approach the time of dispersion by changing their behaviors from predominantly play and social interaction to those of independence. Aggression between littermates increases until it eventually drives the kittens off on their own.

The personality changes of a maturing cat will be obvious to cat owners. Young kittens are full of play and interact socially with people. Gradually the pet becomes less interactive and, in some cases, aggressive. By six to eight months, the owners are disappointed that their cat is just not what they had hoped for. The only way to predict what the personality of a mature cat will be is to know what the personality of the queen and tom were. A friendly sire and dam provide the best hope of having a friendly cat as an adult.

ALSO SEE: *Asocial, Feline Asocial Aggression, Feline Dispersion Aggression*

Female Behaviors

A few behaviors of animals differ by sex, and those are primarily related to reproductive behaviors. There are differences by species as well. Behaviors unique to females occur in estrus, pregnancy, parturition, and maternal behavior.

ALSO SEE: *Automimicry, Courtship, Decreased Sexual Behavior, Epigamic Traits, Estrous Behavior, Fraser Darling Effect, Gestation, Male Behaviors, Maternal Behavior, Mating Behavior, Parturition, Postcopulatory Behavior, Proceptive Behavior, Reproductive Behavior, Sexual Dimorphism, Sexually Dimorphic Behaviors, Silent Heat, Appendix B*

Fence Jumping

Fence jumping occurs as a problem in dogs, horses, and cattle. In order to successfully manage this escape behavior, the motivation should be determined. For dogs it may involve a need for social interaction or exercise. Horses and cattle often jump a fence because of nearby food. A few individuals get out to return to herds of origin or to go to animals in nearby pastures. Apparently, in some cases the behavior itself is rewarding to the animal. Appropriate food, exercise, and social interaction help stop the problem behavior. Initial or permanent use of confinement, electric fences, or taller fences may be a necessary part of breaking the pattern.

ALSO SEE: *Confinement, Escape Behavior, Exercise, Internal Reward, Running Away*

Feral Animal

A feral animal is a member of a large group of animals that have undergone reverse domestication for several generations. The changes that have occurred during the reversal process involve morphologic, physiologic, and/or behavioral traits, where humans have not interfered with the process. The mustangs, wild burros, longhorns, and hog populations in the river bottoms of southern United States are feral populations. A feral animal is not an untamed domestic animal, so stray dogs and cats are rarely feral.

ALSO SEE: *Domestication, Tame Animal, Wild Animal*

Fight It Out

Dominance and intermale aggressions may become serious over time. Dog owners have often compounded the severity of the problem by repeatedly breaking up fights and not allowing dogs to reach their own conclusions.

To finally settle a disagreement between animals, it may be appropriate to let them fight it out to a conclusion. If there is a concern of potential injuries to dogs, muzzling both animals can be helpful. When size differences are great, the dogs do not come to a resolution, or if injuries are a real possibility, this may not be an acceptable alternative.

ALSO SEE: *Dominance Aggression, Intermale Aggression, Muzzle, Separate*

Filial Imprinting

Rapid imprinting that is associated with moving objects is called filial imprinting, and the sensitive period is typically quite brief. This type of imprinting is usually associated with bird species such as chickens and ducks, where the young follow the dam. The behavior has also been called following-response imprinting.

ALSO SEE: *Imprint Learning*

Filing Canine Teeth

As a "treatment" for aggressive dogs, and to a lesser extent cats and exotic cats, veterinarians have filed the canine teeth to the level of the incisors. Following this procedure, the animal has stopped showing aggression. Because the success of this procedure has not been correlated with a behavioral diagnosis, the reason for the success is open to speculation. For some, the loss of the weapons may be intimidating. In other cases, however, the type of aggression may have been nonrecurring anyway, or the pain associated with an exposed tooth nerve may be preventing most oral behavior.

Complete extraction of the canine teeth has also been used to prevent aggression. It is not always successful. In theory, the severity of the injury should be less, but severe damage can be done by the remaining teeth. Success with tooth removal, while extreme, may represent an appropriate treatment in some cases; however, additional studies are needed to identify the types of aggression for which it is appropriate.

ALSO SEE: *Aggression, Biting*

Filters

Filters are physiological and anatomical determinants of whether environmental stimuli are perceived by an animal. Peripheral filters determine whether the stimuli are detected by the animal and central filters determine what is done with the incoming information.

ALSO SEE: *Central Filters, Peripheral Filters, Stimulus Filtering*

Finicky Eaters

There are a number of reasons animals become finicky eaters. Some that do not have large appetites and have owners that want them to eat more may appear finicky, but they are so only relative to owner expectations. Taste preferences are developed while an animal is young. As they get older, animals may be considered finicky because the flavors or textures of food presented are not particularly desirable.

Dogs that are finicky eaters may be so because of taste preferences or an overzealous or overobliging owner. If the dog learns to hold out for flavorful foods, it may be able to convince its owner that it needs encouragement to eat. Eventually it will insist on the special meals, and owners will go to extremes, like cooking special meals or even pre-chewing food, to appease the dog. Overcoming the human-made finicky eater requires the owner simply to present only dog food for 30 minutes once or twice daily. If the dog does not eat, the food is removed until the next mealtime. Within one to five days, most dogs will begin eating, with an occasional dog taking longer. The hardest part is convincing owners of the importance of a balanced diet. It might be necessary to give them special recipes for a balanced diet so they can continue to prepare the dog's meal.

Cats are commonly described as finicky eaters because of their resistance to eating foods with flavors or textures they do not like. This can be carried to the extreme of actual starvation in a few cases. Obese cats that are put on a no-food diet or are anorexic for several days can develop clinical signs of fatty lipidosis and may not start eating again.

Horses may develop particular taste preferences for plain oats or for a sweet feed mixture and may not want to eat other types of food. Some may develop brand preferences.

ALSO SEE: *Diet Change, Eating Behavior, Food Preferences*

Fixed Action Patterns

These are stereotyped movements that are characteristic within a species. They may be a solitary behavior, such as a horse rolling or a wet dog shaking, or part of a complex behavior, such as eating at the end of prey chasing or chin dragging by bulls during the dismount after breeding.

In recent years, the term "fixed action pattern" has been replaced by "modal action pattern."

ALSO SEE: *Male Behaviors*

Flank Sucking

Flank sucking is a behavior problem shown by some Doberman pinschers when they are stressed. The dog will place its open mouth in its flank and hold the position, either standing or lying. Usually the only damage done is a wet and perhaps slightly ruffled haircoat. Flank sucking apparently has a genetic component because the trait can be followed through certain bloodlines within the Doberman breed. It may not become obvious until the animal undergoes stress.

The problem generally stops when the stress is removed; however, if treatment is necessary, it usually involves confinement so that the dog physically is unable to reach the flank. Antianxiety tranquilizers, progestins, and exercise may be helpful for problem animals.

ALSO SEE: *Confinement, Drug Therapy, Exercise, Genetic Problems, Appendix C*

Flehmen

Flehmen is the behavior in which an animal elevates its upper lip. It is most commonly associated in domestic animals with horses (horse laugh) and cattle (lip curl). Dogs, cats (gape, grimace), pigs, and small ruminants also show this behavior, although it is less obvious in these species because the filtrum limits mobility of the upper lip.

Flehmen apparently helps bring odors, primarily volatile fatty acids, into the vomeronasal organ and is usually associated with sexual or social behaviors. Male animals show the behavior most often, apparently while testing for the reproductive state of females, especially through the urine. The behavior is not common in females, although mares do occasionally show the behavior. Horses tend to show flehmen in inappropriate situations more than other animals.

ALSO SEE: *Horses, Male Behaviors, Sniff-Yawn, Vomeronasal Organ*

Flexibilitas Cerea

Flexibilitas cerea refers to the flexibility in the arms or legs of schizophrenic persons as they remain in the position in which they were placed. The condition has been observed rarely in dogs (Fox, 1971).

Flexor Dominance

In animal species where the young are not completely developed at birth, the central nervous system continues to mature, and changes associated with that can be evaluated. When vertebral flexors can overpower the extensors, a neonate will show a limp, tucked posture in response to being held loosely by the neck.

In puppies, flexor dominance will last for the first four days of life. In cats the response can continue, at least partially, for several years, and can be used to immobilize them. Flexor dominance has also been called the limp posture.

ALSO SEE: *Extensor Dominance, Nape Bite*

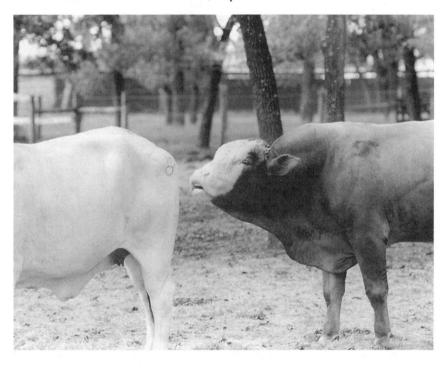

Flehmen. Flehmen is shown by a bull after investigating the cow's perineum (Vet. Med./Small Anim. Clin. 78:579, 1983).

Flight Distance

The social (reactive) distance at which an animal will start to flee from an approaching intruder is called the flight distance. This distance will vary with species and other influences, as discussed under social distance. A cat will run when the approacher is within approximately 6 feet of the animal. For the horse, the distance is approximately 21 feet, and for cattle, it is approximately 18 feet. Taming an animal reduces the flight distance to zero. Animals can be driven in groups or worked in chutes by staying visibly inside the flight distance, but not so close as to provoke an attack. The curved design of cattle chutes allows handlers to use the social distance to their advantage and to minimize the amount of rough handling necessary for working the animals.

ALSO SEE: *Critical Distance, Reactive Distances, Social Distance, Tame Animal, Trailer Loading*

Flightiness

Flightiness is a tendency for certain animals to show mobile alarm more prominently than would be expected in the species as a whole. There may be a genetic component to this, and flightiness should be suspected if the behavior is common in certain strains or bloodlines. It can also be an individual's characteristic.

ALSO SEE: *Mobile Alarm, Reactive Anomalies*

Flooding

Flooding is the continuous application of stimuli to an animal so as to accustom it to those stimuli and desensitize its reactions.

ALSO SEE: *Behavior Modification, Desensitization, Fear of Noise, Habituation Learning*

Fly Snapping

Dogs will suddenly turn and snap at a fly passing by. Some dogs will occasionally show the behavior even though no flying insect is around. This unusual behavior may be a vacuum activity, an attention-seeking behavior, the response to a perceived fly due to the movement of a remnant of the hyaloid artery within the eye, or the expression of a behavioral seizure. Exercise will usually help eliminate the behavior as a vacuum activity. No attention should be given directly to the behavior to ensure that it is not and does not become a method to get attention. The expense and complication of surgery for removal of the arterial remnant do not justify the procedure. If fly snapping represents the only manifestation of seizural activity, it is usually not treated.

ALSO SEE: *Attention Seeking, Exercise, No, No Attention to Behaviors, Obedience Class, Punishment, Seizures, Vacuum Activity*

Follower

Young that are always in close proximity to their mothers are called followers. The behavior is usually associated with species that travel great distances or ones where the young run to escape predators. These young nurse frequently throughout the day, suckling small amounts each time. In domestic animals, the foal is an example of a follower; the wildebeest calf is an example in the wild.

ALSO SEE: *Layer Out, Maternal Behavior*

Followership

Cattle and sheep are strongly attached to a social group, either herd or flock. While dominance and leadership are generally considered important components of a social group, these species are more dependent on an active followership. There is a strong tendency to follow the animal in the front. This behavior can be seen in cattle as they graze; as those in front orient in a particular direction, other members of the herd gradually change directions until most of the herd is facing the same direction. The tendency for sheep to be followers is a useful behavior for working them. Sheep will follow goats trained to lead sheep into slaughter plants (Judas goats) or livestock trailers. A single sheep secured in a trailer also can entice others to enter.

Other group animals show lesser degrees of followership. Horses tend to follow the group, a trait used in pack strings and stables that rent horses for trail rides.

ALSO SEE: *Dominance, Social Behavior*

Following-Response Imprinting

This type of learning is also called filial imprinting.

SEE: *Filial Imprinting*

Food Allergy

Food allergies can be expressed in a number of ways. Classically, in veterinary medicine, they are associated with gastrointestinal signs or dermatologic problems, but they can also be manifested by behavioral changes. The hyper syndrome in dogs can be produced by such allergies, and the general discomfort associated with the allergy increases the likelihood of irritable aggression.

An allergy can develop to any type of food an animal eats. For dogs, the reaction is probably most common to foods with high protein levels or proteins from specific animal sources. Often, by dropping the protein level below 20% or changing the protein sources, the problem is controllable. Other allergies have implicated sugars, carbohydrates, or food additives. Cats are susceptible to red meat allergies, particularly beef. Horses may react to diet additives.

A diet change to eliminate the offending ingredient is the treatment of choice. Just the change during hospitalization may be enough to stop the problem in the patient, although it will generally take several weeks to get the offending material out of the system. Only by selective challenge can an absolute diagnosis be made, and many owners are so pleased with the initial results of the diet change that they are unwilling to try this procedure.

ALSO SEE: *Allergy Workup, Diet Change, Hyper Syndromes, Irritable Aggression*

Food Begging

Food begging is a behavior usually seen in the young of species that depend on the parents to bring food. Pecking of certain spots on the parent or gaping may get the same results for young birds. In canids, submissive vocalizations and mouth licking may stimulate the bitch to regurgitate. The begging behaviors may persist long after they are necessary because they are rewarded with food.

ALSO SEE: *Ingestive Behavior*

Food Imprinting

This is a term that has been used to describe the development of food preferences, although the behavior probably does not represent a true form of imprinting.

ALSO SEE: *Food Preferences*

Food Preferences

Food preferences are learned by the young of all species during the first several months after they start on solid food. This is a time when it is important to offer a variety of flavors and textures to prevent the animal from becoming a finicky eater later in life. This early learning is particularly critical in cats since they can later become aggressive or anorexic when a preferred food is not available. Some horses will not eat foods with additives, such as medications. Others show preferences for sweet feed being added or not added to oats, or for a certain type of hay over their grain. There is even the rare individual that shows a preference for a particular brand of oats.

ALSO SEE: *Anorexia, Diet Change, Feeding Tradition, Finicky Eaters, Food Imprinting, Ingestive Behavior*

Food Provisioning

Food provisioning is the feeding of one animal by another. The most common form is the feeding of the young by its parent. Food can also be shared during courtship or among members of a social group.

ALSO SEE: *Ingestive Behavior*

Food Storage

Certain species store food for use at a later time. Some, such as carnivores, use short-term storage when a kill is more than they can consume at one time. A number of species put food away for times when it is not otherwise available. Food storage, by definition, requires that there is a period of overabundance and that the food remain edible.

Foreleg Kick

Several of the male ruminants will use a stiff-legged, forward-directed kick with their forelimb as a part of the courtship behavior. The forelimb may be raised between the females hindlimbs or to the side of them. The anestrous female will move away from this advance.

Form Analysis

One technique used to study the relatedness of two animal species is to compare the similarities of their behavior patterns. The sameness in sequences can indicate a genetic relatedness, and a divergence may be helpful to determine genetic drift.

Form Constancy

This describes the degree of consistency with which a behavior is performed. It can represent a fixed (modal) action pattern, an instinct, a reflex, a stereotyped behavior, or a rigidly learned behavior pattern.

ALSO SEE: *Fixed Action Patterns, Instinct, Reflex, Stereotyped Behaviors*

Fostering

Fostering is the process of inducing a female to accept and begin to care for young that she did not birth. Orphaned young often can be raised by females that are not their natural mothers. The behavior is most common in females who have recently given birth and are still establishing a mother-infant bond. The other time of best acceptance is when the female is about to start the weaning process, that is, when the female is less discriminatory about the young. Multiparous females are more likely to be receptive to attempts to foster young, and wild ancestors of those species may actually share nursing responsibilities. This is true for wolves and wild pigs. Size and smell of the young are often an important factor as to whether or not an infant is accepted. Ideally, the young animal should be about the same age and size as the female's own young, if she still has them, although it has been suggested that adopted young could be slightly larger. The odor factor can be minimized if the infant spends time crawling with the female's offspring while the female is away. Feces of the female or her offspring have been smeared on the young animal, and skins from a dead offspring have been used as a coat before the infant was introduced to help transfer imprinted odors to the dam.

Bitches are generally receptive to fostering before they imprint on their young and when they begin the weaning process. Care still needs to be used when attempting to introduce a puppy. Most queens will readily accept new kittens, even during the second or third week. By introducing the kitten to the queen's litter first, a new kitten is usually accepted right away. Mares seldom foster another mare's foal, even if put together near the time of birth. Fostering is common in cattle, particularly dairy cows. Many times there is only a partial acceptance, though, because the cow's head may need to be restrained while the calves nurse. Fostering of piglets is relatively easy, especially when piglets are put with a sow before her litter establishes a teat order. If the sow is not confined to a crate, it is usually necessary to let the new piglets acquire the appropriate odors. At sheep ranches, pelts from a recently dead lamb can be fitted onto an orphan before it is presented to the dead lamb's mother. Some ewes are still resistant and must be restrained for a few days until the lamb's feces are a by-product of the foster ewe's milk.

ALSO SEE: *Teat Order*

Fraser Darling Effect

Synchronization of the reproductive state of a group of animals can occur due to social stimulation. This phenomena has been described in women housed in dormitories, and it has been documented in animals, too. The strength of the effect is dependent on group size and/or density.

Fratricide

Fratricide is the killing of one sibling by another. This occurs most commonly among birds of prey where eggs hatch on successive days. The older chick may starve out the younger, push the younger chick out of the nest, or directly attack its sibling. This may represent a strategy for ensuring the survival of one offspring.

This type of infanticide has also been called sibicide and siblicide.

ALSO SEE: *Infanticide*

Frustration

Frustration is the feeling that results from the failure to achieve a certain goal when the attainment of the goal would be gratifying. As a result of this failure to accomplish, the animal may show depression or lack of interest, stress-related behaviors, aggression, a displacement activity, or a behavior directly related to the intended goal. Examples of behaviors that result from apparent frustration in animals include excessive grooming, stereotypies, destructive behaviors, and running away.

Elimination of the source of the frustration or stress is the primary approach to addressing associated problems.

ALSO SEE: *Depression, Destructive Behaviors, Excessive Grooming, Exercise, Psychological Well-being, Remove the Stress, Schedule, Stereotyped Behaviors, Stress-related Behaviors*

Frustration-induced Aggression

This is a form of aggression that seems to result from a frustration. It may be directed toward another animal nearby (thus resembling redirected aggression) or toward nearby objects (a target humans often use). Some believe this type of aggression is similar to pain-induced aggression.

ALSO SEE: *Aggression, Frustration, Pain-induced Aggression, Stress-related Behaviors*

Fun in Location

For certain behavior problems, such as housesoiling in a new baby's room, a change in the attitude of a dog can cause a desirable change in behavior. The owner should decrease interaction with the pet in the usual locations and increase positive interactions in the problem area. Petting, talking, and playing can make marking or other behaviors unnecessary for the dog. If a family is expecting the arrival of a baby, the baby's room can become a fun area for the pet even before the baby's birth. When coupled with a firm schedule of human interaction, problems can often be prevented.

Fun in a location can also be useful in other species. Horses, and to a lesser extent, cats, cattle, swine, and laboratory animals, can become stressed when first exhibited or when put into unusual surroundings. The encouragement of apparently pleasurable behaviors, such as eating or exercising in the show ring before the show, can provide an opportunity for the animal to relax before it must concentrate on appropriate tasks.

ALSO SEE: *New Baby, Schedule*

Fun with Baby

When a new baby arrives in a family, the pet may show aggression toward the infant, a clinging behavior toward the owner, urine marking of the child's toys or furniture, or destructive chewing around the baby's things. New parents then become concerned. Usually what has happened is that the pet's share of attention has been superseded by attention toward the baby. The room may be suddenly off limits. Instead of blocking the dog or cat from activities associated with the baby, the owners should include the pet in the fun sessions. When the child is bathed, the dog should be in the room to receive the gentle voice. When the baby is held, it might also be convenient to pet the dog or cat. Positive experiences in the presence of the infant usually result in a positive relationship for the animal.

ALSO SEE: *New Baby*

Furniture Scratching

Cats condition their claws on available materials, provided they are appropriate in texture, height or length, and location. Cats prefer materials that are loosely woven and have a vertical orientation, allowing the claw fragments to catch and pull free (Hart and Hart, 1985). When the pet is confined to a house, it will use furniture or other available items for this purpose. The behavior is usually limited to a few locations, but a great deal of damage can be done by one cat.

The problem can be controlled in several ways. First, an acceptable scratching post must be placed where the problem usually occurs. The piece of furniture should then be removed or changed in texture, as by covering it with plastic. This re-education procedure can take several months to be completely successful, depending on how long the behavior has been going on.

Owners who want a quick change in behavior or who are not willing to change their home's appearance may want the cat declawed. The problem is most easily prevented by teaching the appropriate behavior to kittens.

ALSO SEE: *Claw Sharpening, Claw Sharpening—Carpet, Claw Sharpening—Curtains, Declawing*

Galactophagia

Galactophagia is anomalous milk sucking, or the sucking of milk from an animal that is not the animal's dam or foster mother.

SEE: *Anomalous Milk Sucking*

Gape

A facial expression in cats that is their variation of flehmen. It has also been called a grimace.

ALSO SEE: *Flehmen*

Garbage Eating

Dogs, cats, and several types of wild animals commonly break into garbage cans and sacks set outdoors. In most areas, the initial culprit is often a dog, with cats and other animals being opportunists once food scraps have been exposed. The damage is both unsightly and time consuming to pick up. It is also potentially dangerous for the animal if it eats discarded items such as chicken bones. The behavior is rewarding because of the success at getting food tidbits, and so it is likely to continue. Prevention is successful only if the animal is physically confined or the garbage made inaccessible.

Garbage eating within a house tends to take two forms. The first is when an item in the garbage attracts the pet by its smell and is accessible. Food scraps, sanitary napkins, and soiled disposable diapers are commonly involved (Beaver, Fischer, and Atkinson, 1992). Other pets take items out of trash cans and scatter them throughout the house, usually facial tissues and other paper products. This type of behavior is a form of separation anxiety, since the items are generally not eaten and instead are scattered and/or shredded. The easiest technique to control either type of tampering with garbage by a house pet is to prevent access to the garbage. It can be shut in a cupboard or room, or kept out of reach on a counter.

ALSO SEE: *Separation Anxiety*

Gate Crashing

Gate crashing is an escape behavior in which the animal hits the gate until it opens or breaks. The behavior is generally learned by trial and error, starting when the gate was left unlatched and the animal accidently pushed it open. The next few times may have been reinforced by a weak latch or rotten boards, so that learning to escape was reinforced. Eventually the animal will hit the gate harder until it can escape. Stopping the behavior requires several unsuccessful attempts at getting out or appropriate punishment as the behavior is attempted.

ALSO SEE: *Escape Behaviors*

Generalization

When lessons or behaviors learned are applied to similar but unique situations, the animal has made a generalization. A gunshot goes off over a dog's head causing a severe startle reaction. The dog may then show an extreme reaction to thunder when the next thunderstorm comes through.

ALSO SEE: *Insight Learning*

Genetic Problems

Although the genetic basis for behaviors has not been well studied in veterinary medicine, a number of normal and abnormal behaviors can have a genetic basis. Several of them can also have an environmental cause or trigger. The exact mode of transmission has not been worked out for many of these behaviors, but there is enough anecdotal evidence to indicate that a hereditary basis exists. A great deal of work still remains in order to identify other behavioral genetic problems and to define the specific modes of inheritance. Normal behaviors that have a genetic basis include the mimic grin; certain personalities, including timidness and dominance; and breed-specific behaviors, such as the tendency to work cattle, hunt, or learn to guard things. Problem behaviors with a genetic basis include personality extremes, fear biting, fear of noise, leash fighting, flank sucking, and wool sucking.

ALSO SEE: *Dominant Personality, Fear Biting, Fear of Noise, Flank Sucking, Leash Fighting, Organizing Behavioral Histories, Rage Syndrome, Tail Chasing, Timid Personality, Tongue Rolling, Wool Sucking*

Genital Presentation

Genital presentation is a behavior that exposes the genitalia and is directed toward potential mates or rivals. In certain primates, the colored sex skin becomes more visible.

ALSO SEE: *Reproductive Behavior, Threat Displays*

Geophagia

Geophagia is soil eating.

SEE: *Soil Eating*

Gestation

Gestation is the time of pregnancy. The length of time varies with the species (see Appendix B), but tends to be longer for larger animals.

ALSO SEE: *Female Behaviors*

Goats

Goats, *Capra hircus*, are some of the earliest domesticated animals. They first associated with humans as *Capra ibex* (ibex) or as *Capra aegagrus* (the bezoar goat), and this early association was valuable to humans for food and for clothing. These animals were browsers with versatile feeding patterns in the mountain ranges of Europe and Asia, allowing them to survive a number of harsh environments. Through gradual selective breeding over the last 9000 or so years, they have developed into the modern goat (Clutton-Brock, 1981).

ALSO SEE: *Appendix B*

Gradual Introduction

There are many situations when the gradual, rather than abrupt, introduction of a new animal or object is beneficial. This is particularly true for cats. When a new cat is brought into a home that already has resident cats, the new individual should be confined to a room by itself with food, water, a bed, and litter box. This will give the resident cats time to get used to the smells and sounds of the newest addition. Eventually the new cat is allowed out for increasing lengths of time.

Any change for an animal should be gradual. New types of litter should be added to the old litter over a span of several weeks. Changes in schedules can also be made successfully if they are gradual.

ALSO SEE: *Housesoiling, Schedule*

Grass Eating

Grass eating is one variation of plant eating. It is a normal behavior in all the domestic species, although it is infrequent in carnivores.

ALSO SEE: *Ingestive Behavior, Plant Eating, Stool Eating—Another Species*

Greeting Behaviors

There are four basic approaches used when two animals come together. The facial approach is a straight on, nose-to-nose approach that is typical of animals that are somewhat familiar with each other. Horses exchange deep breaths if friendly, and humans can use the technique of blowing in a horse's nose to reassure it. There are, however, individuals that do not appreciate the greeting and attempt to bite, just as they would a conspecific.

The inguinal approach occurs when the approaching individual can put its nose to the other's lower flank area. The anal (anogenital) approach has one animal investigating the smells of the perineum of the other. If the approacher presents its side view to the front of the other animal, the approach is called a broadside or lateral threat. This is a distance-increasing silent communication behavior most commonly associated with cattle.

ALSO SEE: *Contact Greeting, Distance-increasing Silent Communication, Lateral Threat*

Grimace

Grimace is a facial expression in cats that is their variation of flehmen. It has also been called the gape.

ALSO SEE: *Flehmen*

Grooming Behavior

Grooming behaviors are types of comfort or self-maintenance behaviors. The types shown are generally restricted in different species based on body flexibility. Grooming includes self-grooming, self-grooming with mechanical assistance, and mutual grooming between conspecifics.

Self-grooming behaviors are quite variable. Licking of the mouth area, body caudal to the neck and distal limbs is one type. The teeth can also be used to relieve itches and groom hair coats. The forelimb may be licked and then rubbed against the face, as cats commonly do, to extend the range of salivary grooming.

The forelimb can also be held forward to rub the face on, a behavior of ungulates. The hindlimbs are used most often to scratch the neck, caudal head, and ears.

The most inaccessible locations, the neck and topline, are usually groomed with assistance. Mutual grooming is one type of assisted grooming with several variations. Two horses will stand parallel, facing in opposite directions to use each other's tail to keep flies off the face. Withers nibbling in horses and picking by primates are other examples of mutual grooming. In addition to a pure grooming function, mutual grooming may have a social function as well. It can be used to strengthen bonds, as in primates, or reconfirm a social order, as in cattle where the dominant cow is usually licked by the lower-ranking cow. The second type of assistance is with a mechanical scratcher, like a tree limb, building corner, or the ground with rolling or dust baths. Dogs seem to roll in particularly foul-smelling substances. While the actual cause is not known, the author has two theories for the behavior. One is that rolling is an attempt to take on an odor that the dog finds pleasurable, much like people put on cologne. The other is that rolling is an attempt to cover the odor with the dog's own smell. Dogs do urinate on animal excreta as well as roll in it.

Shaking the body removes excess water or dust, usually after rolling, and limb flicking in cats seems to have the same function.

ALSO SEE: *Bachelor Groups, Cleaning Symbiosis, Comfort Behavior, Inappropriate Licking, Licking, Limb Flicking, Preening, Rolling, Shaking, Social Grooming, Wallow, Withers Nibbling*

Ground Pecking

Chickens peck at the ground in a number of different circumstances. Feeding is the most common, and a hen often pecks at the ground in an apparent attempt to encourage her chicks to do it. Cocks may use ground pecking to hold hens together or as an apparent method to minimize tensions in the presence of other males.

ALSO SEE: *Ingestive Behavior, Stress-related Behaviors*

Ground Rutting

Cattle and other ungulates rub their horns, antlers, or heads on the ground, typically during the breeding season. The specific purpose is unknown, although it has been speculated that the behavior releases tensions associated with the presence of other males.

ALSO SEE: *Antler Rubbing, Male Behaviors, Stress-related Behaviors*

Group Cohesion

This is the force that allows the continuous, close association between social

group members. It is related to various forms of vocal and silent communication.
ALSO SEE: *Animal Sociology, Distance-reducing Silent Communication, Vocal Communication*

Group Distance

Group distance is the social (reactive) distance that represents the spacing between groups of the same species. Although the home ranges of several groups may overlap, members of the various groups seldom mingle. The amount of separation they maintain is the group distance. Vocal communication, olfactory marks, and timing are used to maintain this distance when visual contact is not possible.
ALSO SEE: *Home Range, Reactive Distances, Social Distance*

Group Effect

Group effect represents the benefits to individuals of living in a group. These include protection against predators, collective defense, cooperative hunting, and shared raising of infants.

Group Predation

Group predation is hunting and capture of prey by groups. This is a common behavior in canids and in the lion. It can also be found in other species, including some ants and birds.
ALSO SEE: *Predation*

Grudge

One complication of behavior problems has to do with the owners. They often carry a grudge against the animal, and this results in a change in the way they interact. Since animals live in the present, they do not remember a specific transgression and do not understand the owners' change in attitude. Elimination of a problem behavior is more easily accomplished if the owner does not hold a grudge against the animal, but assumes instead a positive attitude.
ALSO SEE: *Positive Attitude*

Guarding Behaviors

Guarding behaviors are usually associated with males protecting their females from roaming males trying to establish a breeding group. They can be used to prevent mating by other males to ensure increased reproductive success for the harem male. Guarding also describes the protection of an infant or members of a social group, a behavior associated with canids, among others.

Guilt

Guilt is a human interpretation of what an animal, usually a dog, may be feeling. It is usually accompanied by a statement that the animal "knows he's done wrong because he has a guilty look." This guilty expression is a submissive posture and no more. It is a response to a very dominant posture made by the human and not a response to the memory of an earlier behavior.

ALSO SEE: *Autoshaping, Housesoiling—Defecation*

Gulping Food

Eating food at a rapid rate can be a problem in any species. It is more common in dogs and horses that are fed once daily. If the problem is severe enough to warrant management, several things can be tried. Several small meals can be given during the day, or several small portions can be given during a single mealtime. Food that is nutritional, but bland, may be able to be substituted for the type of food that had been used. Large objects too big to swallow can be added to the food bowl or feed trough to make food more difficult to scoop up. Rocks are commonly used in horse feeders to slow the animal that tends to gulp its food.

ALSO SEE: *Bolting, Ingestive Behavior Problems*

H

Habit

A habit is a learned pattern of behavior that has become as rigid as a reflex. Once established, this pattern is difficult to eliminate. Habits are behaviors of individuals rather than species.

ALSO SEE: *Habituation Learning, Reflex*

Habit Preening

This is a ritualized preening behavior associated with courtship in certain birds, including ducks. It can be a displacement activity or result in a visual change in appearance.

ALSO SEE: *Displacement Activity, Preening*

Habituation Learning

This is a type of operant conditioning in which a stimulus-response is repeated, without a positive or negative reinforcer, until the response no longer occurs. The behavior may reappear if the stimulus is strong enough. Habituation learning occurs in normal animals in response to various noises in the environment. A dog will be alerted by a door slamming, but if that noise is repeated several times, it will eventually be ignored. This is the basis for training some gun dogs. The gun is fired repeatedly until the dog no longer responds to the noise.

Dogs with hyper syndrome conditions, particularly hyperactivity and hyperkinesia, do not undergo habituation to noises. They will respond just as actively the tenth time as they did the first.

Habituation learning, like extinction, can be used to treat certain problems. For the dog that attacks the telephone or doorbell, the repeated ringing without human interaction may be sufficient to stop the problem.

ALSO SEE: *Aggression and Telephones, Desensitization, Destructive Chewing, Extinction, Flooding, Learning, Operant Conditioning, Stimulus-Response Relationship*

Hair Eating

The behavior of eating hair or wool, usually that of associating animals, can become a problem if excessive. Mothers will often ingest some hair from their offspring during normal grooming. Tail chewing in horses is common. It may represent a somewhat normal form of oral exploration by foals; however, if excessive, continuous, or present in older horses, it should be regarded as a problem. Hairballs in cats, rabbits, and calves can result in gastrointestinal blockage, making medical or surgical intervention necessary.

Eliminating the problem requires a critical look at environmental conditions, including diet, exercise, housing, and social interactions. Evaluation of the diet, especially relative to adequate protein, should be made and raised to appropriate levels if low. Crowding, lack of adequate exercise, or other stresses may need to be corrected.

Trichophagia is the term applied to hair eating.

Hair Pulling

Hair pulling is a form of self-mutilation typical of primates. Some caged individuals do not seem able to cope with their environment and will grab handfuls of hair, causing large bald areas. This behavior is generally associated with nonenriched environments. Social groups in large enclosures and environmental enrichment with mechanisms the primate can manipulate tend to prevent or eliminate the problem.

Sheep kept in restrictive environments show a variation of this behavior, wool pulling. Successful management of the problem addresses the diet, pen densities, and general management systems.

ALSO SEE: *Boredom, Environmental Enrichment, Self-Mutilation, Stress-related Behaviors, Wool Pulling*

Halter Breaking

In the behavioral context, halter breaking takes on two meanings. The first is the process of getting horses, cattle, or other species accustomed to wearing a halter and getting them to accept being restrained and tied by the halter. This usually entails one or more tries at pulling back in attempts to get free. Head restraint is a method for dominance control in most animals.

Halter breaking can also be a problem behavior. When an animal struggles against being tied by a halter and the equipment breaks, the animal has won its battle and is more apt to try this technique the next time it is tied. Through trial and error learning, the problem can become so severe with some individuals that they cannot be restrained by tying. Treatment for this problem is discussed under Pulling Back.

ALSO SEE: *Pulling Back, Trial and Error Learning*

Handedness

Handedness is the preference for using the hand (or foot) on either the right or left side. Cats, the best studied of the domestic species, show a preference for the right paw in 20% of individuals, the left paw in 38.3%, with 41.7% being ambidextrous (Warren, Abplanalp and Warren, 1967). Later studies by Tan, Yaprak and Kutlu (1990) indicated a right-paw preference of approximately 51%, with 12% being ambidextrous. They also evaluated differences in handedness by sex and hormone influences.

Hard-to-Read Postures

In some animals, such as dogs, physical restraints may make it very difficult for them to completely express a distance-reducing or distance-increasing posture. A very short tail, pendulous lips and ears, dark eyes, and hairy faces are features that can cause an incomplete expression or misinterpretation of postures. The short tail is difficult to see. Weight of large lips may prevent them from being elevated to show teeth, while large, floppy ears have less mobility for expression.

Hair may cover the stare of a threat.

ALSO SEE: *Distance-increasing Silent Communication, Distance-reducing Silent Communication*

Harem

The harem is a type of relatively stable social group comprised of one male, several sexually mature females, and varying numbers of their juvenile young. The young usually leave as they mature, and the male may occasionally be defeated and replaced by another challenging male. This type of group is well documented in feral horses, with a harem consisting of the stallion and one to five mares with a varied number of foals, yearlings, fillies, and immature colts. This is a highly stable, equine group, with the younger males the most likely to leave. Occasionally more than one adult male may be associated with a harem, as is the case in approximately 10% of the horse groups (Berger, 1986). It is also common in a number of other species, including antelope and primates.

ALSO SEE: *Animal Sociology, Male Behaviors, Multimate Group, Promiscuity*

Head Nodding

Horses are the most common animal to develop head nodding as a problem behavior. In this behavior, the animal flips its nose in an up and down, "yes" motion. Because the behavior often results from a poorly fitting bit or tooth trouble, any diagnostics should begin in the mouth. Over time the nodding can develop into a typical stereotype and no longer be related to the mouth. Facial insects and ear ticks can also initiate this problem. As with any stereotyped problem, stress may contribute.

The longer the problem has existed, the more difficult it is to stop. In all cases, medical causes must be ruled out first. For some horses showing this behavior, pasturing them may be sufficient to reduce the frequency. Another approach is to use a different type of bit or a bitless bridle. Punishment can be useful but only if appropriately used. In some cases, elimination of the problem is not possible.

ALSO SEE: *Head Shaking, Stereotyped Behaviors*

Head Rubbing

Cats may rub and butt their heads on a person or other animal. While this is generally considered a friendly behavior, the rubbing may occasionally have a marking function.

Swine confined to narrow crates for prolonged periods may develop head rubbing as a problem. The behavior is probably a stereotypic response to environmental stress and can be stopped or minimized by using larger pens, pastures, and social interaction.

ALSO SEE: *Distance-reducing Silent Communication, Marking, Stereotyped Behaviors*

Head Shaking

Head shaking is a behavior problem most frequently seen in caged birds, stalled horses, and zoo animals. In this stereotyped behavior, the head is rotated so the forehead moves left to right. The problem can also be related to stress. In horses, problems with the teeth or improperly fitting or used bits are major contributing factors.

Stopping the problem is not always possible, particularly if it has been going on for a long time. It is useful to get the animal into a more natural environment, such as a pasture for the horse. It is usually necessary for a horse to have a long break from the old environment or working conditions before training can resume. Even then, a bit should be avoided if at all possible. Punishment, if properly applied, may help.

ALSO SEE: *Head Nodding, Stereotyped Behaviors*

Hearing

Domestic animals have quite a range of hearing capabilities. Humans hear in an approximate range of 15 cycles per second (cps) to 20,000 cps. Horses, at 55 to 33,500 cps (Heffner and Heffner, 1983), and cattle, at 23 to 35,000 (Heffner and Heffner, 1983), are similar in their ranges. Dogs hear into the higher ranges, from approximately 15 cps to 60,000 cps (Fox and Bekoff in Hafez, 1975). The silent dog whistle and sound repellers are pitched around 30,000 cps frequency. The complete extent of cat audition is not known. The range starts at approximately 20 cps and the upper limits of nerve conduction, 100,000 cps, actually represent the limits of the test equipment (Beaver, 1992). Since mice can make very high-pitched sounds, the 100,000+ cps range is not unreasonable.

ALSO SEE: *Bioacoustics*

Helper

A helper is an individual, usually from the same social unit, that helps the parents raise their young. It may involve bringing food or protecting the young. Helpers are often related to the youngsters. It is theorized that this help to a related individual aids the ultimate survival of a specific gene pool.

ALSO SEE: *Kin Selection, Sociobiology*

Hero

Each year awards are given for heroic acts by animals, usually dogs, but occasionally cats, horses, pigs, or others. Many other animals are considered heroes by their owners. Many canine acts of protection are based on the instinctive protection of higher ranking pack members or on territorial protection. Owners occasionally want to test their dog to see if it will respond in a heroic way. This is not necessary, and the situation set up may not be realistic enough to get the hoped-for response. In general, most dogs will protect their owner if they respect the owner as a higher ranking pack member. One exception might be toy breeds, because they were developed to retain puppy characteristics, and not for pack protection. Terriers are protective of territory; a pack is generally not of major importance to terriers.

Cats can be heroes even though they are regarded as asocial. They are most commonly involved in responding to a fire and waking owners in their attempt to escape. Occasionally cats attack burglars, probably as territorial protection. Snakes have also been attacked.

"Pruscilla," a Texas pig of some fame, saved a person from drowning.

ALSO SEE: *Altruism, Anthropomorphism, Owner Protective Aggression, Territorial Protective Aggression*

Hiding

Cats that are injured, sick, or extremely fearful may go into hiding. This strategy of survival is the way an asocial species can decrease its chances of being caught by a predator. It also decreases the need for food, because less energy is spent moving.

ALSO SEE: *Asocial, Lying Out*

Hierarchy

Hierarchy has a double meaning in behavior. The first meaning is that of a specific social order from number one, or alpha, individual on down.

The second definition indicates the varying degrees of motivation needed before a behavior is expressed. In prey-chasing cats that experimentally have had new mice individually introduced, the cat would initially alert, stalk, pounce, nape bite, and eat. Over time the behavior changed to alert, stalk, pounce, and nape bite. Gradually the cat would alert, stalk, and pounce. Then it would alert and stalk. Alert was the last behavior to go. This hierarchy of behaviors is necessary to ensure that enough food will be successfully caught to supply nutritional needs. The cat that just plays with a mouse does not have enough motivation to continue to higher levels of the behavior.

ALSO SEE: *Motivation, Motivational Energy, Predation, Social Order*

History Taking

The most important part of working with animal behavior problems is getting a complete and accurate history. While medical data, laboratory values, owner-animal interactions, and animal reactions to environments and strangers are absolutely necessary for properly evaluating some situations, the historical information is the most important. Since a good behavioral history takes time to get, one to two hours in some cases, handling problem animals in a veterinary practice requires more than the routine appointment. When a client mentions a problem behavior, it is best to schedule an appointment for an appropriate length of time and then charge the client accordingly. This ensures two things: First, that the owner will be motivated enough to carry out whatever therapy is necessary, whether that is medicating the animal at appropriate times or using a prolonged schedule of behavior modification. Second, rescheduling an appointment prevents the veterinarian from feeling guilty about other clients waiting while the behavior problem is being appropriately diagnosed and treated.

A general behavioral history gathers a lot of information that will determine if more specific details are necessary and in what area of questioning. For some behaviorists, a history form ensures a consistent line of questioning. Others prefer a free flow of conversation. Regardless of preferences in information gathering, there are four primary questions that must be answered. Each generates other more specific questions.

What exactly happens? Vague descriptions of a problem must be clarified. For example, if the complaint is that the dog "messes in the house," does the owner mean it is making a mess by chewing up things, it is defecating in the house, it is urinating in the house, it tracks in dirt and mud, or it does something else entirely?

Where does the problem occur? The first reply is often that it happens "all over the house." In reality, the problem may be confined to one or two rooms, and that information may be helpful in determining the cause of the problem. For example, defecation in one room may indicate the dog has been banned from that room and now marks it whenever an opportunity arises.

When did the problem begin? This question is useful in two ways. The longer the duration of the problem, the longer it can take to eliminate it. A general rule of thumb for many learned patterns of behavior is that eliminating the problem can take as long as the problem has existed. Knowing when the problem began may also be useful in determining what started it. Owners often tie the behavior to an event such as the birth of a new baby, the visit of a relative, a move, or other major occurrence. At other times, the veterinarian may be able to correlate "three weeks ago" with the start of school, a major weather cold front, or the Christmas holidays.

When does the problem occur? Some behaviors are triggered by events that happen at set times of the day or in the presence or absence of the owners. This helps narrow down the events that trigger the behavior.

Specific questions can be used in a history-taking session. They can also be used on a history form, although a rigid approach generally yields less information than one in which the owner freely describes events that have happened. Any history form should have an area where general comments can be noted in addition to specific observations. Housesoiling and aggressive problems require additional information to that taken on a general form.

One type of general history form is shown in Appendix A. The questions on it are described in more detail below.

Signalment. *Age*—Certain problems are more apt to be associated with certain ages. *Sex*—A problem such as urine spraying in housesoiling cats is relatively normal for intact males and difficult to control in the other sexes. Other sexually dimorphic behaviors are also commonly seen as behavior problems. *Species*—Dogs, cats, horses, and other animals generally have species-specific problems because they are limited in the ways they can react. *Breed*—Genetic problems are common, as are breed predispositions for certain types of behavior. For example, Siamese and beagles are vocal, but not all owners recognize this. *Name*—A pet's name can tell the veterinarian a lot about the feelings of the owner toward the animal. This has some value in predicting the owner's expectations and the motivation to treat a behavior problem.

Background information. *Other pets*—The age, sex, species, breed, and names of other pets help define the patient's relationship to the total family. *Family members*—The number of adults and number and ages of children in the household help clarify problems where interactions with family members are inappropriate. *Observation of the problem*—In a multianimal environment, it is important to know which animal is showing the behavior problem. If the owner is not certain, strategies must be devised to determine which is the appropriate animal. *Source of the patient*—Where the owners acquired the animal may be important, particularly for dogs and cats. It can have an effect on the owner's attitude toward the animal, the animal's reactions to various happenings, and the ability to learn more about siblings and relatives. *Age of the animal when obtained*—Early critical experiences can be evaluated if the owners have had the animal since it was very young. *Medical history*—This can be important for coordinating medication or explaining the development of problems. While this information may be in the veterinarian's records, mobility of clients means that it may be necessary to obtain a brief medical history while taking a behavioral history.

What exactly is the problem? Have the owner define the specific complaint, but be alert for other problems that might also be mentioned during the discussion of the problem. These secondary problems may be related to the problem of concern or they may be behaviors that do not concern the client. A dog brought in for chewing expensive houseplants may have been eliminating on the carpets since it was a puppy, but that was not considered a problem by the owner.

When did the problem begin? *Duration*—This is important from the diagnostic and prognostic points of view. *Progress of the problem*—It is important to know if the problem is progressively getting worse or better or if it is staying at the same severity.

When does the problem happen? *Frequency*—Problems that only occur one or two times usually cannot be monitored to determine if a therapy works; however, swift, appropriate punishment for certain behaviors can stop them from becoming ongoing problems. Problems that occur from several times a day to several times a week may indicate that something in the household routine needs adjusting. *Timing of occurrences*—The presence or absence of people can be an important clue to the role they play in triggering the behavior. Even specific timing may indicate a triggering stimulus. For example, the noise of an automatic sprinkler at 7:30 AM may initiate a bout of barking at the same time.

Where does the problem occur? *General location*—The general location helps differentiate an indoor and outdoor problem. *Specific location*—Specific rooms, locations in a yard, or spots in the pasture can point to triggers in that direction. *Specific areas that are involved*—The type of flooring, piece of furniture, plant, or other household item targeted may help design a plan to stop the problem. A cat that gets on cabinets, for example, can be discouraged by having undesirable experiences on the cabinet. *Specific individuals*—If the items targeted belong to a specific person, there may be a negative relationship between the animal and person. That relationship will decline even more unless specific measures can be used to stop it. The specific target can also be the animal itself, as in the various types of self-mutilation.

General information. *Location of the animal during the day*—This information helps give perspective to a problem that happens when the owners are away. *Location of the animal when the owners are home*—The relationship between an animal and the owners is clarified. *Location where the animal usually sleeps*—This also clarifies the owner/pet relationship. *Diet*—The type of food is important if food allergies or excess protein might relate to the problem. *Frequency and time of feeding*—These patterns are particularly relevant for dogs defecating in the house and horses that crib or wind suck. *Formal training*—Dogs with the hyper syndromes are usually obedience school dropouts. Others have been star pupils, but still develop problems. Horses may have been through a series of trainers or none at all. *Guilty look*—While this is a learned response, it may indicate that the owner is punishing the animal at an inappropriate time. *Recent changes*—New pets or family members can cause problems. New cats in a neighborhood or other changes a cat can view may be enough to precipitate spraying or other psychogenic problems.

ALSO SEE: *Appendix A*

Hobbles

Hobbles are a restraint device used on the legs of horses and cattle. There are three primary styles, with a number of variations for each. The one-leg hobble keeps one front foot off the ground. The typical equipment is a figure-8 strap encircling the forearm and metacarpus of the same limb. This technique is useful when working on the opposite rear limb. It can also teach the horse that it can be psychologically controlled by the person that has just taken away the animal's ability to flee. After 15 to 30 minutes, most horses will accept handling that they would not tolerate before.

A pair of hobbles is put just above the metacarpophalangeal or metatarsophalangeal joints. Historically, these have been useful on the forelimbs to keep the cowboy's horse from straying too far during the night. Now they are more often used during trailering to keep a horse from pawing or kicking and during training to prevent kicking.

Breeding hobbles or kick hobbles connect the hocks to the neck and prevent the backward kicking action. They are used on the female to help protect the stallion or bull during natural service.

ALSO SEE: *Kicking, Striking, Trailer Kicking*

Home Range

This is the area an individual or group would normally inhabit. Included within this space are areas for eating, resting, grooming, and mating. For most domestic species, the home range is artificially limited by fences. For wild or feral species, the supply of food often determines how large this area will be. Between groups of the same species, the home ranges may overlap, although there usually is not an intermingling of members.

ALSO SEE: *Group Distance, Reactive Distances, Social Distance*

Homing

Homing is the ability of some animals to find their way back to a certain location, usually a birthplace or a breeding site. There are several theories as to how this can occur, and there are several probabilities that vary with species. In some instances, a learned pattern, a good sense of direction, and/or keen ability of smell can start the individual out correctly. In other situations, there may be help from an internal magnetic compass or instinctive ability to navigate using the sun's position.

ALSO SEE: *Migration*

Homology

Homology is the study of anatomical similarity due to common ancestry and the evolutionary changes that have resulted. The osseous changes in the limbs from *Eohippus* to *Equus* exemplify this area.

Homosexual Behavior

True homosexual behavior is rare in animals. Inappropriate mounting can occur in atypical environments, but when given the choice between an animal of the same sex or the opposite sex, the opposite is almost always the choice.

ALSO SEE: *Inappropriate Mounting, Male Behaviors, Monosexual Syndrome, Mounting, Pseudocopulation*

Hormonal Imbalance Aggression

There are a number of types of aggression that are related to the imbalance of hormones within an animal. Why this aggression appears to the extent it does in some individuals is not always clear, and additional studies with hormonal genetics and chromosomal assays are needed.

Estrous females have been known to increase the amount of their aggression toward females of the same species. This is normal and most noticeable in mares and bitches. Bitches in a false pregnancy may guard objects. Even years after an ovariohysterectomy, a bitch may continue to show cyclic tendencies toward aggression to other females at the same regularity as had occurred before the surgery.

In mares, high testosterone levels have been reported to cause aggression and stallionlike behavior (Beaver and Amoss, 1982).

ALSO SEE: *Interfemale Aggression, Ovariectomy, Pseudopregnancy, Testosterone-induced Aggression in Mares*

Horse Laugh

Flehmen behavior shown by horses is often called the horse laugh.

SEE: *Flehmen*

Horses

Fossil remains of horse ancestors have been traced back 60 million years to *Eohippus*. The civet-sized animal had four complete toes on the forelimb and three on the rear limb, possibly with padded feet. The teeth indicated *Eohippus* probably browsed on small shrubs. Ancestors progressed through, or were associated with, other types as size increased, weight-bearing digits changed, and teeth were modified. These ancestors include *Hyrocotherium, Orohippus, Epihippus, Mesohippus, Miohippus, Hypohippus, Parahippus, Merychippus, Hipparion, Pliohippus,* and *Plesippus.* Within the last million years, a wild horse, *Equus scotti,* roamed the Northern Hemisphere, but it eventually became extinct. Przewalski horse, *Equus ferus przewalski,* is probably not the main progenitor, but there is controversy as to which subspecies did give rise to the modern horse (Clutton-Brock, 1981). By approximately 4000 BC, the horse was being used as a food source; however, this role was probably quickly replaced by its use as a draft animal.

ALSO SEE: *Domestication, Appendix B*

Hot Spots

Hot spots are areas of localized moist dermitis or hypersensitivities, usually occurring over the lumbar area of dogs and rarely on cats. It is a form of self-mutilation. The lesions are usually controllable medically. For those animals in which reoccurrence is a problem, another aspect should be considered. Some individuals internalize environmental stress and redirect it to themselves. Control of the environment with a schedule and exercise is usually helpful for long-term management of the problem.

ALSO SEE: *Excessive Grooming, Exercise, Lick Granulomas, Schedule, Self-Mutilation*

Housebreaking

Housebreaking is a term used interchangeably with housetraining. It is the process of teaching a puppy to eliminate in an acceptable location, usually out-of-doors.

ALSO SEE: *Housetraining*

Housesoiling

Housesoiling is a problem behavior in which dogs, cats, or other pets urinate and/or defecate in unacceptable locations within the house. In some cases, the problem relates to a lack of proper housetraining or litter box training; in other cases it is related to a medical problem. In still other cases there has been some factor in the environment that has changed.

History taking for housesoiling problems needs to be extensive in order to determine the specific diagnosis and appropriate course of action. Once housesoiling is established as the problem, specifics as to whether it is defecation, urination, submissive urination, spraying, or urine marking must be obtained. Each variation of housesoiling has its own cause and treatment considerations.

ALSO SEE: *Added Litter Boxes, Cribbing, Diary, Elimination Behavior,*

Gradual Introduction, Housesoiling—Defecation, Housesoiling—History Taking, Housesoiling—Spraying, Housesoiling—Submissive Urination, Housesoiling—Urination, Housesoiling—Urine Marking, Housetraining, Hydrocephalus, Indoor-Outdoor

Housesoiling—Defecation

Defecation in inappropriate places can be related to a number of factors. For dogs the problem may be related to the animal never having been appropriately housetrained, being physically ill, or not being allowed to completely finish defecation outside. The history should include whether the dog has ever shown acceptable behavior. Puppies that did well eliminating on paper may have difficulty adjusting to a different type of surface. Outdoor dogs have a tendency to use shag carpets and bath mats like they had previously used grass. Dogs that have a chronic history of eliminating in the house, even though they may have at one time been housebroken, may have forgotten their early behavior and need retraining. In all these cases, the owner should redo the lessons of basic housetraining: punish the dog only if it is caught soiling, praise acceptable elimination behavior, and put the dog on a well-defined schedule.

Physical illness as a cause of inappropriate defecation can not always be avoided; however, do not attempt to change the behavior until the illness is over. Then if the housesoiling is still a problem, behavioral modification can be instituted.

A major cause of defecation problems in dogs is the physical prevention of the dog going out to defecate. Feeding just before the owner leaves in the morning or just before bedtime is most likely to cause problems. The dog may even ask to go out, but no one responds. Sometimes by changing the feeding time to late afternoon, the gastrocolic reflex can cause defecation at a more acceptable time. During bad weather, the owner may put the dog outside in the morning and assume it both urinates and defecates. The dog, on the other hand, does not want to get cold or wet and stays close to the door. It comes back in the house, and the owners leave. As the morning continues, the pressure to defecate increases until the dog eliminates indoors. If this situation continues over several days, the owners may punish the dog when they get home, since the dog looks guilty and "must be doing it on purpose." The owners may also begin to have negative feelings about the dog and decrease their contacts with it. The animal may learn that it can get attention for housesoiling and continue to do the behavior. Negative attention becomes better than none at all. The owners need to develop a positive attitude, not punish the dog unless it is caught defecating, and return to basic housetraining, including going out with the dog so they are sure it does eliminate outside, and they can praise appropriate behavior.

Defecation as a problem for cats tends to have one of two relating factors. The first is an acquired aversion to the litter box. This can occur because the box was not cleaned often enough, an abrupt change of litter was made, or pain was associated with the litter box. Cats generally dislike dirty litter boxes, with some individuals being fussier than others. Ideally, in multicat households, there should be at least the same number of boxes as cats. While most people completely change the litter every 3 to 7 days, more frequent changing may be necessary. Abrupt changes of litter types, especially from plain clay to odor-added types, will cause 50% of cats to stop using the box, although half of these will start back again in a few days. All introductions to new types of litter should be made gradually over the course of four to eight litter box changes. Cats apparently blame any pain of defecation (or urination) on the location and will stop using the litter box if it hurts to go there. This is most obvious with cases of lower urinary tract disease, however, it is common for painful defecation as well. The pain may be related to a physical illness, injury while defecating, or very hard feces. Careful evaluation of the diet (dry food) and the character of the feces can be helpful in the history. Appropriate treatment is useful for medical causes. Hard feces can be softened by additives or a diet change.

The second factor for cats not defecating in a litter box is its location. Cats, and especially kittens, that have to travel to the back bedroom of a three-story house from the living room on the first floor just will not bother. The box must be conveniently located from the cat's perspective. Access should not be accidentally shut off either. The litter box must also be of an appropriate size. Many big cats get in the litter box but the anus hangs over the edge so the feces are outside. A high-sided or a covered box is very useful. If defecation occurs in one location outside the box, an additional litter box can be added at that location. While this may not be convenient to the owner, if the cat can learn to defecate in the new box, the box can later be moved, an inch a day, to a more acceptable location. Confinement with food, water, bed, and litter box can be helpful for the chronic problem in which the cat chooses a remote location to defecate. This confinement can be limited to the specific times that defecation normally occurs, or it may be constant. The use of confinement to manage feline defecation problems must be continued for a long period of time, usually about as long as the problem has been occurring. A few days shut in a bathroom does not allow enough time to unlearn the undesirable behavior and relearn the acceptable one.

ALSO SEE: *Added Litter Boxes, Feeding Schedule Change, Grudge, Guilt, Housesoiling, Housesoiling—History Taking, Housetraining, Indoor-Outdoor, Positive Attitude, Praise, Punishment, Remote Punishment, Retrain to Eliminate, Schedule*

Housesoiling—History Taking

A general history is important for basic information about the problem pet, but additional information is necessary when housesoiling is involved.

If the pet is a dog, the following information may be helpful.

Normal patterns. *Location*—Where the dog normally eliminates is important for a comparison to the location of the problem. *Frequency*—Timing of trips outside may be a clue to the problem. It may also indicate that a hurried owner or bad weather causes a timing problem. *Posture for urination*—A difference between the normal posture and that used during the problem behavior occasionally occurs.

If housesoiling is the problem with a cat, additional information is important. Particularly important to determine is if the owner has seen the cat show the problem. If not, urination and spraying must be differentiated by whether the urine hits a vertical surface, horizontal surface, or specific item. When housesoiling occurs in a multicat household, it is important to know which cat is eliminating inappropriately. Other historical information will come from the following questions.

Litter box use. *History of use*—Determine if the cat ever used the litter box. Some did not and probably will not. *Current use*—When and for what does the cat use the box? Have the owner provide information about whether the cat currently uses the litter box at all.

Litter box management. *Number of boxes*—In general there should be one litter box for each cat. *Location of box*—The current location of the box should be compared to the location of the problem and accessibility for the cat. A small kitten will not travel to the distant corner of a basement if all the normal activity is on the first floor. *Litter type*—Some cats do not like certain types of litter, especially the scented varieties. *Recent changes in litter type*—Abrupt changes in litter type will cause 50% of cats to stop using the box. *Feces patrol*—The frequency of removing feces can affect a cat's desire to use the box. It is best if feces are removed at least daily. *Complete changeouts*—Litter that is too wet or dirty may drive a cat off, so patrol or changeouts become important. *Age*—Older litter boxes may take on undesirable odors of their own, so an occasional new box should be phased into use.

Other information. *Cleaning products*—Odor elimination is more for the owner than the pet; however, products with strong odors of their own and those with ammonia may worsen the situation.

ALSO SEE: *Aggression—History Taking, History Taking, Appendix A*

Housesoiling—Spraying

Urine spraying is a form of urine marking. It is often a normal behavior; however, when urine is sprayed inside a home, it is usually regarded as a problem by the owner. In working with cat owners who find urine outside the litter box, it is important to determine if the cat sprayed the urine or if it urinated in an unacceptable location. The question is easily answered if the owner has actually seen the cat spray urine from a standing posture. The diagnosis of *Housesoiling—Spraying* is more difficult if the elimination has not been seen. Then questions to determine if the urine is found on vertical objects such as walls, doors, curtains, and chair legs are necessary. If so, the cat is spraying.

Cats normally spray to mark their territory, and the frequency increases with an invasion or stress within. The location sprayed is usually related to the source of the stress. While many things can be perceived as an invasion of a territory, roaming cats outside a window or door are the most common. The owners may be aware of the stranger cats, or they may not. Regardless, spraying of curtains, windows, doors, or furniture from which the cat observes the outside is strong evidence of stray cats. Other territorial stresses such as multicat households, guests, major changes in a cat's schedule, minimal hiding spots, and negative attitudes toward the cat also trigger the problem.

Spraying is a normal behavior for tomcats and estrous females. Since it is a sexually dimorphic behavior, castration is a good recommendation for intact tomcats. Of neutered males though, approximately 10% will spray under certain conditions. In spayed females, 5% will spray. These numbers can be cut in half with appropriate treatments (Hart and Hart, 1985).

To stop cats spraying, the ideal solution is to eliminate the source of the stress. If a new cat recently joined the household, it may need to be removed. Schedules should be reestablished. When roaming cats are involved, it may not be possible to control them, so other measures can be used. Closing the curtains, using draw shades (even on the outside of the window), or confining the animal away from the area are often acceptable alternatives. These techniques may be needed only to get through the feline breeding season, when cat roaming peaks. Antianxiety tranquilizers may be useful at the beginning but should not be depended on for long-term control. Remote punishment may also be helpful.

If the history indicates a certain person is being targeted for urine—dirty clothes, pillow, favorite chair, shoes, or person—the likely diagnosis is *Housesoiling—Spraying*. Regardless of the posture described, this is evidence that the cat is sending a message. Obviously, if the behavior goes on very long, the person is going to send his or her own message, and a negative relation gets worse. To stop the negative cycle, the targeted individual should feed the cat and give it the majority of petting. Most cats will quickly stop the marking behavior.

For the problem cat that is part of the resistant 2.5 to 5%, making it an indoor-outdoor animal may be a workable alternative. Olfactory tractotomy has been used for the resistant cat for which nothing else has worked (Hart and Hart, 1985). The procedure is currently not in wide use.

ALSO SEE: *Drug Therapy, Housesoiling—History Taking, Housesoiling—Submissive Urination, Housesoiling—Urination, Housesoiling—Urine Marking, Indoor-Outdoor, Intention Spraying, Olfactory Tractotomy, Remote Punishment, Sexually Dimorphic Behaviors, Spite, Temper Tantrum, Urine Spraying*

Housesoiling—Submissive Urination

Dogs that show active or passive submissive distance-reducing postures may urinate as one sign of submission. This behavior is not done as an elimination behavior, and punishment is not effective, since the animal is already submitting. In fact, punishment tends to make the animal more prone to show submissive urination. It is important for an approaching person to look as unthreatening as possible. Over time it may be possible to increase the dog's confidence so that it does not feel such a strong need to show the extreme submissive behaviors.

ALSO SEE: *Avoid Excitement, Decrease Body Threat, Increase Pet's Confidence, Passive Submission, Psychogenic Urinary Incontinence, Submissive Urination*

Housesoiling—Urination

Dogs and cats may urinate in the house. While some people do not seem to mind the behavior, most do. Of those who have tolerated this urination, often for years, the replacement of a carpet or a move may focus attention and make the behavior a problem. *Housesoiling—Urination* must be differentiated from other problems involving urine. This is normal urination in an unacceptable location. Most times housesoiling begins as a normal response when the urge comes but access is blocked to the outside or to a litter box. One occurrence should not cause great concern because an occasional accident is inevitable. In a few cases, the animal never was housebroken at all. This is an important piece of historical information, since housebreaking or retraining may have to be a major part of the recommendation.

For dogs, the schedule of going outside and proper rewards for eliminating are important. It is also important that owners do not assume that the dog is showing the behavior to "get even," and that they understand that "guilty" looks are not associated with any particular behavior. Negative attitudes and grudges must be stopped so that the motive for the soiling does not change from one of elimination to one for getting attention, even negative attention. Positive interactions, including play, grooming, obedience work, and lots of praise, break the negative cycle, while a good schedule helps stabilize elimination patterns.

When cats urinate outside the litter box, the problem must be critically evaluated. This may be the first sign of onset of lower urinary tract disease. Apparently cats "blame" pain on location, so if it hurts to go one place, they go somewhere else. An outdoor cat could go anywhere. An indoor cat does not feel any more restricted. Appropriate diagnosis and treatment of feline urologic syndrome (FUS) usually stops the problem. For some cats, urinating out of the box can be controlled by modifying their diet to acidify the urine. This can be done with commercial foods or by simply adding a few tablespoons of tomato juice to the food. Even with a clinically normal urinalysis, some cats respond well, perhaps indicating a subclinical manifestation. Probably the most common cause of cats not using their litter box is that the box is too dirty. Some cats are particularly fastidious, and others change as they get older. In multicat households, it is recommended that there be at least one litter box for each cat. Abrupt changes in the type of litter will cause 50% of cats to stop using the box, and only half of those will slowly accept the change. The introduction of a new type of litter is best made gradually over several changes.

If one spot is used for urination, the addition of a litter box to that spot is often adequate. This can work even for multiple spots. Bowls of food on problem areas have also been used and can be used in combination with added litter boxes. After a period of time, approximately equal to as long as the problem has been occurring, the litter boxes can be inched daily to a more convenient location. When there are several spots in several rooms, it is generally more convenient to confine the cat to a small room with food, water, a bed, and a litter box. A gradual reintroduction to more of the house can be made after an appropriate length of confinement. It is important for the owner to realize that a few days of confinement for a several-week problem will not stop the problem. An old pattern must be unlearned and an acceptable one relearned.

The location of the litter box is important. It should be readily available at all times. Young cats will not go to the back bedroom on the third floor to eliminate if all their activities are centered around the first-floor living room. Physical barriers, such as closed doors, can precipitate the problem, as can psychological ones, when other cats stay nearby. Abrupt changes in location of the box may confuse the animal.

For the cat whose owners have lost patience, gradually making it an indoor-outdoor animal may be an acceptable alternative, even for the declawed cat. In combination with acceptable alternatives, remote punishment may be worth trying, so that the cat is punished for approaching the unacceptable areas. Olfactory tracts can be severed in severe cases (Hart, 1981; Hart, 1982); however, the technique is not commonly done and may be more significant relative to urine spraying.

ALSO SEE: *Added Litter Boxes, Grudge, Guilt, Housebreaking, Housesoiling—History Taking, Housesoiling—Spraying, Housesoiling—Submissive Urination, Housesoiling—Urine Marking, Indoor-Outdoor, Olfactory Tractotomy, Remote Punishment, Retrain to Eliminate, Spite*

Housesoiling—Urine Marking

Male dogs use urine as messages for those who follow. It can apparently communicate who, when, sex, rank, and other subtle messages. Dogs, particularly males, will mark things in a home if they perceive a need to assert their presence. This behavior, then, parallels urine spraying in cats, which is a form of urine marking.

When urine is found in inappropriate locations, it is important to differentiate submissive urination, urination, and urine marking. Marking is often directed at items associated with a particular person or location. This might be a baby's toy, a new carpet (when the dog is no longer allowed in the room), a favorite chair, or a guest's clothing.

Treatment for *Housesoiling—Urine Marking* involves efforts to minimize the stress. Fun can be centered around times when the baby is there. The old dog may again need to have access to all parts of the house. New people can be included in fun or feed times.

ALSO SEE: *Housesoiling—History Taking, Housesoiling—Spraying, Housesoiling—Submissive Urination, Spite, Temper Tantrum, Urine Spraying*

Housetraining

Teaching a dog to eliminate in an acceptable location, usually outdoors, is called housetraining or housebreaking. The concepts discussed here can be used for dogs of all ages; however, the lessons may be easier for puppies. Persistence and consistency are important. The basic concept uses three natural tendencies of canine elimination. The first is to eliminate in group locations; the second is to eliminate at certain times; and the third is to avoid soiling the sleeping area. While both praise and punishment techniques have been successfully used, the dog's social nature makes praise alone successful in most young dogs. Housetraining may begin as soon as the puppy can consistently remember, generally around eight weeks of age.

Three major components are needed to housetrain a puppy. The first is patience. While some puppies learn the lessons in a few days, never to have an accident again, other normal dogs may take weeks or even months of patience, consistency, and effort to become successfully trained. Patience is also needed because occasional mistakes will occur, some of which are actually the owner's fault.

Confinement is the second major consideration in housetraining. Since dogs do not normally soil their bed area, confinement to that area takes advantage of that instinct and it discourages activity, which in itself can stimulate eliminations. However, the owner's lifestyle must also be considered. If he or she is gone for short periods of time, confinement to a small area such as a crate is appropriate. If the owner must be gone for 8 or 10 hours at a time, eliminations may occur because the bladder capacity is exceeded. If this is a possibility, the area of confinement should be large enough for the puppy to move away from its bed to use a corner of a small room or kennel. There should not, however, be enough area to encourage exercise.

Schedule is the third major factor in housetraining. It is important to take puppies to the elimination area, either a specific area outside or to the papers inside, at times when eliminations normally occur. These include after waking up, after exercise, after eating, and before going to sleep. Since puppies eat, sleep, and exercise several times in a day, the frequency of going out is more than four times daily. For young puppies, an extra trip outside in the middle of the night helps ensure they do not soil their bed area and meets the puppy's needs as dictated by a small urinary bladder capacity. Going out should be a time of business, so play is inappropriate. The area the puppy goes to may be more stimulatory if smells of excreta are already there. As soon as the puppy begins urinating or defecating, it should be praised by the owner to reinforce the behavior.

Other species can be trained to eliminate in certain locations within a house or to go outside. These include cats, rabbits, ferrets, and swine.

ALSO SEE: *Confinement, Praise*

Howling

Howling is a form of vocal communication most dogs have in common with other canine relatives. The tone and intensity vary with the purpose for which it is used. The sound is used primarily as a threat or warning, although it can be expressed by an apparently lonely individual or as a show of pack affinity.

When an intruder is heard approaching a wolf pack, the alerted wolf will start to howl. Other wolves in the pack will join in. Dogs generally howl for the same reasons. An "intruder" can be a strange noise, such as a wailing siren or a noise maker. Joining in with vocalizing is seen in domestic dogs when they howl as a person sings or plays a musical instrument. The standard explanation that "it hurts the dogs ears" has not been shown to be true by behavioral observations. Noise that dogs do not like usually causes a crouched, submissive posture as the animal tries to get away from it, or a restless attitude with attention directed toward the sound.

Since dogs tend to be more vocal than their canine cousins, the howl and bark can be more easily elicited. It is also easy to couple a "sing" command to the behavior, via classical conditioning, to get the animal to howl with an appropriate cue.

ALSO SEE: *Barking, Boredom, Excessive Vocalization—Howling, Vocal Communication*

Huddling

Huddling is a contact behavior in which individuals try to gain as much contact as possible. It is used to conserve body heat and may also have an important social function, particularly in swine.

ALSO SEE: *Contact Behavior*

Human-Animal Bond

Humans have historically shared their lives with animals and have formed strong bonds with certain individuals. While that interaction is typically thought of relative to dogs and cats, it certainly is a great deal broader. Horses, cattle, swine, goats, sheep, birds, snakes, and numerous others have been included in this human-animal relation. The human-animal bond is diverse, ranging from humans who have no like for animals at all to those with an intense pathologic relationship. This subject area is receiving a great deal of attention and research.

ALSO SEE: *Bond*

Hydrocephalic Aggression

This is a nonaffective aggression associated with the increased intracranial pressure of hydrocephalus. Hydrocephalic aggression should be suspected in any small dog, especially under 10 pounds, presented for aggression. Other descriptions in the history could include words such as "stubborn," "stupid," or "not housetrained." Diagnosis and treatment are typical for that of the more classic forms of hydrocephalus. There is some evidence that nontypical breeds may also have the condition. Certain lines of St. Bernards, Rottweilers, and perhaps other breeds with a rounding of the cranium have shown evidence of slightly dilated ventricles.

ALSO SEE: *Hydrocephalus, Nonaffective Aggression*

Hydrocephalus

Hydrocephalus is an increased volume of cerebrospinal fluid within the brain. While this has many causes, ranging from the congenital predisposition in small breeds with large skulls and brachycephalic breeds to that acquired from later obstructions, the results are a change in behavior and neurologic reactions. Ventricular dilatation will increase pressure gradually throughout the brain, so the types of signs are numerous. Specific behavior problems associated with hydrocephalus include hydrocephalic aggression, housesoiling, hyperactivity, "stubbornness," tail chasing, and poor learning ability. In any susceptible breed, hydrocephalus should be at the top of the differential list until proven otherwise.

ALSO SEE: *Housesoiling, Hydrocephalic Aggression, Hyperactivity, Medical Problems, Tail Chasing*

Hyperactivity

Hyperactivity is both a general term used for an overactive individual and a specific term used to describe a specific type of overactivity. In the general sense, the word has been used interchangeably with hyperkinesis, which adds to the confusion of these subjects.

In the specific sense, this author uses hyperactivity to describe one type of hyper problem. The hyperactive dog is usually a relatively young animal that does not undergo habituation learning. Loud noises continue to startle the animal, and obedience classes may have been tried unsuccessfully. These dogs tend to bark a lot and jump up on people or objects. Owners may notice that the dog sleeps very little compared to a normal dog. The definitive diagnosis is made by response to therapy after hyperthyroidism and food allergies have been ruled out.

A hyperactive dog will return to normal behaviors with standard tranquilizers, such as those in the phenothiazine group. Once normal behavior is established, the dog should go into obedience training. As it begins learning, the dog often can get by on gradually reduced doses of the tranquilizer. Eventually some dogs no longer need drug therapy.

Quantification of the extent of hyperactivity is desirable. While hospitalized, the dog is placed in a run, and its activities are monitored for 15, 20, or 30 minutes. After the first treatment begins to take effect, the activities are again counted or videotaped. Periodic reevaluation with this same procedure is helpful in maintaining control of the problem with minimal amounts of drugs.

ALSO SEE: *Drug Therapy, Habituation Learning, Hyperkinesis, Hyper Syndromes*

Hyperesthesia

Hyperesthesia is a hypersensitivity to tactile stimuli, often associated with a burning or tickling sensation. Central filters may modify the perception of stimuli, resulting in an abnormal reaction (Fox, 1971). This phenomenon may explain why some dogs develop a reluctance to being touched.

ALSO SEE: *Central Filters, Hypoesthesia*

Hyperkinesis

The terms hyperkinesis and hyperactivity are often used interchangeably to apply to any hyper behavior. This author uses hyperkinesis in a more specific sense—to describe a hyper behavior that is treatable with stimulants.

Behaviorally, hyperkinetic and hyperactive dogs act the same. The typical presentation is a relatively young dog, usually 1 to 2 years old, that is so active that the owners can no longer cope. The dog does not undergo habituation in various situations and is often an obedience class dropout. Affected dogs tend to bark a lot and seldom sit or lie for more than a few seconds. The diagnosis of hyperkinesis is made by response to therapy after hyperthyroidism and food allergies have been ruled out. The hyperkinetic dog does not respond appropriately to standard tranquilizers. The animal may calm down, but the effects are short lived, or the dog may get worse in activity levels, even becoming aggressive. Stimulants, on the other hand, calm the hyperkinetic dog. Dextroamphetamine was originally used for treatment, but it has a short duration of action. Methylphenidate became more popular because of its longer duration. For either drug, the animal's response dictates the next dose. It is desirable to find the lowest dose needed to control the behavior. Once under control, the dog should start obedience training, since learning is now possible. The dose of the stimulant can generally be reduced over time if training is done, and some dogs can eventually be taken off medication.

For some hyperkinetic children, caffeine is used to modify the behavior. Unfortunately, in dogs this stimulant does not decrease the activity level.

In diagnosing and evaluating the response to therapy, it is advisable to establish quantitative information while the dog is hospitalized. This can be done by counting the types and frequency of active behaviors such as barking, jumping, and running for a 15, 20, or 30 minute time period when the dog is in a run. Data collection is repeated after the stimulant has been given and had time to take effect. Because stimulants are controlled substances, it is easier to eliminate hyperactivity as a diagnosis first by testing with a tranquilizer. Then, if the hyper behavior remains, the stimulant can be tried. It is recommended that the progress be reevaluated by taking the patient off the stimulant every 4 to 6 months and then measuring the pre- and post-medication activities as was initially done. This procedure is necessary to quantify the true extent of the problem and to help prevent misuse of a controlled substance by a client.

ALSO SEE: *Drug Therapy, Habituation Learning, Hyperactivity, Hyper Syndromes, Appendix C*

Hyperphagia

Overeating and rapid eating are the abnormal behaviors of hyperphagia. These are shown by animals that bolt their food down. Many were nutritionally deprived as youngsters; others have been on restrictive diets. When a horse gets access to large volumes of a preferred food such as grain, it can develop grain overload and laminitis as a result of overeating. In other species, rapid eating does not allow food to get completely to the stomach, so regurgitation can follow.

Prevention of hyperphagia can be accomplished in several ways. Grain can be widely spread in a thin layer, or large smooth stones can be put in the trough to slow uptake by the problem horse. Increasing the frequency of feeding, feeding several small meals, and feeding hay before grain are other techniques that may be useful.

ALSO SEE: *Bolting, Excessive Food Intake*

Hypersexuality

Hypersexuality is the showing of sexual behavior to an extreme degree. The most common forms of this behavior are inappropriate mounting and masturbation.

ALSO SEE: *Atypical Sexual Behavior, Buller Steer Syndrome, Inappropriate Mounting, Masturbation*

Hyper Syndromes

In animals, as in people, some individuals seem unable to slow down to a normal rhythm of activity. The hyper syndromes have several causes. In making an appropriate diagnosis, it is important to rule out a normal animal that has not been allowed to get rid of its energy. Active dog breeds that are confined to a house or apartment and horses on high-energy rations that are confined to a stall should be considered normal and allowed to get appropriate exercise.

Animals affected by any of the hyper syndromes should first be evaluated medically and then behaviorally. Included in this broad category are food allergies, hyperthyroidism, hyperactivity, and hyperkinesis, as well as combinations of these and other conditions not currently understood.

Except for hyperthyroidism, the hyper syndromes are most well defined in dogs. There is no reason to assume they do not occur in other species. They probably have been overlooked and problem animals disposed of.

ALSO SEE: *Exercise, Food Allergy, Hyperactivity, Hyperkinesis, Hyperthyroidism*

Hyperthyroidism

The behaviors of hyperthyroidism are those usually associated with an increase in metabolic activity. The behaviors include a high level of activity, polyphagia, increased vocalization, and polydipsia/polyuria. Aggression has also been associated with the condition.

ALSO SEE: *Aggression, Polydipsia, Polyphagia, Polyuria*

Hypnosis

Hypnosis is a state of tonic immobility that occurs during close proximity of potential danger. The opossum is the best known user of this state. The catatonic state in cats, fainting by humans, and shock are similar in function and may be variations of hypnosis.

ALSO SEE: *Catatonic Reaction*

Hypoesthesia

Decreased sensitivity to touch and/or pain stimuli is called hypoesthesia. In humans, the condition is associated with psychotic and hysteric reactions, and perhaps similar reactions occur in animals (Fox, 1971).

ALSO SEE: *Hyperesthesia*

Hyporexia

Hyporexia is a decreased appetite when compared to normal. The physical presence of a very dominant individual can cause hyporexia in subordinates.

ALSO SEE: *Social Order*

Hypothermia

Very young puppies, kittens, and piglets can not maintain or regulate their body temperatures and must depend on shared warmth from the dam, littermates, and external sources to prevent hypothermia. Geriatric animals also tend to lose their ability to control body temperature. Old dogs may shiver or dig inside the house. Cats may seek the warmth of a radiator, heat vent, electric blanket, or sun spot for increasing lengths of time. Horses may shiver in weather that had not presented a problem to them a few years earlier. Appropriate attention must be given to the young and aged to prevent medical or behavioral problems from developing.

ALSO SEE: *Digging—Indoors*

Hypothyroid Aggression

This is a type of aggression associated with hypothyroidism. Both dogs and cats have been presented where aggression was the only complaint, and where there were no other signs of classical hypothyroidism—no loss of hair, thinning of skin, or lethargy. The history indicates the gradual onset of an irritable or crabby disposition with resentment to handling or attention. The pet may sleep in bed, but not want the owner to share a sofa. It may bite if the owner tries to walk through a door at the same time. Laboratory results show a low level of T_3 and T_4. Treatment is thyroid replacement with drugs such as levothyroxine.

ALSO SEE: *Competitive Aggression, Irritable Aggression, Nonaffective Aggression*

Hypotonia

Hypotonia, tonic dyskinesia, tonic immobility, and submissive inertia are other terms for catatonic reactions.

SEE: *Catatonic Reaction*

Hypoxia

Hypoxia is an oxygen deficiency within the body. Because low oxygen levels affect oxygen-sensitive tissues first, the brain is one of the first organs affected. In the past, aggression in dogs was not differentiated into types, and many techniques were tried to manage the problem. Some were successful, but most were not. Prolonged, deep, barbiturate anesthesia was one technique that did produce behavior changes, more often on post-surgical feline patients than on clinically aggressive animals. Bloodletting is another technique that produced behavior changes. It is probable that the changes in both procedures resulted from non-select cerebral hypoxia rather than from the techniques.

ALSO SEE: *Aggression, Anesthesia, Bloodletting*

Hysteria

Hysteria is a behavior of flight in poultry associated with a reactive anomaly. Without an apparent stimulus, a hen will suddenly fly around, squawking. There is an apparent relationship between this behavior and flock density. While toenail removal had been advocated for decreasing the degree of hysteria, reduction of the number of hens in a given space is generally more successful. Hysteria may represent an extreme form of mobile alarm.

ALSO SEE: *Mobile Alarm, Reactive Anomalies*

I

Idiopathic Aggression

Most causes of aggression can be determined, provided there is an adequate history and medical workup. In a low number of cases, a cause cannot be determined, and idiopathic aggression is the appropriate diagnosis. During a 15-month period, 21 cases of idiopathic aggression were diagnosed from 542 cases of canine aggression worked up at Texas A&M, a rate of 3.9%.

ALSO SEE: *Affective Aggression, Aggression, Aggression—History Taking, Nonaffective Aggression*

Imprint Learning

Imprint learning is a specialized type of learning that has restrictive conditions and time periods. One form of imprinting is species identification. This is when an animal learns what species it belongs to, which then affects mate selection in later life. Imprinting to its own species is instinctively given the highest priority in a learning situation when access is available to its own and another species.

Imprint learning can also occur in special bonding situations. The most well-defined of these are the paired imprinting of a dam to her offspring and the neonate to the dam. While the timing is slightly different between the two, the two-way relationship is critical in prey species.

Imprinting to a location for later return, such as with salmon, is called place imprinting.

ALSO SEE: *Erroneous Imprinting, Filial Imprinting, Learning, Operant Conditioning, Place Imprinting, Sensitive Period*

Improper Socialization

When taking a behavioral history, it is important to learn about the early exposure of the animal to others of its kind and to different species. Improper socialization is one of the four major causes of behavior problems seen, especially in dogs and cats. Without any socialization, the individual is leery of an approacher. When early exposure is limited, the animal develops the isolated syndrome and is generally regarded as handicapped in a social situation.

ALSO SEE: *Fear of People, Improper Socialization Aggression, Isolated Syndrome, Organizing Behavioral Histories, Socialization*

Improper Socialization Aggression

When a puppy or kitten is poorly socialized to other species, it is stressed when forced to interact. In many cases where the contact is intense, the animal may respond aggressively in an effort to escape. Even retention in a location that is stressful can result in a high degree of irritability and aggression. The aggression that results from the stresses of close social contact or locations is a variation of irritable aggression.

ALSO SEE: *Improper Socialization, Irritable Aggression, Isolated Syndrome, Socialization*

Inappetence

Inappetence is usually termed anorexia. The short-term loss of appetite is relatively normal; long-term anorexia may require treatment.

SEE: *Anorexia*

Inappropriate Elimination

When an animal eliminates in an inappropriate location, the behavior may not be appreciated by the owner. If the problem elimination occurs inside the home, it is called housesoiling. Inappropriate eliminations generally include normal elimination behaviors, such as urination or defecation, in an inappropriate location. Marking behaviors are usually not included.

ALSO SEE: *Displacement Activity, Housesoiling, Housesoiling—Defecation, Housesoiling—Urination*

Inappropriate Licking

Licking is a normal part of self- and mutual-grooming behavior in domestic animals. There are times when the behavior is considered inappropriate. Dogs and cats probably lick humans or occasionally each other as an extension of mutual grooming or social interaction. Cats and dogs may self lick excessively

I

and horses have been known to lick handlers when they were nervous. Both situations can be a displacement activity. Licking can also be directed toward objects. This can occur from apparent boredom, from nutritional deficiencies (particularly salt), or as environmental exploration as is common with the young. Taste or smell aversion can control some of the problems, if external influences are also controlled. For some reason, cats that are feline leukemia virus positive may develop an exaggerated licking behavior of unusual objects such as floors, bricks, or carpets. Aversion techniques are less successful for those cats than confinement away from selected areas.

ALSO SEE: *Boredom, Displacement Activity, Excessive Licking, Grooming Behavior, Licking, Loud Licking, Smell Aversion, Taste Aversion*

Inappropriate Mounting

Inappropriate mounting can occur in any species, and it can take any of six forms depending on the individual involved and other external factors.

Mounting by females is usually done by estrous females, most commonly in cattle and swine. Mounting is a male sexually dimorphic behavior, so it is most commonly shown by males; however, females also demonstrate the behavior. On the scale between masculinity and femininity, the ovariectomized female is slightly more masculine than the intact female. Mounting by ovariectomized females does occur, particularly in dogs.

The second type of mounting problem, excessive mounting by males, is usually related to territory, dominance, and age. Dogs will often mount subordinates in a pack, and tomcats will mount other cats within their territory. These are normal. Environmental disturbances, such as new animals in an area or the odors or sounds of an estrous female, may result in the dog or tomcat showing excessive mounting of nearby animals. Excessive mounting is also a common behavior in juvenile males nearing puberty. While this is a nuisance for dog and cat owners, it can be very disruptive and potentially injurious in livestock. Young stallions, in particular, need to be around other horses of their age or older in order to be disciplined for their biting and mounting behaviors.

The third type of inappropriate mounting, inappropriate mounting behavior during mating, is usually a function of age. Learning is a component of mating behavior, so inexperienced males may not get the sequence correct initially. Dogs and tomcats have been observed to mount the head of the female. More commonly in all species, the male mounts the female from the side and will either dismount and try again or move along the female to a more caudal position. Observational learning has been shown to shorten the learning for young bulls.

Multiple mountings, mounting of young animals, and mounting of other species or objects are the last three types of inappropriate mounting. They are most commonly associated with males without access to estrous females. The threshold stimulus for mounting decreases with time if the behavior does not occur. Eventually a minimal stimulus triggers the behavior. Many times the stimulus or the response will seem inappropriate. Excitement, such as may be associated with visitors in a house, may be enough to trigger a pet dog to mount an owner (a pack member), a wadded-up rug, a cat, or another dog. Since these forms of inappropriate mounting are most commonly shown by intact male pets, they provide a strong argument for castration as the treatment of choice. Exercise before events that are likely to trigger these behaviors can also be used to decrease the incidence.

ALSO SEE: *Atypical Sexual Behavior, Buller Steer Syndrome, Damming-up Theory, Male Behaviors, Masturbation, Monosexual Syndrome, Mounting, Observational Learning, Sexually Dimorphic Behaviors*

Increase Pet's Confidence

Dogs that are extremely submissive and those that are submissive urinators need to increase their confidence about the social situation that precipitates the problem. Owners must become deliberately less threatening. Useful behaviors include avoiding eye contact (the stare), squatting down rather than leaning over, presenting the side view instead of the front view, and encouraging the dog to come instead of reaching to get it. The voice should be high pitched, soft, and coaxing.

ALSO SEE: *Housesoiling—Submissive Urination, Psychogenic Urinary Incontinence, Submissive Urination*

Indirect Punishment

Indirect punishment is a form of punishment for a particular behavior that is associated with the environment or an event rather than with the presence of an individual. This is usually called remote punishment.

ALSO SEE: *Direct Punishment, Normal Behavior, Punishment, Remote Punishment*

Individual Distance

Individual, or personal, distance is the social (reactive) distance immediately around an animal into which preferred associates ("friends") are allowed. If others enter this space, the animal tries to move away.

By way of example, if strangers approach to ask directions, you get an uneasy feeling if they get close enough to invade your individual distance. In a veterinary office, touching, taking temperature, and examining an animal are invasions of the individual space. It may be necessary to take a little extra time to let the animal accept your close presence.

ALSO SEE: *Distance Animals, Pawing, Personal Distance, Reactive Distances, Social Distance*

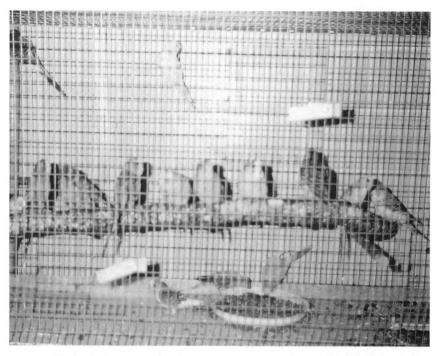

Individual Distance. Birds sitting on a limb or wire will space themselves at the outer limit of the individual distance (start of the social distance).

Individualized Group

This is a social group in which members know each other individually. Domestic animals belong to this type of group.

ALSO SEE: *Animal Sociology, Anonymous Group, Social Group*

Indoor-Outdoor

Cats that are housesoiling with defecation, urination, or spraying may show the behavior a long time, even years, before the owner presents it as a problem. At that point, the cat may have learned to eliminate anywhere, or the owner may have lost total patience, making different solutions impossible. If housing considerations, such as apartment living and heavy traffic nearby, are not factors, the problem may be made more tolerable by making the cat an indoor-outdoor pet. The owner gradually increases the amount of time the cat spends outdoors, but maintains a feeding schedule inside. Most cats adapt very well, even declawed ones. For many owners, keeping the cat outside is a more humane alternative than euthanasia, even if it may not be their ideal solution.

ALSO SEE: *Housesoiling, Housesoiling—Defecation, Housesoiling—Spraying, Housesoiling—Urination*

Infanticide

The young of a species may be killed by adults of that species for several reasons. It may occur in dogs, cats, and pigs where the female kills the runts. Males may also kill young. In many species of animals, nursing of young prevents estrus and ovulation. When a new breeding male enters a group structure, he may kill some or all of the infants. This behavior brings the females into estrus sooner and increases his chances of passing on his genes to another generation.

Cronism refers specifically to the parent eating its own young. Fratricide is the killing of a sibling.

ALSO SEE: *Cannibalism, Cronism, Fratricide, Sociobiology*

Infantile Behavior

The term infantile behavior is used to describe juvenile patterns being used by adult animals. These behaviors are often associated with courtship or with appeasement displays.

ALSO SEE: *Appeasement Behavior, Courtship, Early Ontogenetic Adaptation, Juvenile Characteristics*

Ingestive Behavior

Ingestive (eating) behavior can be divided into four main components: nursing, transitional phase, adult patterns, and drinking. Nursing, or suckling, behaviors are seen first and gradually change during the transitional period to a combination with adult eating patterns. At weaning, the adult patterns persist alone, although some parts may not be perfected yet. Drinking is the remaining type of ingestive behavior. Adult ingestive patterns are discussed here; the other three are described elsewhere.

The dog evolved with a feast-or-famine eating pattern. Because wolves do not have a source of food readily available, they have times of plenty after a successful hunt and times of lean before the next kill. When there is a kill, pack members share in the large food supply, eating as much as they can physically hold, if available. Dominant members get the most if there is any shortage. The domestic dog has retained the feast-or-famine eating pattern and often develops obesity as a result of an over-generous food supply. While food preferences develop in all species to some degree, they are a particular problem for dog and cat owners. Given appropriate time, dogs will gradually switch to a less-favored food.

Cats, on the other hand, evolved from small felids that ate rodents. Because their eating behaviors center around several small meals each day, free-choice feeding is less likely to result in obesity. Only recently have commercial cat foods became calorie dense, thus contributing to the problem of overweight cats. Food preferences commonly develop in cats and can become a significant problem. Cats will literally starve themselves to death if an acceptable food is not available. This makes it extremely important for owners to feed kittens a wide variety of flavors and textures. Even in predation, flavors tasted as kittens are still favored by adults, both in types of prey hunted and in catches actually eaten.

When grazing, the horse will cut off grass with its incisors, taking one or two mouthfuls before moving on to another step. The pastures are very long in areas where the horse eliminates because it will not eat there. Other spots may be overgrazed. Horses normally spend half their day grazing; however, management styles may limit access to food. When access to grazing is limited, a number of problems can follow. Medical complications revolve around the need for a relatively constant supply of roughage, so a minimum of two meals including hay or grass is recommended. When less than 1 pound of hay is fed for each 100 pounds of body weight, wood chewing becomes extreme. Other stereotypies, such as cribbing and weaving, can result from the extra time available to a stalled horse and the energy it retains from not having to find its own food. Lack of salt and exercise should be considered if aggression becomes a problem.

Cattle show a very different eating pattern because of their ability to ruminate. Grazing is still important but occurs for 4 to 9 hours daily, usually in cycles that peak near sunup and sunset. Rumination occurs between eating periods and takes approximately 75% of the time of grazing, in periods lasting between 2 and 60 minutes. The remastication lasts about 1 minute per bolus. Most of the time, cattle are lying during rumination, although some stand. Any type of stress can stop rumination, with potentially serious consequences.

Pigs are omnivorous, with very flexible ingestive behaviors. The time spent eating can be as long as 6 to 7 hours if they are on pasture, to less than 10-15 minutes if fed from a trough. Food and taste preferences are well-studied as are the influences of crowding, competition, and dominance (Signoret, Baldwin, Fraser and Hafez in Hafez, 1975; Syme and Syme, 1979; Beaver, 1989). In pastures and when unconfined, pigs root up underground food items to eat. It is this tendency, along with their keen sense of smell, that has led to their use in finding truffles.

Specifics on taste preferences by the various species are found elsewhere.

ALSO SEE: *Aggression, Appetitive Behavior, Burying Food, Drinking, Feast or Famine, Feeding Ceremony, Feeding Tradition, Food Begging, Food Preferences, Food Provisioning, Grass Eating, Ground Pecking, Hypothalamus, Ingestive Behavior Problems, Nursing, Obesity, Polyphagia, Predation, Stereotyped Behaviors, Taste, Transitional Phase, Weaning*

Ingestive Behavior Problems

A number of problems are associated with eating behaviors or patterns. The most obvious is obesity. Others in this group of problems involve eating things not normally considered to be part of a diet, using the mouth to grab things, or not eating. Specific problems are discussed under their individual titles.

ALSO SEE: *Aerophagia, Anomalous Milk Sucking, Anorexia, Body Pecking, Coprophagia, Cribbing, Cronism, Destructive Chewing, Dysphagia, Egg Eating, Excessive Food Intake, Feather Eating, Galactophagia, Grass Eating, Gulping Food, Hair Eating, Hyperphagia, Hyperthyroidism, Ingestive Behavior, Lip Curl, Obesity, Pica, Pollakidipsia, Polydipsia, Polyphagia, Soil Eating, Urine Drinking, Wind Sucking, Wood Chewing*

Inhibited Bite

There are numerous instances in which one animal bites another, but purposefully does not bite as hard as possible. The severity of the bite is inhibited. The nape bite of sexual behavior in cats, dogs, and horses is one example. Queens and bitches carry their young using an inhibited bite, and the warning bite of a fearful animal also fits this category.

ALSO SEE: *Fear-induced Aggression, Maternal Behavior, Nape Bite*

Inhibition

When a specific behavior by one animal prevents the expression of an expected behavior by another, it is said to inhibit the behavior. Appeasement displays inhibit aggression. A displacement activity may be used for the same reason. Inhibition may also result in redirection of the expression of aggression.

ALSO SEE: *Appeasement Behavior, Displacement Activity, Redirected Aggression*

Innate Learning

Innate learning is another name for latent learning—learning that is not immediately obvious.

SEE: *Latent Learning, Learning, Operant Conditioning*

Innovation

Innovation is insight learning.

SEE: *Insight Learning*

Insight Learning

Insight learning is generally equated with thinking and reasoning. Thus, it is regarded as the highest form of learning. There is a debate as to whether any animal species can reason through certain situations. Tool making by chimpanzees fashioning twigs to probe termite mounds is cited as one example of planning. Roger Fouts reported that his chimpanzee "Washoe" signed the words "hard berry" for the first nuts she saw. In studies done at Texas A&M, researchers have seen horses and beagles stop in the middle of a maze, look back and forth between two options, and then make a choice. Whether this is reasoning or happenstance, we may never know.

ALSO SEE: *Intelligence, Learning, Thinking*

Instinct

This is a stereotyped series of actions that are similar in all members of a species. Most instinctive behaviors are easily evoked by simple stimuli. Examples include bird migration, maternal behavior, and earth-raking by cats.

ALSO SEE: *Damming-up Theory, Habit, Reflex, Vacuum Activity*

Instinct-Training Interlocking

This is a concept, initially introduced by Konrad Lorenz as "drive-training interlocking," that says certain innate programs must interact with certain environmental factors to provide the complete expression of a behavior. Kittens can pounce and stalk in play, but they must interact with natural prey to perfect the skills needed for successful hunting as adults.

Intelligence

Intelligence has a broad range of meanings, including the ability to learn from the environment, mental ability, or measured success at a task. Measurements of "intelligence" are biased by the design, the application, and the limits of the test group. Human tests that involve reading are already biased against the blind, uneducated, and dyslexic.

Testing for "intelligence" within a species has been done, and tests are marketed for dogs and for cats. While these are generally fun to try, it is important to understand they are measuring many things besides the intangible "IQ."

There are rankings of "intelligence" among animal species, but these are flawed as well. First, the various tests try to measure something that is poorly defined relative to humans, much less animals. Then these tests are biased in outcome based on the type of response asked for. Elephants, sea lions, horses, and chickens would score high on a test requiring nose pushing. Cats and primates would do poorly. Horses will outperform cattle in a timed maze, but will score more poorly if the maze test counts movement into squares not on the path of the shortest distance between start and finish.

ALSO SEE: *Cognition, Insight Learning, Learning*

Intention Movement

This is an introductory behavior of a behavior sequence that is expressed without completing the rest of the series. It is used to communicate a motivational state. In bulls, a shift of weight to the forelimb closest to another animal is a mounting intention. In courtship, the same movement tests the readiness of the female. It can also serve as an increase in aggression during an agonistic encounter between bulls.

ALSO SEE: *Distance-increasing Silent Communication, Male Behaviors*

Intention Spraying

Cats may assume a spraying posture by standing backed up near an object, with a vertical, twitching tail, but no urine is actually sprayed. Intention spraying, then, is the behavior of feline urine spraying, without the urine. The significance of the behavior is not completely understood since it often occurs when spraying would not be appropriate.

ALSO SEE: *Housesoiling—Spraying, Urine Spraying*

Interfemale Aggression

Intrasexual aggression occurs most commonly between males of a species; however, threats and fighting can occur between females as well. When this aggression is associated with the physical presence of another female, regardless of dominance, territory, and other stimuli, the behavior is considered to be interfemale aggression.

ALSO SEE: *Dominance Aggression, Hormonal Imbalance Aggression, Intermale Aggression, Intrasexual Aggression, Territorial Aggression*

Intermale Aggression

Intermale aggression is a male sexually dimorphic behavior most typically expressed by an intact male threatening or fighting another intact male. Fighting can occur at any time, regardless of dominance rankings of the individuals, the presence or absence of the owner, or the presence of a female. It is considered one type of affective aggression and is also a type of mobile aggression. In certain free-ranging species, intermale aggression is common, at least seasonally, whenever males get too close to each other. For some species, fighting does not occur unless there is a female in heat. In others the male presence alone is significant. In dogs, intermale aggression is common in certain breeds, such as the terriers, German shepherds, Dobermans, and Rottweilers. Tomcats will tolerate other toms in their territory if they are more or less permanent residents. Stallions and bulls can be kept in this manner unless females, anestrus or in estrus, are around. Free-ranging boars tend to remain solitary until the breeding season arrives.

Since intermale aggression is a male sexually dimorphic behavior, it is partially dependent on testosterone. In some species there is also a learned component, so castration or progestins will not completely eliminate the problem.

This behavior must be differentiated from competitive (dominance) aggression.

ALSO SEE: *Affective Aggression, Castration, Competitive Aggression, Dominance Aggression, Drug Therapy, Fight It Out, Interfemale Aggression, Intrasexual Aggression, Mobile Aggression, Separate, Sexually Dimorphic Behaviors*

Internal Reward

Many behaviors, including some unacceptable ones, have a built-in reward system for the animal, such that the outcome is "rewarding" or the behavior "enjoyable." The prey-chasing behaviors fulfill an instinctive drive in dogs and cats. Stereotyped behaviors are self-rewarding because they get rid of stress and perhaps release endorphins. Escape is its own reward.

Such behaviors can be difficult to eliminate because the motivation is internally driven. That internal reward must be eliminated, or it must become insignificant, usually relative to the simultaneous punishment. In some cases, the unacceptable behavior can be prevented only by physical barriers. Dogs that chase cars or livestock can be chained up or penned. Horses that are stall weavers or pacers have been managed by hobbles. It is better to both address the initiating cause of the problem and to minimize the reward. Narcotic antagonists may be useful to minimize the perception of "enjoyment."

ALSO SEE: *Ankle Attacks, Car Chasing, Chasing Cars, Chasing Livestock, Cribbing, Drug Therapy, Excessive Vocalization—Barking, Feces Throwing, Fence Jumping, Jumping on People, Livestock Chasing, Masturbation, Motivation, Prolonged Sucking Syndrome, Running Away, Stall Kicking, Stereotyped Behaviors, Stereotyped Pacing, Stereotyped Weaving, Tail Chasing, Wind Sucking*

Interspecies Communication

Interspecies communication is very limited. When multiple species gather in an area, as occurs on the plains of Africa, the alarm or flight response when one species sights a predator may also result in a response by other species. In general, though, humans are the only species capable of understanding the more complex messages of other species, especially in regard to signals without a self-preservation message. A great deal of research is being conducted on chimpanzees, gorillas, and dolphins to explore their nonverbal language skills.

ALSO SEE: *Communication Behaviors, Distance-increasing Silent Communication, Distance-reducing Silent Communication, Interspecific Releaser, Vocal Communication*

Interspecific Releaser

This is a behavior that serves as a communication between species. Often it is a warning, expressed vocally or by an action. Certain mammals may use bird warning calls or running by hoofed species to increase their own awareness of potential danger.

ALSO SEE: *Interspecies Communication, Mixed-Species Group*

Intimate Distance

The intimate distance is another name for the space immediately surrounding an individual—the personal distance.

SEE: *Personal Distance*

Intrasexual Aggression

Intrasexual aggression is aggression between individuals of the same sex. Not restricted to males, this aggression can occur between two females, two neutered females, or two neutered males, but the frequency of occurrence is greatly reduced. The fights are generally quite serious, ritualized, and difficult to break up.

ALSO SEE: *Interfemale Aggression, Intermale Aggression, Mobile Aggression, Mouth Play, Separate, Sexually Dimorphic Behaviors*

Intromission Impotence

Primarily associated with bulls and rams, intromission impotence is an abnormal behavior of male reproduction. There is active mounting and clasping, but little thrusting, and a persistent intromission failure.

ALSO SEE: *Male Behaviors*

Investigative Behavior

Investigative behaviors include any of the distance-reducing silent communication postures and actions that indicate curiosity. These include directing attention by looking, smelling, and moving toward the object or individual with ears forward and a cautious approach. Animals usually use multiple senses to interact with an object, including licking and chewing it. Care must be used so that these oral exploratory behaviors do not get the animal in trouble. Plastic bags eaten by calves have been fatal.

Young animals go through a period when they investigate other animals. Once this socialization is completed, they usually go into a period of peak environmental exploration. While the actual time period for this varies with species, the behaviors of the young are very much directed at interacting with things around them.

ALSO SEE: *Licking of Objects, Neophobia, Socialization*

Investigative Distance

This is a social (reactive) distance where the animal shows interest in an approacher. The animal becomes aware of the approach at the perceptive distance, but now shows an interest by intently watching the approacher. At some future time, the animal will decide to flee, attack, or accept this individual based on sensory information gathered.

ALSO SEE: *Perceptive Distance, Reactive Distances, Social Distance*

Irritable Aggression

Irritable aggression is aggression that results from a lowering of the threshold that triggers an episode. Animals that are in pain (often chronic), uncomfortable, or under stress often lash out aggressively at episodes that should not normally initiate aggression. An analogy is the ease of triggering aggression in a person with a headache or toothache. It is important to clear up the underlying medical problem or to control it with analgesics in order to reverse this form of aggression.

ALSO SEE: *Avoid Excitement, Drug Therapy, Food Allergy, Improper Socialization Aggression, Kennelosis, Nonaffective Aggression, Pain Relievers*

Isolated Syndrome

The isolated syndrome is part of the deprivation syndrome in which the individual has limited exposure to an enriching environment. This condition is most noticeably manifested in dogs, and it is usually relevant to their interactions with people. If the dog had a limited introduction to people of all sizes and shapes as a puppy, it may not respond in an acceptable manner as an older dog. This response, when forced, tends to take on one of two extremes. The dog is fearful and hides, or it aggressively tries to ward off the approacher.

Dogs can also develop an isolated syndrome relative to places. If raised in a kennel, a dog is stressed later when forced to live in a home environment or in a large yard. They may pace, show aggression, or retire to one small area.

Once the isolated syndrome has developed, there is little that can be done to change the dog. The socialization period ended a long time before and the environmental exploration period is over. The most humane thing for the animal is to keep its environment as constant as possible and minimize social contact. Once owners understand the socialization process and how its incomplete application caused the actions they see in their pet, they are usually willing to minimize stress for the dog.

The isolated syndrome at its extreme produces a "Kaspar-Hauser" animal. This is an animal raised under such restricted conditions that it has no opportunity to achieve any normal behavioral development. The condition is named after a German child who was extremely retarded developmentally and could only remember living in a dark room.

ALSO SEE: *Deprivation Syndrome, Fear-induced Aggression, Fear of People, Improper Socialization, Improper Socialization Aggression, Kennelosis, Socialization*

J

Jaw Chomping

Jaw chomping is a distance-reducing behavior shown by young horses at times of greeting. While there is some disagreement, the behavioral context is probably submissive. For this behavior, the lips are pulled back, the mouth is partially open, and the mandible is moved up and down without the teeth making contact. Foals show this behavior most commonly when approached by an older horse; however, yearlings and occasionally older horses will use jaw chomping when approached by an older, dominant horse.

The terms jaw chomping, snapping, and teeth clapping have been used to describe this behavior.

ALSO SEE: *Vacuous Chewing*

Jumping Fences

Jumping fences as a behavior problem is described under fence jumping.

SEE: *Fence Jumping*

Jumping on People

Some dogs jump up on people by rearing on their hind feet and placing their front feet as far up on the person as they can. The behavior usually starts in puppies and continues because owners encourage it, do not discourage it, or do not use consistency to stop it. Jumping up probably begins with the puppy's attempt to get to and lick the face of its higher ranking pack members—the owners. As the dog gets older, jumping may take on another meaning—that of dominance over the person. Just as a dominant dog may stand on the shoulders of lower ranking pack members, the same behavior can be used to show dominance over a person. Young wolf cubs show the same behaviors toward pack leaders. While licking may not always occur, the jumping may continue.

To change the behavior, every attempt should be punished or corrected. Success is an internal reward, so elimination of the problem requires consistent negative interactions or the use of a substitute behavior that is mutually exclusive, such as having the dog sit when it starts to jump.

ALSO SEE: *Internal Reward, Licking, Normal Behavior, Punishment, Substitute a Behavior, Time-Out*

Juvenile Characteristics

Juvenile characteristics are those that distinguish young from adults. The differences are generally physical, although behavior can also be included. Typical juvenile characteristics include different hair or feather coat, different markings, a disproportionately large head, large and prominent eyes, a different gait, unique vocalizations, and a high degree of exploratory behavior.

These differences serve to camouflage the young, permit some types of social contact that would otherwise not be tolerated, and minimize aggression toward the young.

ALSO SEE: *Exploratory Behavior, Infantile Behavior*

Kennelosis

A dog raised in a particular environment can develop an attachment for that type of environment such that placement in another situation can be very stressful. A dog kept in a kennel for several years may do well on the show circuit, but be unable to do well when later put into a home environment. The reverse can also occur when a house-raised dog, even one accustomed to being around a lot of other dogs, does not adjust to a kennel environment if boarded. The coping response might be irritable aggression, anorexia, or hiding.

ALSO SEE: *Anorexia Nervosa, Irritable Aggression, Isolated Syndrome, Place Imprinting, Socialization*

Kicking

Kicking is a distance-increasing behavior shown by many of the ungulate species as a threat or attack. The animal lifts one or both of its rear feet. While picking up a foot serves as a warning, thrusting it rapidly backward is more typical of an aggressive behavior. An animal may also move the limb forward to get at a fly or other pest under its abdomen. Cattle, donkeys, and a few horses can abduct the pelvic limbs in a sideways ("cow") kick.

For protection from a horse's kick, it is best for a person to remain close to the animal and immediately lateral to the pelvic limb. Children are most likely to be hurt running up behind a horse, and experienced horsemen are apt to forget caution when working underneath, as when they polish hooves.

Kicking by horses can become a problem behavior. Some horses turn their rear ends toward a person entering a stall as the only sign of aggression. Others turn their rears and then kick or threaten to kick. That behavior is particularly dangerous because the person may be trapped against the side of the stall, compounding the severity of the blows. The nonaggressive animal that only faces in the opposite direction may spontaneously stop turning away when it learns that the person means no harm. Each move to face the approacher can also be rewarded (Skinnerian shaping). The more aggressive animal may also be punished with a single, quick stroke with a whip or rope for each approach that is met with a rear view. Horses quickly learn to watch the approacher.

Kicking by horses can also be directed at stalls or trailer gates. This, of course, places a great deal of stress on the legs of the animal and can result in injury if the barrier breaks. Hobbles and kick chains can be useful. Hobbling two limbs together can prevent the kicking behavior. A single leg hobble that holds the carpus flexed can also be used to gain psychological control over an aggressive horse. The kick chain hits the horse when it kicks out with its limb, serving as an immediate punishment.

Because cattle can kick sideways, treating them can be more difficult. The safest method is to restrain them in a chute so there is a physical barrier. If giving an injection, stand on the side opposite the injection site. Cows typically lash out in the direction of the pain.

ALSO SEE: *Distance-increasing Silent Communication, Hobbles, Skinnerian Shaping of Behavior, Stall Kicking, Striking, Trailer Kicking*

Kinesis

Kinesis is the movement of an animal away from danger or unfavorable areas of its environment and toward favorable ones. This can be further subdivided into klinokinesis, in which the direction of travel changes in direct proportion to the severity of the stimulation, and orthokinesis, in which the speed of movement away is in direct proportion to the stimulus severity.

ALSO SEE: *Locomotion*

Kin Recognition

This is the ability of an animal to recognize or differentiate between relatives and those not related to it. This helps minimize inbreeding.

Kin Selection

Kin selection is the use of behaviors by an individual that helps the survival of animals closely related to it, and thus favors the survival of a specific gene pool. Although parental care of offspring is generally not included in the definition, altruism and helper animals are associated. Kin selection is an aspect of sociobiology.

ALSO SEE: *Altruism, Helper, Sociobiology*

Kleptogamy

Kleptogamy is mating by males that normally would not have an opportunity to mate because they lack a territory, are subordinate, or do not belong to the group. The term literally means "to steal a mate."

ALSO SEE: *Male Behaviors*

Kleptoparasitism

This is the stealing of food or other items from members of other species, or on rare occasions, from one's own species.

ALSO SEE: *Ingestive Behavior*

Klinokinesis

When an animal is escaping an undesirable location or situation, the direction of travel changes in direct proportion to the severity of the stimulus.

ALSO SEE: *Kinesis*

Latent Learning

Latent learning occurs without a recognized reward and when the learning is not immediately obvious. For example, veterinarians who were raised around a lot of animals are aware of the behaviors of elimination or reproduction because they have seen them. Discussions of these behaviors are "obvious" because of the previous learning, even though no conscious effort was made to learn initially. Animals apparently can also experience latent learning. Puppies raised in environments rich in exploratory opportunities tend to learn other lessons faster than those raised in a barren area.

Latent learning has also been called innate learning.

ALSO SEE: *Exploratory Behavior, Isolated Syndrome, Learning, Operant Conditioning*

Lateral Threat

One posture used as a distance-increasing message places the threatening individual at a 90° angle from the potential victim. This broadside stance may be subtle, as in cattle and many other ruminants, because there are few other signs to emphasize the posture. In cats, the lateral body position is part of the defensive threat; however, the other signs, like piloerection and the arched back, emphasize the broadside view.

ALSO SEE: *Defensive Threat, Direct Punishment, Distance-increasing Silent Communication*

Layer Out

This is a term used to describe the young that lie in hiding while their mothers graze. They are also said to be hiding or lying out.

ALSO SEE: *Lying Out*

Learned Aggression

Learned aggression takes advantage of the animal's instinct for protection of self or group and couples it with a reward so that specific situations can trig-

L

ger the aggression. It can be divided into trained aggression, as with guard dogs, and unconsciously learned aggression.

ALSO SEE: *Affective Aggression, Trained Aggression, Unconsciously Learned Aggression*

Learned Excitement

In certain situations, the excitement of an event can be transferred between animals. This induction of mood is most common for group behaviors that are associated with survival, such as the herd reaction to flee that follows the sighting of a predator. In domestic animals, horses and dogs show learned excitement most commonly. The shying of one horse to an object that startles it often results in a flight reaction by others nearby, particularly those following.

Learned excitement in dogs has a different connotation from that in horses. Owners often unconsciously encourage a behavior through rewards or by creating a great deal of excitement around an event. A group of children that races to answer a phone or doorbell can produce a dog that associates excitement with a specific stimulus. As a result, the dog becomes responsive to the stimulus even when an external excitement is not present and the ringing of the telephone may be enough to trigger an inappropriate response.

ALSO SEE:: *Aggression and Doorbells, Aggression and Telephones. Classical Conditioning, Sympathetic Induction of Mood*

Learning

Learning is a process that modifies an individual's behavior or knowledge as the result of interaction with the environment. How this interaction takes place defines the various types of learning. The presence, absence, or type of motivating factors can affect the process too. The consistent ability to learn gradually develops after birth rather than being fully developed at birth. For puppies, the consistency in learning starts at approximately 3 weeks. It probably occurs about the same time for kittens. Foals and calves are born in a more highly developed state, so learning begins within the first few days. The first lessons may come the easiest of all because the animal is naive. Subsequent lessons building on those already learned are also relatively easy because of the "learning to learn" phenomenon. The most difficult lessons occur when previous techniques or learning must be negated first.

ALSO SEE: *Classical Conditioning, Cognition, Habituation Learning, Imprint Learning, Innate Learning, Insight Learning, Latent Learning, Learned Aggression, Learned Excitement, Learning Capacity, Learning Disposition, Local Enhancement, Motivation, Observational Learning, Operant Conditioning, Pavlovian Conditioning, Prenatal Learning, Prompting and Fading, Puzzle Box, Skinnerian Shaping of Behavior, Training, Trial and Error Learning*

Learning Capacity

Learning capacity is the amount of information that an individual can learn. It is related to how, what, when, and where this learning can take place. The limit is called the learning disposition. While learning capacity is not really measurable, the concept is generally well-accepted. The capacity increases in the animal kingdom relative to the species position on the phylogenetic scale. There is also individual variation.

ALSO SEE: *Learning, Learning Disposition*

Learning Disposition

The learning disposition of an animal is the limit of its learning capacity. This limit is probably governed by genetic factors, varying with the type of lesson to be learned. Lessons that are critical to an individual's survival are rapidly learned, while those that are insignificant to the animal are harder to teach.

ALSO SEE: *Learning, Learning Capacity, Motivation*

Leash Fighting

Leash fighting by dogs can be related to two factors. For some dogs there apparently is a genetic component because the problem has been seen in association with certain family lines. The specifics of the heritability have not been worked out. When genetics seems to be involved, the problem is often obvious in the puppy. These are youngsters that show extreme reactions when a collar and leash are put on. A great deal of behavior modification is needed to lessen the frantic reactions because habituation is relatively ineffective. Older dogs can also show leash fighting. These dogs start fighting when they realize the limits of their freedom because they are not accustomed to wearing a collar or to being restrained by a leash.

ALSO SEE: *Behavior Modification, Dog Collars, Genetic Problems, Stress-related Behaviors*

Legal Concern

In problem cases, especially with aggression, some animal owners either do not comprehend the potentially serious outcome of the behavior or they are seeking information about the complete scope of the problem. Veterinarians have an obligation to mention that there may be legal ramifications for an animal's behavior once the aggressive tendency for it is known. Specifics of an owner's legal responsibilities should be given by the client's attorney, since laws vary between cities and states.

Certain general rules exist. All animal owners are expected to take reasonable precautions for confinement of their animals to prevent the general public from being hurt. Dogs are often given a "one bite" chance so that there is greater assumed responsibility once the first injury has occurred. This "one bite" exemption has been denied for certain types of dogs and for dogs where the first attack caused major human injuries.

ALSO SEE: *Aggression*

Lick Granulomas

These are localized areas of moist dermatitis usually located on the paws or forelimbs of a dog. The lick granuloma, also known as acral lick dermatitis, acral pruritic nodule, and neurodermatitis, is a form of self-mutilation. There may be multiple causes for this type of problem. For those cases that are not responsive to traditional medical treatments or recur, stress should be considered as a contributing factor. Dogs that internalize stress often direct the effects of this stress to themselves. A few chew their nails. More often, however, the dog begins to show excessive licking. If continued long enough, a lesion develops. Long-term management of lick granulomas includes control of the dog's daily schedule and exercise. Drug therapy may be helpful initially to reduce stress. If the owner can detect the onset of the problem early enough, increased exercise and more attention to minimizing changes in the human-canine interaction times are usually sufficient to stop progression.

ALSO SEE: *Excessive Grooming, Exercise, Hot Spots, Schedule, Self-Mutilation, Appendix C*

Licking

Licking is a behavior common to several species and used in a variety of situations. It involves the animal wiping its tongue across an object, such as itself during grooming; a conspecific, as in mutual grooming; or food, particularly salt. Licking behaviors can occur at other times, too. For dogs, licking represents a form of passive submission shown by subordinates to higher ranking pack members. Cats lick their owners apparently as a variation of mutual grooming. Feline leukemia virus positive cats may lick inanimate objects, but the reason is unknown. The prolonged sucking syndrome of cats may involve licking as well. Horses and cattle sometimes lick their human handlers in efforts to get salt or to relieve stress.

ALSO SEE: *Excessive Licking, Grooming Behavior, Inappropriate Licking, Jumping on People, Licking of Objects, Mutual Grooming, Passive Submission, Prolonged Sucking Syndrome, Tongue Play, Tongue Rolling*

Licking of Objects

The young of many species may lick various objects as part of their environmental exploration. Occasionally an individual shows an excessive desire for licking unusual objects, such as an owner's hand, floors, or bricks. Salt deprivation in livestock can cause them to lick or chew places where salt may have been deposited from sweat. This problem is easily correctable. Cats that are feline leukemia virus positive have been known to show excessive licking of floors, fireplace bricks, and other unusual objects. The specific cause of the behavior is unknown, but it is nonresponsive to most therapies. Dogs, too, have been known to lick unusual objects. In some cases, it is an attention-getting behavior, which can be extinguished by the owner not showing attention to the behavior or by substituting an acceptable response for a specific command. Other dogs apparently lick as a displacement activity during times when there is nothing else to do. An occasional horse, dog, or cat licks its owner or handler in an attempt to reduce internal stress, such as when at a show.

Licking of objects should not be confused with pica, destructive chewing, or the prolonged sucking syndrome. Taste aversion, preventing access to the object (including the use of a muzzle), and/or confinement are the most successful techniques to stop excessive licking.

ALSO SEE: *Attention Seeking, Confinement, Licking, Muzzle, No Attention to Behavior, Pica, Prevent Access, Prolonged Sucking Syndrome, Taste Aversion*

Lignophagia

Lignophagia describes the wood chewing behavior common in horses confined to stalls and paddocks.

SEE: *Wood Chewing*

Limb Flicking

Limb flicking is a behavior shown by cats when they get their paws wet. Each wet limb is quickly shaken in turn. This represents a local variation of shaking. An occasional cat will show the behavior even though the paw is not wet. The reason for the atypical behavior is not understood, but some cases may be a form of behavioral seizure.

ALSO SEE: *Seizures, Shaking*

Limp Posture

This is another term for flexor dominance.

SEE: *Flexor Dominance*

Lip Curl

The common name used to describe flehmen in cattle is lip curl.

SEE: *Flehmen*

Litter (Bedding) Eating

Confined animals may develop a behavior of eating their bedding, even after it has become soiled. Over time the behavior can become preferential, particularly for horses and poultry. In birds, litter eating is usually a result of crowding at feeders, and there may be a genetic component as well. Nutritional, medical, and stress factors should be evaluated.

ALSO SEE: *Coprophagia*

Livestock Chasing

Livestock chasing is a variation of prey chasing (predatory aggression) by canids and large felids. It is similar to dogs chasing cars, bicycles, or joggers. Livestock chasing is difficult to eliminate in dogs because the behavior is internally rewarding and each attempt to chase must be defeated. Complete success can be accomplished only by confinement away from or preventing access to livestock. Any other type of treatment using the most diligent attempts to change the behavior has no more than a 50% chance of success. Each attempt to chase must be punished as it begins, as when the owner can grab a long rope trailed by the dog and inflict verbal punishment as the animal is pulled back. Extremely negative experiences associated with chasing bouts can also be tried. Dogs have been made to carry killed chickens or lambs tied around their necks or in their mouths until the carcass disintegrates. Emetics injected into a killed carcass usually work too slowly to be associated with the actual chase. Remote-controlled shock collars have also been tried, but are no more successful than other techniques. All are dependent on the long-term motivation of the owner to outlast the problem.

ALSO SEE: *Aversive Conditioning, Car Chasing, Internal Reward, Predatory Aggression, Prevent Access, Reinforcement Schedules, Shock Collars*

Local Enhancement

Local enhancement is a type of learning that combines trial and error with observation. To achieve a goal, such as finding food or mating successfully, the animal uses trial and error. However, because the animal watched another accomplish the behavior, the number of attempts is less than expected based on pure trial and error learning. Young bulls have used local enhancement to achieve intromission sooner. Horses have learned to negotiate "T" mazes for grain in a bucket more rapidly with this process.

ALSO SEE: *Learning, Observational Learning, Trial and Error Learning*

Locomotion

Locomotion is the way an animal moves. While there are a number of differences throughout the animal population, the general arrangement of foot-fall patterns is similar.

The walk is a four-beat gait, meaning each foot lands at a separate time. The gait is also described as symmetrical because the second four pattern of feet on the ground mirrors the first four. Unlike in the slow walking speed, the fast walk does not have a phase in which all four feet are on the ground at one time. Visually, the diagonal limbs seem to move at almost the same time.

The amble is also a four-beat, symmetrical gait with the same foot-fall patterns as the slow and fast walk. The timing is different, however, so that the visual perception is that the limbs on one side are moving forward at almost the same time.

The trot is a two-beat, symmetrical gait in which the diagonal limbs move forward at exactly the same time. In the slow trot, all four limbs are on the ground briefly at the same time. At the fast trot, there is a suspension phase with no feet touching the ground.

The pace has the same two-beat, symmetrical rhythm as the trot; however, ipsilateral (same-side) limbs move forward at exactly the same time. Since the entire center of gravity shifts to the one side, the animal can generally move faster at a pace than at a trot. In some species or breeds, the pace is not considered a desirable gait.

The gallop has several different patterns depending on speed. It is a four-beat gait, but not symmetrical. The faster the speed, the more likely there will be one or two suspension stages. Animals that have a great deal of flexibility in their backs, such as cats, can show the double suspension as they reach for the next stride, after pushing off with their hind limbs, and after a push with the forelimbs as the rear limbs reach forward. Since this is an exhaustive behavior, it is usually reserved for serious matters. Long travel is generally at a trot or walk.

Many forms of locomotion use these same movements. Swimming and climbing are walking movements. Jumping is a gallop.

There are a number of references that deal specifically with locomotion (Hollenbeck, 1971; Gambaryan, 1974).

ALSO SEE: *Climbing, Stotting*

Long-Term Pair Bond

Long-term pair bond describes a mated pair that remains as a single reproductive unit over several reproductive periods. Some species of birds, such as geese and swans, have a long-term pair bond that lasts the lifetime of the partners.

ALSO SEE: *Reproductive Behavior*

Loud Licking

Dog owners and occasionally cat owners may complain about their pet's loud licking behavior. The problem usually occurs at night when the owner is trying to sleep. Licking is a normal grooming behavior, but the situation makes it undesirable. Since the behavior cannot be stopped, alternative solutions must be found. For example, if the owner and pet sleep in separate rooms, the pet may groom without bothering the owner.

ALSO SEE: *Inappropriate Licking, Licking*

Lunar Periodicity

Physiological rhythms of animals living in tidal zones are often synchronized to those of the tides, and thus, moon phases. These recur in approximately 29.5-day cycles.

ALSO SEE: *Biological Rhythms*

Lying Down

The three basic techniques an animal can use to lie down or to get up are thoracic limbs first, pelvic limbs first, or both ends at the same time. While there are numerous combinations possible for both lying down and getting up, the following are the most common variations. Cattle lie down by tucking their forelimbs under them and with their rear end touching first. They get up by elevating their hindquarters before the chest comes off the ground. Dogs and cats are quite flexible in their variations, although the dog and cat tend to touch the ground and rise with both fore and rear halves of the body moving in approximately parallel units. Horses, swine, and some dogs will lie down so that their chests contact the ground first and get up with pressure on the forelimbs elevating the chest first; continued pushing then forces the back half up, too.

ALSO SEE: *Locomotion, Resting Behaviors*

Lying Out

Lying out is the name given to a young ungulate's behavior of lying in hiding while its mother grazes. Immobility is the defense against predators. After a period of time, the mother will return, and the infant will get up to interact with her. As exemplified by calves, the young suckle large quantities during a few nursing bouts each day. The behavior is often misunderstood by people who think deer fawns have been abandoned. The young have also been called hiders and layer-outs.

ALSO SEE: *Follower, Hiding, Layer Out, Lying-out Period, Maternal Behavior*

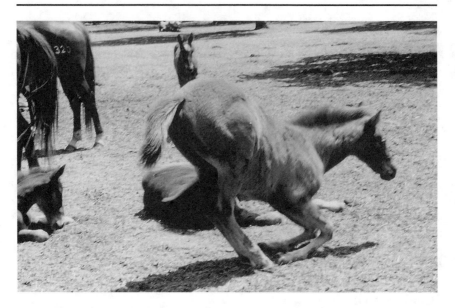

Lying Down. This foal shows the typical behavior of a horse starting to lie down by lowering its chest first.

Lying-out Period

The time when a juvenile ungulate rests in concealment while its mother grazes some distance away is called the lying-out period.

ALSO SEE: *Lying Out*

M

Macrosomatic Animals

Macrosomatic animals are those with a well-developed sense of smell. While this is a relative definition, most mammals are considered macrosomatic, with the exception of the primates and some others.

M

ALSO SEE: *Microsomatic Animals, Scent Marking, Smell*

Male Behaviors

Around the time of birth, male animals experience a testosterone surge that is responsible for masculinizing certain parts in the brain. Without that priming, the brain would continue to develop as feminine. The infants of both sexes mature similarly until the time of puberty, when the testosterone from the developing testicles triggers the development of behaviors generally associated with males of the species.

Behaviors typically associated with maleness are related to mating, marking, and roaming.

Selection for individuals that perform well in showing or on the race track may actually be selection against those that will do well as sires. While libido is not related to fertility, individuals that demonstrate interest in females often do not perform maximally. Then they will be less favored as sires. Those that do perform successfully may not have an interest in females or may be reluctant to show interest in females because of previous punishment for doing so. Following retirement, most males can be encouraged to express their natural behaviors again.

ALSO SEE: *Caterwauling, Coolidge Effect, Courtship, Decreased Sexual Behavior, Epigamic Traits, Estrous Behavior, Experienced Male, Fainting, Female Behaviors, Flehmen, Ground Rutting, Harem, Intention Movement, Kleptogamy, Masturbation, Maternal Failure, Mating Behavior, Mounting, Nape Bite, Postcopulatory Behavior, Rank Mimicry, Reestablish Dominance, Refractory Period, Reproductive Behavior, Sexually Dimorphic Behavior, Somnolent Impotence, Territory, Weaving*

Male Care

This is parental care of the young by males. The term is usually interpreted broadly to include any type of interaction between the male and the young, except aggression. While sucking does not result in a milk meal, some males will allow a juvenile to suck on them. An old gelding may allow a foal to suck on his prepuce without showing aggression, or a male dog may allow puppies to attempt to suckle his nipples.

Marking

Marking is a behavior used to call attention to an individual, area, or object. It can take on many forms, but they all depend on the senses to be distinguished.

Visual marking involves altering the terrain in such a way as to call attention. Humans might put up a flag or sign. Animals paw holes (bulls) or scrape the ground (dogs).

Vocalizations are another method used for marking. These are most commonly used in areas with dense growth to mark the location of one group of animals to avoid accidental interaction by others. Tomcats also vocalize to help delineate a territory.

Most marking is olfactory and thus involves chemical cues. Urine is one of the most widely used substances, as is well known for dogs, cats, and horses. Dogs urinate as information and on territorial boundaries. Cats mark territory and objects. Stallions urinate and/or defecate on the excreta of other horses after smelling it. In fact, several species develop dung heaps as a result of similar behavior. Normal body products such as sweat and saliva also are used for marking. Cats use the corners of the mouth to leave salivary odors on objects. Other body areas can have active modified sebaceous glands that serve the same functions. In tomcats, the feet, chin, and base of the tail are useful for marking. Special scent glands, such as carpal, periorbital, tarsal, and anal glands, produce unique odors that are sprayed or directly applied to objects like grass. The olfactory boundaries can be so strong as to stop an animal at a territorial edge as surely as a fence.

ALSO SEE: *Claw Sharpening, Head Rubbing, Scratching, Smell, Urination, Urine Spraying*

Masturbation

Masturbation is the behavior of self-stimulation of the genital area. In animals, the behavior is most commonly seen in bulls, stallions, dogs, and primates that have not had recent exposure to females. The behavior is learned and has its own internal reward, which increases the repeatability.

As a behavioral complaint, masturbation is reported more in dogs. The behavior can be initiated by licking of the penis or by rubbing against objects like a wadded-up rug or an owner's leg. In some cases the dog owner may be aware of a nearby estrous female, and her scent has triggered the lowest threshold—that for sexual behaviors. Masturbation occurs. Recommendations to manage the problem dog include avoiding excitement, increasing exercise before events that are likely to be exciting, and castration. Punishment is seldom successful because of the internal reward; however, diverting the dog's attention from this behavior may help.

Masturbation is a relatively common behavior in singly housed male laboratory primates. It is one of several behaviors, including the stereotypies, that may be coping behaviors used to minimize the perception of environmental stress.

Female animals can also masturbate. In dogs and cats, the animal raises itself from a sitting position with its forelimbs and swings like a pendulum.

ALSO SEE: *Atypical Sexual Behavior, Castration, Damming-up Theory, Divert Attention, Excessive Sexual Behavior, Exercise, Inappropriate Mounting, Internal Reward*

Material Protective Aggression

The protection or guarding of objects such as food, toys, or facial tissue is material protective aggression, a form of affective aggression. Since the behavior is self-rewarding, some animals make a game of it and use this success to climb in dominance. Material protective aggression is often a part of competitive aggression and hormonal imbalance aggression, particularly in pseudopregnancy.

ALSO SEE: *Affective Aggression, Competitive Aggression, Dominance, Hormonal Imbalance Aggression, Protective Aggression, Pseudopregnancy*

Maternal Aggression

Females with young show a strong protective reaction toward their offspring. This instinctive reaction is facilitated by the post-parturient hormonal state and the physical presence of the young. Neonatal distress vocalizations readily trigger maternal aggression, but the mere approach of a person or animal may be enough to initiate the response. The intensity of the reaction decreases with time because of changes in hormone levels and infant size. In females giving birth to a litter, any youngster's distress vocalization can excite the behavior. In horses and cattle, the call for help is responded to only when it is from the female's own offspring.

If it is necessary to temporarily separate the young from the dam, it is best to avoid as much stress as possible and keep the youngster between the handler and the dam. Few females will endanger their own young just to attack the intruder.

Maternal aggression is considered one type of nonaffective aggression. It is also regarded as a type of mobile aggression.

ALSO SEE: *Distress Call, Mobile Aggression, Nonaffective Aggression*

Maternal Behavior

Maternal behavior is the type of parental care given by a mother to her offspring. It begins with parturition and continues until the youngster goes out on its own. Much maternal behavior revolves around feeding the infants and giving them time to develop tastes and skills that allow them to survive to adulthood. Attention to the neonate varies between species. In dogs and cats, licking is important to stimulate respiration, remove the fetal membranes, and eventually orient the youngster toward the mammary area. In large domestic animals, mothers are attentive after the birth, and licking is useful to help the female imprint on a particular foal or calf. Wild species show an even greater maternal variation. At one extreme are turtles, which show no interest in the young; at the other are primates with their close mother-infant attachment.

Infant rejection occurs for a number of reasons. First, it is a normal behavior of weaning. It is also associated with environmental factors such as lack of food or water, new males, inappropriate scents on the young, or congenital anomalies. Stress within the area, improper hormone levels, and lack of maternal training are also factors. In many domestic species, maternal behavior was not a selection criteria during domestication or breed development, and it actually may have been selected against accidentally because of other criteria.

Maternal Failure

Maternal failure is a persistent negative reaction toward a newborn, primarily by not allowing it to nurse. There is a failure of milk let-down.

ALSO SEE: *Maternal Behavior, Rejection of Neonate*

Mating Behavior

Mating behavior is the intermediate phase of reproductive behavior, between the courtship and postmating phases. Mating begins with the mount and ends with ejaculation, and includes pelvic thrusts and intromission. Multiple mounts are common before intromission occurs.

Dogs show the most variation of this phase. Once intromission occurs, the male's bulbus glandis is held in place by the female's constrictor vestibuli muscles to form the tie. For 10 to 30 minutes, the two dogs are unable to separate. Also during the tie, the male dog will dismount, raise one hind limb over the back of the female, and twist so that the dogs are standing in opposite directions while still tied together. Females have been known to thrash around so much that they throw the male on the ground without the tie being pulled apart.

Boars also have a long ejaculation time (3 to 20 minutes, averaging 4 to 5 minutes); however, they do not form a tie.

ALSO SEE: *Courtship, Female Behaviors, Male Behaviors, Mounting, Postcopulatory Behavior, Reproductive Behavior, Appendix B*

Mating March

Mating march describes the close moving of a male and female associated with courtship behavior. The term was originally associated with ungulates where the stiff gait of the male resembled the goose step.

ALSO SEE: *Courtship*

Mating System

This describes the type of mating system used by a population or a species. Monogamy and polygamy are the most common types.

ALSO SEE: *Monogamy, Pair Bonding, Polygamy, Promiscuity, Reproductive Behavior*

M

Maturation

Maturation can be used to describe behavioral, physical, or neurological development over time. It usually implies changes from juvenile to adult characteristics. Behavioral maturation in its purest definition includes changes in behavior unrelated to learning, exercise, or physical changes. One example is leg raising by male dogs for urination, since this appears when testosterone levels are great enough. Physical maturation includes the loss of juvenile features, such as when head size becomes relatively smaller due to body growth. Neurological maturation can be followed with changes in reflexes and senses. For example, puppies at first show a crossed extensor reflex and eventually lose it. This reflex in an adult is considered abnormal.

ALSO SEE: *Increase Pet's Confidence, Juvenile Characteristics*

Mechanical Communication

Communication between conspecifics that uses noise produced external to the body and vocal apparatus is called mechanical communication. This includes sounds made by rubbing body parts together, as in clapping or leg rubbing, as well as hitting an object, as in pecking on wood or hitting a log with a stick.

ALSO SEE: *Communication Behaviors*

Medical Problems

One major category of causes of behavior problems is medical problems. While veterinarians ordinarily recognize such things as polyuria and polydipsia as associated with specific medical problems, that they can be primary behavior problems is an important concept. The reverse is also true. A significant number of behavior problems have a medical basis. A medical workup for a behavior problem is an important step in arriving at a specific diagnosis and developing an appropriate treatment protocol. It also may encourage the discovery of as yet unknown medical-behavior links.

ALSO SEE: *Atypical Narcolepsy, Catatonic Reaction, Coprophagia, Drug Therapy, Epileptic Aggression, Feces Eating, Food Allergy, History Taking, Hormonal Imbalance Aggression, Hydrocephalus, Hyper Syndromes, Hyperactivity, Hyperkinesis, Hyperthyroidism, Hypersexuality, Hypothyroid Aggression, Lick Granulomas, Medical Workup, Mental Lapse Aggression Syndrome, Narcolepsy, Organizing Behavioral Histories, Polydipsia, Polyphagia, Polyuria, Rolling Skin Syndrome, Seizures, Sex-related Aggression, Sexually Dimorphic Behaviors*

Medical Workup

Any animal presented for a behavior problem should first be evaluated medically, as subtle medical changes can be significant behaviorally. Increased aggression between family dogs may relate to retinal atrophy. Cervical pain can be presented as anorexia because the pain is too great for the animal to reach down to the food bowl. Specific problems related to medical conditions must also be eliminated before other courses of action are tried.

Detailed history taking is an important part of any medical workup, including one with behavioral overtones because it can help guide the way to a problem source. For example, the "funny look in its eyes" can indicate seizures, and a refusal to go out at night may signal a visual loss.

ALSO SEE: *History Taking, Medical Problems*

Mental Confusion

Apparent mental confusion is observed most commonly in animals immediately after a seizure, whether it is a classical form of seizure or a behavioral form. Dog owners recognize the post-ictal phase as confusion or as a contradictory personality in which the dog is biting during the seizure and seeking attention in the post-seizural phase. Cerebrovascular accidents and senility as a cause of mental confusion are not well documented in veterinary medicine.

ALSO SEE: *Epilepsy, Senile Aggression*

Mental Lapse Aggression Syndrome

This is a type of aggression in which a dog that has been a good family pet suddenly turns aggressively on family members and friends. The behavior change is dramatic and usually consistent. The typical history is that of a 1.5- to 2-year-old dog from one of the more popular breeds that has suddenly become very aggressive. On electroencephalograms (EEG) of anesthetized animals, this syndrome shows up as a low voltage-fast activity pattern. Since the EEG pattern is more like that of a wild animal than a dog and since the patient has no fear of humans, the dog represents a potentially serious danger to all humans. There is no known treatment, and the recommendation is euthanasia.

Mental lapse aggression syndrome should be differentiated from other types of aggression, especially dominance aggression which is much more common and not as consistent. Both types of aggression can coexist.

ALSO SEE: *Dominance Aggression, Euthanasia, Nonaffective Aggression, Rage Syndrome*

Microsomatic Animals

These are animals with poorly developed olfactory senses. Birds and primates are generally considered microsomatic.

ALSO SEE: *Macrosomatic Animals, Smell*

Middening

Midden means a dungheap. In behavioral terms, middening has been used to describe uncovered defecations by cats either outside the litter box or outdoors.

ALSO SEE: *Housesoiling—Defecation*

Migration

Migration is travel by a group of animals between locations, usually separated by a relatively great distance. This is most often associated with changes in the season. Types of animals range from insects, to birds, to mammals. Navigational aids are subject to a great deal of speculation.

ALSO SEE: *Homing*

Migratory Restlessness

At times when migratory animals begin their travel, there is a general restlessness within the group until the actual journey begins. This restlessness can also be observed in confined individuals.

ALSO SEE: *Migration*

Mimic Grin

The mimic grin is a canine facial expression associated with distance-reducing, friendly communications. In this expression of passive submission, the lips are pulled back showing the teeth. When first observed, the behavior is startling because of its similarity to the bared-teeth expression of aggression, but careful observation of the other body signs indicates that they are all distance reducing. For many mimic grinners, the behavior is directed only at the owner and a few other friends, and the grin may be used only when the dog is very excited.

ALSO SEE: *Distance-reducing Silent Communication, Passive Submission*

Mimicry

Some species that are not particularly dangerous have developed color patterns, a shape, or a behavior that mimics that of more dangerous species. The alternating colored bands of red, black, yellow, black, red of the Arizona king snakes are similar to the red, yellow, black, red bands of the poisonous coral snake. Mimicry also is used to attract food. The angler fish uses a wormlike projection to attract smaller fish within striking range.

ALSO SEE: *Stimulus Model*

Mixed Motivation

Mixed motivation occurs when more than one message is communicated at a time. An example is the mixture of growls and whines by a wolf to show dominance, but not too much, when greeting a cub. Ambivalent postures of canine body language, as with fear biters, also form a mixed signal, probably indicating internal uncertainty.

ALSO SEE: *Ambivalent Postures, Conflict*

Mixed-Species Group

This is a group of animals of several species existing in the same general location. The vast herds of animals of the African plains are a classic example, but the group could be as simple as a dog, a cat, and human, or horses, cattle, chickens, robins, and cottontail rabbits. From a defensive perspective, the variation in sensory abilities among the animals may increase mutual warning capabilities.

ALSO SEE: *Interspecific Releaser*

Mobile Aggression

Mobile aggression is a reactive anomaly shown toward a perceived threat, as in dogs where the animal moves aggressively toward an approaching individual. This type of response represents one of several types of normal forms of aggression. A cow shows maternal aggression in protecting her new calf. Geese may protect their territory. A dog may bite out of fear. Intrasexual aggression is also a common form of mobile aggression.

ALSO SEE: *Aggression, Fear-induced Aggression, Intrasexual Aggression, Maternal Aggression, Reactive Anomalies, Territorial Protective Aggression*

Mobile Alarm

Sudden flight from approaching potential danger can be termed mobile alarm. This is a common response in animals normally considered prey or those evolved from such animals. In domestic animals, much of the tendency to flee has been bred out; however, with prolonged confinement, individuals tend to accumulate energy and overreact to small stimuli. Exercise is useful for these animals. Some individuals will show a tendency to flightiness even when management systems are appropriate. In poultry the extreme of mobile alarm is called hysteria.

ALSO SEE: *Flightiness, Hysteria, Reactive Anomalies*

M

Modal Action Pattern

The modal action pattern is a more recent term applied to a fixed action pattern.

SEE: *Fixed Action Patterns*

Monogamy

Monogamy describes the mating system whereby a single male is mated with a single female. This pair bond may last through one reproductive cycle, several, or until the death of one of the pair.

ALSO SEE: *Mating System, Polygamy*

Monomorphism

Animals that show monomorphism have no differences in appearance or behavior within the species. This includes includes the lack of differences in appearance between males and females.

ALSO SEE: *Polymorphism*

Monosexual Syndrome

This is the sexual mounting of males by males to the exclusion of females. This term has been used to describe inappropriate mounting in bulls, rams, boars, and feedlot steers.

ALSO SEE: *Buller Steer Syndrome, Excessive Sexual Behavior, Homosexual Behavior, Inappropriate Mounting, Male Behaviors, Mounting*

Mood

Mood is a feeling or state of mind that can affect where a behavior occurs and how the sensory input will be processed. Mood and motivation are generally considered to interact with each other, although for some the two terms are equivalent.

ALSO SEE: *Central Filters, Motivation, Motivational State*

Mood Induction

Mood induction is the changing of an animal's mood. One animal can change from grazing to flight because of the flighty reaction of a nearby individual.

ALSO SEE: *Social Facilitation, Sympathetic Induction of Mood*

Mother-Infant Attachment

This is the strong bond between a mother and her young. The relationship is often associated with the mammalian bond, especially that of primates. The mother-infant attachment is important for infant care, feeding, protection, and learning. The longer the association between the dam and her offspring, the greater its relevance to juvenile learning. There are instinctive components that become greater or lesser depending on maturation of juvenile characteristics, changes in hormonal status, and nutritional factors. Once the bond is formed, separations before the normal transitional phase begins are stressful to both mother and infant. Separation at the end of weaning is generally well-tolerated, and the individual's recognition of the other thereafter varies. In most species there is no recognition. In others, the younger animal stays with the group and is occasionally disciplined or groomed by the mother.

ALSO SEE: *Maternal Behavior, Transitional Phase*

Motivation

Motivation is the desire or inner drive that causes an animal to do something. There are obvious connections with most behaviors that an animal exhibits, from hunting to play.

Motivation also has a direct influence on the rapidity of learning. An animal's motivations to get a specific reward, even an internal or poorly defined reward, or to avoid a punishment are important in the learning process. The degree of motivation varies among individuals. As a result, tests always have some degree of variability based on the desire of individual animals to get to the outcome. Food rewards are more acceptable to animals that have been held off food; however, for some individuals, food is not a strong motivational tool. The success of any learning project may depend on finding the strongest motivating factor for each individual.

ALSO SEE: *Drive, Hierarchy, Internal Reward, Learning, Learning Disposition, Mood, Praise, Priming Stimulus, Punishment, Reward*

Motivational Energy

Motivational energy refers to the amount of motivation needed before a behavior is expressed. The term hierarchy has also been used. The initiation of a single behavior or a series of behaviors has been well studied in several species. Cat predation on mice requires higher levels of motivational energy for killing the mouse than for stalking it in the first place. Newly introduced estrous cows are more likely to renew a bull's interest in breeding.

ALSO SEE: *Hierarchy, Motivation, Refractory Period*

Motivational State

This term is intended to describe the sum of the physiological and perceptual factors that influence an animal's reaction. The intent is to avoid the single-directional definitions associated with terms such as drive.

ALSO SEE: *Drive, Mood*

Mounting

Mounting is a behavior in which one animal raises the cranial part of its body on top of a conspecific. The behavior is usually associated with males mounting females for copulation. More than one mount may be necessary before intromission is achieved, and in some species, the nape bite precedes the actual mounting.

Several variations of mounting are associated with reproductive behavior. Pubertal and inexperienced males may mount several times without successful reproduction. They also may have an inappropriate orientation during these mounts, trying a side or even head approach. Animals not allowed access to females may begin to mount other males. This homosexual mounting usually stops when females are present. Young animals mount as a form of play, and estrous cows will mount other nearby cattle. Animals that are well socialized to another species and do not get to interact with their own kind may attempt to mount the other species, particularly when excited. This is particularly true for dogs and to a lesser extent for cats.

Mounting can also be associated with nonreproductive behaviors. Dogs mount (or stand on the shoulders) as a sign of dominance, and cats often mount other cats within their territory.

ALSO SEE: *Coital Misalignment, Excessive Sexual Behavior, Inappropriate Mounting, Male Behaviors, Monosexual Syndrome, Nape Bite, Pseudocopulation*

Mouth Play

The young of most species will play bite, nip, or mouth body parts of others nearby. This form of play probably serves to teach how to use the mouth aggressively and defensively in later life. It also is a time when the animal learns jaw pressure, the lesson that a specific amount of pressure causes pain. If a puppy bites its littermate, the littermate will yelp and stop play when it feels pain. If owners tolerate the pain of the puppy's playful bite "because it is cute," the dog learns that it takes a lot of pressure to cause pain. It will continue to bite harder than necessary as an adult.

Mouth play can also be a serious problem for people who work with yearling horses, particularly stallions. These horses are testing skills that will be useful for aggression as an adult.

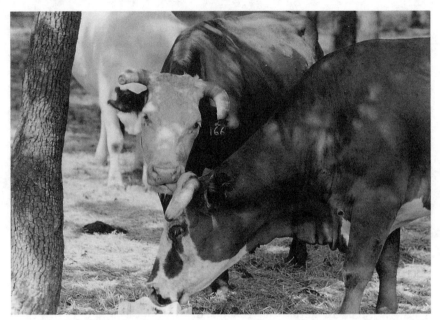

Mutual Grooming. While one cow licks a salt block, a second, lower-ranking cow licks the head of the first.

ALSO SEE: *Intrasexual Aggression, Male Behaviors*

Multimate Group

The multimate group is a social unit in which sexually active males and females live together. This is in contrast to the harem group with its single male. Primates have several variations of multimate groups.

ALSO SEE: *Harem, Reproductive Behavior*

Mutual Grooming

Mutual (social) grooming, also called allogrooming, is a behavior in which one individual grooms another. This probably occurs for several reasons. First, it serves a grooming function by caring for body areas that the individual has difficulty caring for by itself, typically the neck, head, or back. Primates often groom the backs of their conspecifics. Cats lick the necks of preferred associates, and horses use withers nibbling. A second function is social. In cattle, social order plays a role as to which animal does the grooming and which is groomed. Cows are generally groomed by lower-ranking ones. A third reason mutual grooming can occur is to defuse aggressive potential. A mutual grooming soliciting posture, presented by an animal that is the target of redirected aggression,

may help stop the attack and give the aggressive animal time to calm down.
ALSO SEE: *Cleaning Symbiosis, Grooming Behavior, Preferred Associate, Redirected Aggression, Social Behavior, Social Grooming, Withers Nibbling*

Muzzle

A muzzle is a device used to cover the mouth or prevent the jaws from being opened. It is used most commonly to keep dogs from biting. The cage or box-type muzzle can be used to prevent major injury by dogs while settling a dominance dispute, to stop self-mutilation by dogs or horses, to prevent destructive chewing by dogs or horses, and to decrease the chances of injury to the handler by a nippy yearling stallion.
ALSO SEE: *Cribbing, Licking of Objects, Pica, Wind Sucking*

Nape Bite

The nape bite is a bite directed at the dorsal neck. It can be an inhibited bite that does not penetrate the skin and is usually associated with sexual behaviors. Tomcats, dogs, and stallions bite the skin on the neck of the female just before or shortly after mounting. Territorial cats may also mount and use the nape bite on other cats that enter their territory. Queens and bitches use this inhibited bite to carry their young.

The term "nape bite" is also applied to the directional killing bite of a cat on its prey. The bite is aimed at a constriction between two wider areas, usually the head and shoulders. In the domestic cat, the kill is achieved when the canine teeth penetrate the spinal cord (Beaver, 1992).
ALSO SEE: *Death Shake, Extensor Dominance, Flexor Dominance, Male Behaviors, Maternal Behavior, Neck Bite, Predation*

Narcolepsy

Narcolepsy is a neurological disorder of the normal sleep mechanism, typically expressed as a sudden collapse (cataplexy) or sleeping of the animal. It has been diagnosed in humans, dogs, cats, horses, and cattle. The EEG is typical of REM sleep, and the EMG shows no recordable muscle tone. The reticular activating system is probably the region of the brain involved, and problems with a neurotransmitter are suspected.

ALSO SEE: *Atypical Narcolepsy, Drug Therapy, REM Sleep, Somnolent Impotence*

Neck Bite

Neck bite applies to (1) the aggressive bites used in fights between canids, (2) the bite used in prey killing, particularly by felids, (3) the grip used by male carnivores and birds during reproductive behavior, and (4) the hold used to carry young by their neck. The nape bite is a neck bite directed at the dorsal aspect of the neck.

ALSO SEE: *Nape Bite*

Neck Shake

For dogs, throat control in a fight is victory, since a prolonged struggle could result in suffocation. Humans can grab the skin on either side of a dog's neck or use a choke collar to transmit the same canine message. The neck shake has two advantages when working with dogs. It does not hurt them physically and thus cause pain-induced aggression, and it sends a message that is well understood.

ALSO SEE: *Distance-increasing Silent Communication*

Necrophobic Behavior

Necrophobic behavior is the carrying of bodies of conspecifics after they have died. The behavior is common in ants, as they remove the bodies from the nest. It is also used by some primate mothers after the death of their infant.

Negative Reinforcement

Negative or aversive stimuli become negative reinforcers when removed if they increase the probability of a behavioral response. The termination of pain or fear is a negative reinforcer and can be associated with aggression or escape. When a dog escapes through a window in response to thunder the level of fear may decrease. If the dog anticipates the thunder by sensing the ozone or barometric change, it may seek to come in before the storm arrives, thus using avoidance to end the negative stimuli. If a person steps on a dog's tail and the dog responds to the pain by biting, the aggression is a negative reinforcer if it ends the pain to the tail.

Negative reinforcement is distinct from punishment, although punishment may result in the expression of negative reinforcement.

ALSO SEE: *Positive Reinforcement, Punishment, Reward*

Neophobia

Neophobia is the fear of novel situations or objects. The degree of fear tends to decrease as familiarity increases. Thus, a new environment or object in that environment will gradually become less fearful to the animal. Curiosity and neophobia are conflicting.

ALSO SEE: *Investigative Behavior*

Neoteny

Neoteny is the general slowing of development relative to sexual maturation within a species and is a process that occurs over many generations. This could be expressed as delayed closure of epiphyseal plates, loss of deciduous teeth, or weaning relative to the onset of puberty.

Paedomorphosis, the retention of juvenile characteristics by an adult, is the extreme end of neoteny. Speeding up sexual development (progenesis) is similar to neoteny in the relative proximity of development and puberty but with a different approach.

ALSO SEE: *Paedomorphosis, Progenesis, Appendix B*

Neuroethology

Neuroethology is that part of behavioral physiology that studies the relationships between the central nervous system and behavior. This includes the senses, the brain's relation to specific behaviors, learning, and memory.

ALSO SEE: *Behavioral Physiology*

Neutral Object

This is the object toward which a behavior is redirected. When an animal is prevented from getting something that it is strongly motivated to get, the goal may be redirected toward a neutral, nonrelative object. This is common in redirected aggression, but can also be seen in the use of novel items for nesting materials or in puppy substitutes during pseudopregnancy.

ALSO SEE: *Pseudopregnancy, Redirected Aggression*

New Baby

A new baby in the family can be upsetting to a pet. The main problem usually begins shortly after the baby comes home, when the novelty of the infant is strongest. As a result, the schedule of human interaction with the dog or cat changes drastically, and the animal responds to the change by marking its territory or seeking attention. The animal's actions may be misinterpreted by the new parents, resulting in the pet being isolated even more. There are several ideas that can be implemented by the expectant parents. The pet should be gradually shifted to a schedule that can be maintained after the baby arrives. Let the animal have fun with the owner in the baby's room, rather than making it off-limits. Get it accustomed to the smells of the room.

If the baby is already home when the client seeks help, the parents can schedule fun time in the baby's room and lots of interaction and fun with the baby present.

The child's safety is paramount, so protection is best ensured by not leaving the pet and the baby together unsupervised. Cats do not "suck the baby's breath." A cat may show interest in the milk-breath smell. It might be possible for a large cat to stop a tiny infant from breathing by lying on the baby's chest. More commonly, however, the cat goes into hiding when the infant cries and only gradually learns to associate with the new family member. With a dog and an infant, the danger increases when the baby starts crawling and can grab an ear or handfuls of hair. The animal may respond instinctively with pain-induced aggression. Another behavior should concern a dog owner. Some dogs become nervous when a baby cries loudly and either begin pacing back-and-forth between the owner and the baby or try to escape to a distant corner of the house. Parents sometimes interpret this as protective behavior, as if the dog is trying to tell them that the baby is upset. In reality the dog is upset and is seeking comfort from the owner. If it does not receive that comfort, it may eventually attack the source of the noise. That dog should be removed from the household or strictly shielded from the stressful events.

ALSO SEE: *Schedule*

New Home

Behavior problems are not always solvable in a given set of environmental conditions, and mismatches in personalities between owner and animal may not be correctable. In such cases, an appropriate recommendation might be to place the animal in a new home. The suggestion could be one of several given when the timid person is matched with a more dominant dog. If the animal is likely to be a problem for the new owners (such as the chronically housesoiling cat, a fear-biting dog, or a horse with a dominant personality), this is not a valid recommendation.

Nidicolous Nestlings

Bird chicks that remain in the nest for extended periods of time and are dependent on parental care are called nidicolous nestlings. They are altricial young.

Nidicolous nestlings are the opposite of nidifugous ones.
ALSO SEE: *Altricial Animals, Nidifugous Nestlings*

Nidifugous Nestlings

Baby birds that are generally well-developed when hatched and rely on their parents primarily to lead them to food are called nidifugous nestlings. Domestic poultry are included because of their precocial nature.
ALSO SEE: *Nidicolous Nestlings, Precocial Animal*

No

"No" can be a magical word when used with certain types of behavior problems. When coupled with a leash jerk, a tug on the halter rope, or some other form of reprimand, an undisciplined animal may suddenly be made aware of the wishes of its owner. The owners have been telling the dog that it should not be doing a particular thing, but their tone of voice and petting actually reinforce the undesirable behavior. An obedience class or some other appropriate instruction in correct training methods should follow to teach the animal how to respond and the owner how to give commands.
ALSO SEE: *Aggression and Telephones, Direct Punishment, Dog Collars, Dominance Aggression, Establish Dominance, Obedience Class, Reestablish Dominance*

No Attention to Behaviors

By trial and error, animals can learn to use a particular behavior to get an owner's attention. An outdoor dog barked one night because it heard a neighbor's dog bark. The owner yelled at the dog, giving it attention. After a few similar episodes, the dog would bark to get attention. A cat's meow in the middle of the night results in the owner filling the food bowl. Soon, the owner is unable to sleep through an entire night. When owner attention, food, or other reward is involved, the problem often can be stopped by simply not giving the reward. At first the animal may try even harder; however, it quickly learns the game plan has changed, and the behavior decreases. This technique is called extinction.
ALSO SEE: *Extinction, Learning, Trial and Error Learning*

Nonaffective Aggression

Aggression can be categorized in a number of different ways. The simplest format consists of two divisions—affective and nonaffective, based on physiological parameters. Nonaffective aggression represents a broad category of aggression without autonomic activation. Subdivisions are clinically more practical. Those of nonaffective aggression are often, but not always, characterized by an attack without warning. In some cases, the victim did not notice the appropriate signs. Included within this category are play aggression, maternal aggression, predatory aggression, sex-related aggression, and several medical types.

ALSO SEE: *Affective Aggression, Maternal Aggression, Play Aggression, Predatory Aggression, Sex-related Aggression*

Nonverbal Communication

Nonverbal communication includes the use of body position, facial expressions, odor secretion, piloerection, and tail position to indicate particular signals. It is the use of body language and is also called silent communication.

ALSO SEE: *Body Language, Distance-increasing Silent Communication, Distance-reducing Silent Communication, Pheromone*

Normal Behavior

Understanding normal behaviors is the first important criteria for working with behavior problems. There are many complaints about an animal's behavior that are the result of the person not recognizing what is normal for that species or breed. In a differential diagnosis list, the veterinarian must separate not only objectionable from unobjectionable, but also normal from abnormal. Client education and minor adjustments can minimize the negative aspects of the normal but objectionable situation. For example, the dog that is licking too loudly at night can be made to sleep in another room.

Complaints for loud licking, jumping on counters, or not coming to an extremely dominant person are common, and they are often made by owners who do not truly recognize that animals are different from humans. Some of the animals may even be rewarded for some of these behaviors.

Treatment consists of finding an alternative the owner can use. Loud lickers may need to spend the night in another room. Countertops may have to be booby trapped to allow indirect punishment, as long as there is another more acceptable location for the behavior.

ALSO SEE: *Indirect Punishment, Jumping on People, Loud Licking, No Treatment, Organizing Behavioral Histories, Trial and Error Learning*

Nose Rubbing

Nose rubbing is a behavior problem shown by swine, and occasionally by dogs and cats. Called snout rubbing in pigs, it seems to be associated with crowding, and may represent a stereotyped behavior. An individual dog or cat may rub its nose for a prolonged time on the carpet, floor, walls, dirt, or other object, even until it bleeds.

ALSO SEE: *Snout Rubbing, Stereotyped Behavior, Testosterone-induced Aggression in Mares*

No Treatment

Normal behaviors that are not understood or appreciated by the owners may not require treatment. Instead, client education is the most appropriate course of action. It may also be possible to find a slight modification in lifestyle that will allow the normal behavior to continue, but no longer be considered a problem. For example, a dog that sleeps on the bed may groom itself at night, but the owners consider the licking to be too loud. Moving the dog to another room at night can be a workable solution.

ALSO SEE: *Normal Behavior*

Nursing

Nursing has two behavioral definitions. One is the maternal behavior of allowing the young to suckle. Included are the behaviors that call the young to the dam, the presenting postures, milk let-down, and the behaviors while the young eat.

Ingestion of milk by the young from a mammary gland is the other definition of nursing. Sucking allows the young to get milk as their primary source of nutrition until they can develop physically or learn what is necessary for adult-like eating patterns. The gradual change between nursing and eating occurs during the transitional phase.

Puppies nurse while the bitch is lying down, and they use their forelimbs to knead the mammary region. The kneading and sucking alternate. Two theories have been proposed for kneading. One is that it helps stimulate milk flow. The second is that it pushes the mammary tissue out of the puppy's face, making breathing easier. There is probably some validity to both theories because of variations in the behavior with age. The transitional stage in which solid foods and nursing exist together begins around 3 weeks.

Kittens also knead while nursing. The behavior begins at a slightly older age than in puppies and may be associated more with milk stimulation. Feline kneading behavior is usually retained into adulthood, when it becomes associated with times considered to be "pleasurable" to the cat. Within the first 5 days after birth, sucking may be limited to a specific one or two teats per kitten, resulting in a characteristic hair pattern around the dam's nipples. The sense of smell is used by the kitten to help locate its specific teat. The transitional stage begins around 5 weeks.

Foals nurse a mare by standing parallel to her but facing in the opposite direction. The foal lowers and stretches its head and neck to allow it to grasp a teat. Nursing is initiated by the foal approximately twice each hour, with each period lasting less than 2 minutes.

Since calves do not follow their mothers as foals do, the number of nursing periods is fewer (4 to 5 times daily), and the duration is longer (10 minutes or more). Variation occurs between beef and dairy calves, probably because of the difference in the dam's milk production compared to the needs of the growing calf. While the cow must be standing for suckling to occur, the calf's position is more variable than that of the foal. The sucking reflex helps close the rumino-reticular groove to help shunt the milk directly to the abomasum, bypassing the rumen. When calves drink from a bucket instead of nurse, the groove does not close, and the milk goes into the rumen.

Nursing piglets show some unique behaviors. The teat order is the most outstanding because it is associated with teat preferences, differential growth, and social orders. Unlike cats and dogs, sows do not randomly nurse individual piglets. When one or more indicate an interest, the sow will grunt for all to take their position as she positions herself. After a minute or two nosing phase, a short quiet period precedes the brief, true sucking. Sucking by neonates occurs approximately hourly, but the intervals increase as the piglets get older.

Non-nutritional sucking can be a problem in any species. It is generally associated with orphans or with youngsters that do not suckle. Pendulous body parts, such as the prepuce, scrotum, vulva, ear, or lip, are sucked most commonly. Although non-nutritional sucking is usually directed toward littermates or others, the behavior can be self-directed too. Prolonged sucking in cats is one variation. Resulting problems include hairballs and retarded growth.

ALSO SEE: *Presentation, Prolonged Sucking, Teat Order, Transitional Phase*

Nursing Position

This is the body position taken by the young while they suckle. In general, species that typically have a large number of young require the mother to present her abdomen, so lying is the typical nursing position. Ungulates have few offspring nursing at a time and the udder is confined, so the young usually stand to nurse, facing caudally. In a few species, mainly primates, the young grasp the mother and hang on to nurse.

During the transitional stage of nursing, as carnivores start the weaning process, the position of the young may have to change to sitting or standing.

ALSO SEE: *Negative Reinforcement, Transitional Phase*

Obedience Class

Obedience classes may be given with a trainer working the dog or with the dog owner learning how to give a command and to follow through. Both types teach the dog how to respond appropriately to a command. Other lessons are more subtle, such as how to respond even with other people and dogs around. There are several techniques used to accomplish the same general goal. Some types of courses are extremely physical. Others work the dogs off leash or with collars other than the usual chain choke collars. Still others use food rewards with praise for motivation. No one way is right or wrong. Each will be right for some types of dogs and wrong for others. Advanced obedience classes involve retrieving, jumping, and tracking.

Many problem behaviors occur because a dog has been allowed to do what it wants. In some cases, dominance is not clearly established. If young dogs are taken through an obedience class, the number of problems later in life may be reduced. However, the fact that a dog has been through an obedience class does not guarantee that problem behaviors will never develop.

ALSO SEE: *Dog Collars, Dominance Aggression, Establish Dominance, No, Reestablish Dominance*

Obesity

Obesity is the condition of having an excessive amount of body fat. This results from not expending enough energy to use up the calories eaten and/or the intake of an excessive number of calories relative to body needs.

Dogs and cats on modern commercial diets have an increased tendency for obesity. These diets are generally very palatable and calorie dense. Livestock show judges have tended to emphasize "bloom," and consumer taste has favored excessive amounts of fat, so obesity in large animals is actually promoted.

Neurologically, the hypothalamus contains both the hunger and the satiety centers. Destructive or irritative lesions in either area can have a profound effect on how much an animal eats.

ALSO SEE: *Brain, Excessive Food Intake, Ingestive Behavior, Polyphagia*

Observational Learning

Observational learning occurs when one animal watches another animal show a particular behavior and then performs the same behavior when given the opportunity. Studies in domestic animals indicate observational learning does occur. One kitten, raised with a German shepherd male, would lift his leg by a tree when he urinated (Beaver, 1992).

ALSO SEE: *Learning, Local Enhancement, Operant Conditioning*

Obsessive Compulsive Disorders

According to the American Psychiatric Association (1987), an obsession is a persistent idea, thought, impulse, or image that is experienced, at least initially, as intrusive and senseless. A compulsion is a repetitive, purposeful, and intentional behavior performed in a stereotyped fashion in response to an obsession. The compulsion functions to neutralize or prevent discomfort and is clearly excessive. Attempts to resist the compulsion result in mounting tension, which is immediately relieved when the compulsive behavior is again performed. Obsessive compulsive disorders severely interfere with normal routine, including social relations.

ALSO SEE: *Psychomotor Agitation, Stereotyped Behaviors*

Offensive Threat

Offensive threats are distance-increasing silent communication postures shown by cats that approach with the intent of having the other cat leave. It is a direct approach, with a stare and open mouth. One forepaw may be raised or swung and growling may be voiced.

ALSO SEE: *Defensive Threat, Distance-increasing Silent Communication, Pariah Threat*

Olfactory Tractotomy

Surgically removing caudal parts of the olfactory bulbs and severing the olfactory tracts from the rest of the brain have successfully stopped inappropriate urination and spraying in a few very refractory cats (Hart, 1982). Although the procedure is not frequently done, it does offer an alternative to euthanasia for the desperate cat owner.

ALSO SEE: *Housesoiling—Spraying, Housesoiling—Urination*

Open-Field Test

The open-field test is a method used to quantify variables such as locomotion or level of anxiety. It usually is done in a contained "field" that has been divided visually into units of space for the purpose of being able to count the times each unit is entered. An open-field test has been used to monitor responses after varying periods of confinement in different stall types, a concern to the veal-calf industry and laboratory animal facilities.

Operant Conditioning

Operant (instrumental) conditioning is a type of learning based on initial studies by E. L. Thorndike and later work by B. F. Skinner. A behavior is primarily influenced by its effects. Skinner described the response in terms of the positive or negative reinforcer that either preceded or followed. Traditionally, trial and error learning is equated with operant conditioning; however, habituation, latent, imprint, observational, and insight learning are also included in the broadest definition.

ALSO SEE: *Habituation Learning, Imprint Learning, Insight Learning, Latent Learning, Learning, Negative Reinforcement, Observational Learning, Positive Reinforcement, Skinnerian Shaping of Behavior, Trial and Error Learning*

Organizing Behavioral Histories

Once the history of a problem has been obtained, the information must be organized to help put the problem into perspective. The behavior is objectionable to the owners, since that is the nature of their concern; however, it is common during history taking to learn of other abnormal behaviors that are not considered objectionable. For example, a dog may be presented for eating expensive plants, but it may also be eliminating in the house.

Another determination that is important is whether the problem is a normal behavior that the owner does not recognize as normal, whether it is an inappropriate behavior for the circumstances, or whether it is "abnormal." Since animals have only a limited number of behaviors they can express, problems are most commonly the inappropriate expression of a normal behavior. Barking is normal, but barking for eight hours is inappropriate. Grooming to the point of self-mutilation is also inappropriate. Normal behavior cannot be eliminated, but alternatives can be sought that will satisfy the owner. Loud licking can be tolerated if the pet stays in another part of the house. Litter flung out of the litter box can be controlled by using a box with a cover or higher sides. The "abnormal" behaviors may be subdivided into genetic problems, medically related problems, improper socialization, and "frustration" or stress-related problems. Each of these can be subdivided more specifically.

ALSO SEE: *Aggression—History Taking, Frustration, Genetic Problems, History Taking, Housesoiling—History Taking, Improper Socialization, Medical Problems, Normal Behavior, Stress-related Behaviors, Appendix A*

Orientation

The ability of a plant or animal to orient its body with respect to an environmental stimulus is called orientation. The actual movement is a taxis, with a positive taxis being a movement of the head toward the source of the stimulus, as with nursing by a foal. The type of stimulus, such as light or gravity, can also name the taxis (phototaxis, geotaxis).

Migration uses orientation, although the stimuli may be very complex.

ALSO SEE: *Migration*

Orienting Reflex

When a sharp noise sounds or a bright light flashes, individuals will orient toward it. It probably serves some role in alerting an animal to potential danger so that flight or fight reactions could follow. The orienting reflex develops in infants at a rate parallel to that of the nervous system. Puppies are not born with reactions to sights or sounds; however, within several weeks puppies will orient to these stimuli. Foals respond within hours.

Orthokinesis

Orthokinesis is when an animal escapes an undesirable location or situation and the speed of movement away is in direct proportion to the severity of the stimulus. Initially the speed is fast, but as the animal moves away and the conditions improve, the rate of movement slows.

ALSO SEE: *Kinesis*

Ovariectomy (Ovariohysterectomy)

The surgical removal of ovaries from a female animal is called an ovariectomy. An ovariohysterectomy is the removal of the ovaries and uterus.

Behavior changes associated with removal of ovaries are variable. Certainly, the female shows neither pregnancy nor estrous cycles. (There are, however, a few exceptions to this last point relative to biological/circadian rhythms.) For animals such as cats, the resulting consistency in behavior is noticeable, while for species such as cattle, the change is almost imperceptible. In dogs, the behavior change is minimal, affecting only the few weeks each year when estrogens would have caused a slight increase in activity. The lack of an estrous discharge is also obvious.

Although an ovariectomy or ovariohysterectomy results in minimal changes for a behaviorally normal individual, the procedure is indicated to prevent pregnancy and to treat pseudopregnancy. In cases of testosterone-induced aggression in mares caused by ovarian involvement, removal of the ovaries also is indicated.

Approximately 47% of female dogs and 31% of female cats have undergone an ovariohysterectomy (Wilbur, 1976). The main differences between the species that contribute to the discrepancies are the inconveniences of estral bleeding in the bitch and the tendency in the past for many female cats to be outdoor pets.

ALSO SEE: *Biological Rhythms, Pseudopregnancy, Testosterone-induced Aggression in Mares*

Over-Grooming

In general, the term over-grooming is used for excessive grooming or excessive licking.

SEE: *Excessive Grooming, Excessive Licking, Self-Licking*

Overshadowing

The simultaneous reduction in the influence of multiple stimuli by working on one is called overshadowing. When a problem behavior has a single overpowering stimulus among several, minimizing the influence of the one stimulus can also decrease the effect of the other stimuli as well. A fear of thunder can lead to an associated fear of barometric pressure changes, ozone, or other stimuli related to storms. By working on the thunderphobia, the other fears are lessened at the same time.

ALSO SEE: *Fear of Thunder*

Owner Protective Aggression

Owner protective aggression is a form of affective aggression in which the animal protects its owner in a situation that the pet perceives as dangerous.

In dogs, the reaction is considered instinctive for the protection of a pack member. In the wild canids, pack members will protect higher-ranking members to ensure survival of the pack. Since humans are generally regarded as higher ranking by their dogs, protection is likely if the dog perceives danger for the person. Concern for protection has caused people to "test" their animal, often resulting in confusion or disappointment with the results. The situation may not be real enough to elicit the hoped-for behavior since the odors of fear were not present, or there may have been confusion if the family members were fighting among themselves. In that case, the dog usually sides with the highest-ranking person. This protective behavior may be reserved for the owners only or generalized to all people. In either case it produces our dog heros. Some dogs, however, should not be relied on to show owner protective aggression. Included in that group are puppies, toy dog breeds (because they were developed to retain puppy characteristics, including behavior), and terriers (because they are more catlike in their independence and territoriality). Owners inadvertently have taught dogs to show aggression to all visitors and then worried that the dog will bite friends. This does not represent true owner protection aggression, but rather a learned aggression.

Cat heroes do exist even though the species is considered asocial. Cats that save an owner from a burning building are usually trying to ensure their own escape. However, cats have been known to protect people by attacking snakes, intruders, or other aggressive cats.

ALSO SEE: *Affective Aggression, Asocial, Hero, Protective Aggression, Unconsciously Learned Aggression*

P

Pack Response Aggression

This is an aggressive behavior seen in some dog colonies and in multi-dog households in which dogs that have been together a long time suddenly turn on one individual in their pack and kill it. In the colony situation, the animals have been geriatric, so senility may be a factor. A second possible explanation is that this type of attack is a method of protecting the pack. If an individual yelps in severe pain, it might trigger a pack response to kill, so that large predators are not attracted to the distress cries. In some cases, there is evidence that the dog that was killed had been caught in a fence, making this theory possible.

ALSO SEE: *Cannibalism, Senile Aggression*

Paedomorphosis

Paedomorphosis is the retention of juvenile characteristics by adults. Toy dog breeds have been selectively bred to retain puppy features. Underdeveloped physical features include the relatively large, rounded heads (often with cranial fontanelles that do not close), poor cranial muscle development, and retained deciduous teeth. Learning patterns can also be affected, since toy breeds can be more difficult to housebreak. (Certain other factors may also result in difficult housebreaking as well.)

Paedomorphosis is the extreme of neoteny.

ALSO SEE: *Child Schema, Juvenile Characteristics, Neoteny*

P

Pain-induced Aggression

Pain can cause an animal to react aggressively, especially if there is no easy method to escape. A few individuals are stoic and will not respond aggressively; however, this is probably more of an exception. The actual attack is often inhibited, representing a warning rather than an attempt to do harm.

Around the eighth week, puppies experience the beginning of stable learning. At this time they are particularly vulnerable to a traumatic experience. A painful experience, which could include a vaccination, can result in a dog that wants nothing to do with an associated person or environment. A shock of static electricity from the hand of a little girl reaching to pet a puppy could cause the puppy to "hate that little girl," "hate all little girls," "hate all children," "hate all people," or have no effect at all. If severe enough, trauma at a later age for the dog can produce similar results. Since young children tend to pull themselves up by grabbing a dog's hair, ear, or tail, pain-induced aggression toward them is common.

Prevention of the painful experiences is the only sure way to prevent pain-induced aggression. Since dog owners are particularly concerned about repeated aggression, it is important for them to understand that each episode involving pain is an isolated event and not indicative of the animal turning on them.

ALSO SEE: *Affective Aggression, Aversion-induced Aggression, Frustration-induced Aggression, Socialization*

Pair Bonding

Pair bonding describes the attraction between members of a mated pair. It can be short term, as during a single mating, or can extend as long as the partners live.

ALSO SEE: *Bond, Dissociation, Harem, Long-Term Pair Bond, Mating System, Monogamy, Polygamy, Reproductive Behavior*

Pandiculation

Pandiculation is the combined behavior of a group when several members stretch at the same time. It appears as if the stretching by one member triggers the behavior in the others. This form of coordinated stretching is also noted in humans.

ALSO SEE: *Stretching*

Paradoxical Sleep

Paradoxical sleep is another term used to describe rapid eye movement (REM) sleep.

SEE: *REM Sleep*

Parental Care

Parental care is the care of juveniles by the mother and/or the associated male. In general, this care includes all types of interactions except aggression. While maternal care is the general rule, individual males may spend large amounts of time tending the young. Male birds often are involved in feeding the young. Extremes are shown by brooder fish males, which protect fertilized eggs by keeping them in the mouth, and by sea horse males, which hatch the eggs in their own brood pouch and go through parturition.

ALSO SEE: *Male Care, Maternal Behavior*

Parental Investment

This term is used to describe the amount of time and effort used by a parent for its young. The mother generally has a greater amount of time invested in her young as compared to the father. It has been theorized that the greater the investment, the greater the likelihood that the infant will survive and ultimately reproduce.

ALSO SEE: *Maternal Behavior, Parent-Offspring Conflict, Sociobiology*

Parent-Offspring Conflict

In sociobiology, parent-offspring conflict has been used to describe the potential friction that can occur between a mother's (or father's) needs and the interests of the young. This conflict has been used to describe the onset of the transitional phase of ingestive behavior and weaning, with food gathering becoming too difficult both to sustain the parent and meet the youngster's needs.

ALSO SEE: *Parental Investment, Transitional Phase*

Pariah

Cats do not have a dominance order such as that typically found in social species. Instead, their relationship is related to territory. A territorial tomcat is the primary owner of a space and may be considered the top-ranking cat when in that space. Most of the other cats would be in more or less equal middle positions, and one or two cats would be of very low rank, the pariahs. The pariahs are stressed in the presence of the territorial cat and show a crouched threat posture to him. If there is too much interaction between the high- and low-ranking cats, the pariahs may choose to leave the territory.

ALSO SEE: *Asocial, Dominance, Pariah Aggression, Pariah Threat*

Pariah Aggression

A pariah responds to the approach of the territorial tomcat with a pariah threat display. The encounters are brief if the pariah can leave, but when it cannot, the pariah cat may increase the threat to aggression. Complaints about feline aggression should include information about the cat's posture. When aggression is directed toward the owner, the history of the cat showing a crouched posture before the aggression indicates that the cat is treating the owner as it would a territorial tomcat. Since owners do not recognize this as a threat posture, they continue the interaction until the cat must lash out to end the encounter. Pariah aggression is best managed by decreasing the amount of direct interaction between the cat and the other cat or person that triggers the pariah response.

ALSO SEE: *Pariah, Pariah Threat*

Pariah Threat

This is a lateral, crouched posture used by the cat to indicate distance-increasing silent communication. The eyes usually stare at the intruder, and the ears are usually flattened. Growling or hissing may also occur. Piloerection and the arched back are not seen with this type of threat.

ALSO SEE: *Defensive Threat, Distance-increasing Silent Communication, Offensive Threat, Pariah, Pariah Aggression*

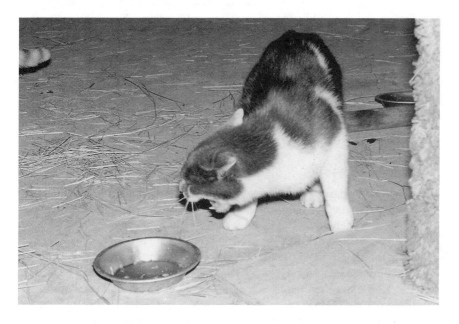

Pariah Threat. The cat is showing the lowered body posture of the pariah threat as the territorial cat approaches.

Parturition

The birth process can be divided into four phases. The contraction phase is the time when uterine contractions begin and increase in frequency and duration. Externally, the behaviors are normal except that there is a general increase in restlessness. Dogs, cats, pigs, and other species that give birth to several young may show a great deal of attention to their nests.

The emergence phase is generally brief, since it is the time when the young enters the birth canal. The chorioallantois breaks from the pressure of the narrow space, allowing a watery fluid to be expelled.

Delivery is the third phase, when the actual expulsion of the young occurs. How the amnioallantois is opened so the newborn can breathe varies somewhat by species. The hooves of young ungulates usually break the membranes during passage through the birth canal. Bitches and queens will bite the membrane open as they clean the infant. The umbilical cord can be broken by the dam (dog and cat), during passage through the birth canal (cattle and sheep), or by the actions of the young (horses and pigs). Foals can recover a considerable volume of blood from the membranes during the time between birth and breakage.

The placental phase is last. There is usually a delay after delivery of the neonate until the placenta is shed. For species that give birth to multiple young, a second or third delivery can occur before the passage of one or more of the placentas. The females in some mammalian species will then eat these membranes. For species that stay in the birth area (dogs, cats, swine), the placenta can provide nourishment, since they cannot go after food for themselves. For species such as cattle, consumption of the placenta provides a means of protecting the hiding area from predators. Foals are rapidly mobile so there is little value for the mare to eat the placenta.

Specific durations and intervals relative to parturition are listed in Appendix B.

ALSO SEE: *Maternal Behavior, Appendix B*

Passive Submission

Passive submission is one type of distance-reducing silent communication used by dogs. An individual uses one or more species-specific body postures to communicate a friendly message. While these postures are well defined and tend to occur in a given order, they do not have to occur in that order. Diverted eye contact is the simplest and usually the first sign shown. Head position includes flattened, lowered ears with a lowered head and neck. The tongue may be flicked in and out, or it may be used to lick the other animal. Thus, licking is a sign of submission. The tail is down, even between the legs, and it may be wagged or held still. The dog will show a lowering of its body. This may range from a slight crouch to complete lying down. Rolling over probably represents ultimate submission, since it exposes the abdomen, which is the only vital part of the body that lacks bony protection. Submissive urination is another behavior associated with passive submission.

A note of caution about two of the body postures: The lowered head, neck, and ears are also associated with a threat in canine distance-increasing silent communication. Motion in the tail can also be deceiving since a very rapid or deliberate back-and-forth flagging is a threat that can be misinterpreted as tail wagging.

When working with a dog showing passive submission, a person should not show excessive dominating, distance-increasing signs. The very submissive dogs may become fearful and bite if a threat such as eye contact continues. For these dogs, it is important to decrease the body threat to prevent fear biting and to gain the dog's confidence.

ALSO SEE: *Appeasement Behavior, Decrease Body Threat, Distance-increasing Silent Communication, Distance-reducing Silent Communication, Fear-induced Aggression, Licking, Submissive Behavior, Submissive Urination, Tail Wagging*

Pavlovian Conditioning

Pavlovian conditioning is the type of learning also known as classical conditioning. It involves the pairing of a conditioned and unconditioned stimulus until the conditioned stimulus produces the same result as the unconditioned one.

ALSO SEE: *Classical Conditioning*

Pawing

Pawing is the swing-forward, draw-back motion of a forelimb. Under natural conditions, animals use the behavior to uncover food. Grazing animals, in particular, paw to remove snow from grass.

Pawing can also be preliminary to aggressive behavior. In that context it may serve as a threat or as a mechanism to relieve tension when an actual bout cannot occur or is undesirable. In the latter situation, pawing would be considered a distance-increasing behavior or a displacement activity. Bulls often paw and rub their horns to form dirt wallows, frequenting these places when aggressive tensions are high.

Pawing has a third meaning. Horses paw during times of apparent anticipation or impatience. This is commonly associated with waiting to be fed or turned out, or with being tied in one location such as to a trailer or in the alleyway of a barn.

ALSO SEE: *Displacement Activity, Distance-increasing Silent Communication, Scratching, Stress-related Behaviors*

Peak Approach Period

This is a period of time during an animal's socialization period when it will actively approach members of its own or other species. While this behavior is generally recognized, it has been best defined in puppies (Fox, 1965), where the peak approach period is between 5 and 7 weeks of age.

ALSO SEE: *Socialization*

Peak Avoidance Period

During the socialization period, an animal is relatively interested in interacting with other animals. Once this individual has completed this period, interaction with strange animals is avoided. This is the beginning of the peak avoidance period. After a while the extreme avoidance is gradually minimized. Environmental exploration generally increases during this time as well.

In puppies, the peak avoidance period begins at approximately 12 weeks of age (Fox, 1965), while in kittens it is closer to 9 weeks (Beaver, 1992).

ALSO SEE: *Socialization*

Peck Order

Peck order is a term that refers to the social order of a group of individuals. Peck order is most appropriate when it refers to the ranking within a group of birds.

ALSO SEE: *Social Order*

Perceptive Distance

The perceptive distance is the point at which an animal is aware of an approacher. For both predators and prey, this awareness is usually triggered by movement. The reaction following perception depends on factors such as what is approaching, distance, speed of movement, location, and "mood." This is one of the social (reactive) distances.

ALSO SEE: *Investigative Distance, Reactive Distances, Social Distance*

Peripheral Filters

Peripheral filters are an individual's senses. These filters determine which environmental stimuli can enter the body to be evaluated. While human vision does not include the ultraviolet spectrum, insects or birds that can perceive that range have a different view of the world. So do insects with compound eyes, those with good low-light vision, and blind individuals. If something in the environment cannot be perceived, it cannot be acted upon.

ALSO SEE: *Central Filters, Filters, Hearing, Smell, Taste, Vision*

P

Peripheral Male

This is another term for satellite male.

SEE: *Satellite Male*

Personal Distance

An animal's personal distance is a space immediately surrounding the individual within which are allowed preferred associates. For other individuals who approach but do not have this close relationship, the inward boundary of the social distance is the limit of approach. When a stranger violates personal distance, the animal may react by moving away, pushing the intruder back, or attacking the stranger. Consider your own reaction to a stranger moving in closely.

A veterinarian must work within an animal's personal distance in order to make an examination. Thus, it is best to take a little time when approaching to let the animal become acquainted and accepting.

ALSO SEE: *Individual Distance, Intimate Distance, Preferred Associate, Social Distance*

Personality

A personality is a deeply ingrained pattern of behavior that includes all aspects of how an individual relates to the environment. Individual animals have unique personalities, just like people. While there are many variations, at least some are genetically determined. The full extent of timidity, aggression, fear biting, and other traits is currently not well understood. The classic work by J. P. Scott and J. L. Fuller (1965) gave a glimpse at how involved the genetics of behavior might be.

ALSO SEE: *Aggressive Personality, Demanding Personality, Dominant Personality, Timid Personality*

Pet Names

The feelings for a pet can be reflected in its call name and this may be useful to a veterinarian in understanding the human-animal bond (Antelyes, 1973). There are many ways to classify these in an unscientific exercise. Names can come from: (1) the location where found ("TC" for trash can); (2) physical description ("Red" for a red cat, "Fifi" for the poodle, "Spot" for a dalmatian); (3) anthropomorphism ("Baby," "Cutie Pie," "Sally"); (4) a sense of humor ("Tiny" for the Great Dane, "Blackie" the white cat); (5) the portrayal of status ("King" or "Duke" for the German shepherd, "Napoleon" for the borzoi); (6) the portrayal of power ("Killer" for the Rottweiler or "Fang" for the German shepherd); (7) feelings of dislike ("Dumb-Dumb" the dog); and (8) attempts not to form an attachment (numbered animals).

When children name the animal, they may do it for reasons that are not immediately obvious. A horse was named "Twoie" because, as the three-year-old child said, "It did a big number 2."

ALSO SEE: *Human-Animal Bond*

Pheromone

A pheromone is a substance resembling a hormone, produced by an exocrine gland, and excreted to the outside of the body. These substances may serve as a means of chemical communication between individuals of the same species (such as sex attractants) or as hormones (such as the pheromone queen bees produce that inhibits other queens from developing).

ALSO SEE: *Scent Marking, Sex Attractant, Warning Behavior*

Phobia

A phobia is a persistent and excessive fear of a specific stimulus from something or some situation. Exposure to or anticipation of the stimulus results in an immediate anxiety response. In animals this often takes the form of the fear of a noise, although other phobias are possible. Fear of thunder is the most common in dogs. More unusual phobias include fears of an automatic lawn sprinkler, of direct sunlight, and of walking on a new carpet.

Dealing with phobias of rapid onset can be diagnostic challenges. A careful search may reveal a specific, but hidden reason for the reaction. Phantom voltage around a milking parlor or stall may quickly teach an animal to avoid a certain location, as might certain smells detectable only by the animal. Removal of this specific source may stop the problem before it gets out of hand.

Behavior modification is the most appropriate way to deal with phobias in general, and results can often be enhanced with drug therapy.

ALSO SEE: *Behavior Modification, Car Phobia, Desensitization, Drug Therapy, Fear, Fear of Environment, Fear of Gunshots, Fear of Loud Noise, Fear of Noise, Fear of People, Fear of Thunder*

Phoresy

Phoresy is the behavior of one animal carrying another. Most often, it involves the use of a carrier to go between food sources. Ticks carried on deer, birds riding cattle, and humans on horseback are examples. The transporting of young by the mother is often excluded from this definition.

Pica

Pica is an abnormal craving to eat unusual or unnatural foods. While coprophagy makes up a major portion of pica presented as problem behaviors, other items can be targeted. Pica should not be confused with destructive chewing, wool sucking, or cribbing. In some cases, pica may be caused by abnormalities within the brain, such as tumors or irritations affecting the hypothalamus. Nutritional imbalances are common causes of pica in livestock species. Salt deprivation causes animals to chew on unusual objects. It can also result in an increased irritability to the animal's personality, causing a normally placid individual to show aggression with little provocation. Wildlife have been known to chew tool handles to obtain salt deposited through human sweat. Horses on a protein-deficient diet may eat the tails of herd mates, and those on a roughage-deficient diet chew wood. Efforts should be made first to eliminate the underlying cause, such as providing salt or addressing nutritional requirements. Taste aversion can be a useful technique to protect objects that are not supposed to be eaten. Preventing access and muzzling can also be useful.

ALSO SEE: *Brain Disorders, Coprophagia, Cribbing, Destructive Chewing, Hypothalamus, Muzzle, Polyphagia, Smell Aversion, Soil Eating, Tail Chewing, Wool Sucking*

Piloerection

Piloerection is the hair standing out from the body because of contractions of the arrector pili muscles. This occurs to help an animal conserve body heat and as a warning behavior. In aggression, piloerection may be restricted to a certain part of the body, such as the shoulders and rump of the dog, or may occur over the entire body, as seen in the feline defensive threat. Piloerection can cause the illusion of a rapid increase in size.

In birds, the equivalent behavior is called feather ruffling.

ALSO SEE: *Distance-increasing Silent Communication, Feather Ruffling*

Place Imprinting

Individuals may develop a strong association for a particular location as the result of an early experience. This can affect homing patterns, most well known in salmon and sea turtles. In domestic animals, stress reactions of moving kennel-raised dogs into a home environment indicate the effects of place imprinting. Kennelosis is the name given to this relationship.

ALSO SEE: *Imprint Learning, Kennelosis, Socialization*

Plant Eating

While plant eating is a normal behavior for the large domestic animals, it is considered unusual for dogs and cats. Actually, the behavior is a variation of normal in these species. Their ancestors ate large ungulates, in the case of the dog, and rodents, in the case of the cat. In the process, the digestive tracts, except perhaps the rumen, were also eaten. The vegetable matter in partially digested form provided certain nutrients for the carnivores. When a modern diet was developed, vitamins and minerals were supplemented to a meat diet, and dogs and cats began to seek vegetable matter. Microbial action in the rumen or cecum breaks down the beta-bonds of cellulose to glucose, which is converted to volatile fatty acids for absorption. Since carnivores lack these microbes, they cannot process the raw grass or plant material (Beaver, 1992). Spring grasses seem favored by many, probably because the dry winter grasses have little appeal. Plant matter tends to stay in the stomach and if in a large enough quantity, irritate the stomach to cause vomiting. Apparently some dogs and cats learn to associate eating plants with vomiting and seek out plants when not feeling well.

Plant eating can be controlled by providing plant material in the diet. A few cooked vegetables are usually sufficient. Cat owners can have lawn grass growing in a flower pot to provide a constant vegetable source for their pet.

ALSO SEE: *Destructive Behaviors*

Play Aggression

The nonaffective aggression shown primarily by young animals is play aggression. During this play, lessons of jaw pressure and acceptable social interactions are learned, and motor skills for defense are tuned. When young animals show play biting, they are learning how much jaw pressure is needed to cause pain, such as when the animal being bitten stops play or shows aggression in return. Since play aggression is one form of play, it helps ease the development of social orders between the youngsters and within a group at the appropriate time. Older animals teach respect for the social order by responding aggressively to the youngsters play biting and kicking. Horses that do not have the benefit of this instruction from herd mates can become difficult to handle.

ALSO SEE: *Antiaggressive Puppy Training, Nonaffective Aggression, Play Behaviors*

Play Behaviors

Play behaviors take on a number of forms in animals. They are seen mostly in the young and represent a method for them to get rid of excess energy, practice brief behavior patterns necessary for later survival, and exercise various muscles. Thus, the majority of play behaviors used by young animals are parts of patterns that might be used by them as adults. Owner reaction is also interesting. Most play behaviors are accepted as such, even though there is growling by puppies, rearing by foals, butting by kids, or even leg climbing by kittens. Many owners do have problems with play behaviors that later are part of sexual behavior. Mounting and pelvic thrusts by an eight-week-old puppy may be called behavior of an oversexed dog, while growling or garden-hose pulling is well tolerated.

Play behaviors generally occur in two forms. Solitary play has the animal interacting with objects in its environment or with itself. This type is proportionately more frequent in adults. Social play allows a youngster to interact with others and will gradually decrease as the animal gets older. In cats, social play is gradually replaced with aggression as the individual becomes more solitary (Beaver, 1992).

In addition to general types of behavior practiced as play, a few postures are specifically related. In dogs, the front-end-down and rear-end-up is a play posture even in adults. Kittens have eight categories of social play: belly-up, stand-up, side step, pounce, vertical stance, chase, horizontal leap, and face-off (West, 1974). Their individual play has been termed mouse, bird, rabbit, and hallucinatory (Beaver, 1992).

Pollakidipsia

Pollakidipsia is an atypically frequent thirst. The total daily volume of water consumed may or may not be abnormal.

ALSO SEE: *Polydipsia*

Pollakiuria

Pollakiuria is abnormally frequent urination. The total volume urinated may or may not be abnormal. This is a typical sign for certain medical problems, including urinary tract infections.

Polyandry

Polyandry is a rare variation of polygamy in which an individual female has several males to mate with. This mating system occurs in a few species of bird.

ALSO SEE: *Polygamy, Polygyny*

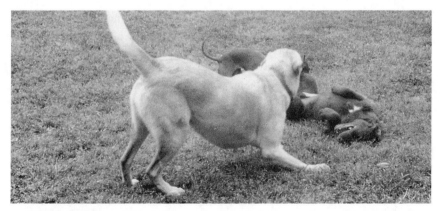

Play Behaviors. This dog shows the front-end-down and rear-end-up species-typical play posture.

Polydipsia

Polydipsia is a prolonged, excessive thirst that usually results in excessive intake of liquids. There are a number of medical problems associated with this behavior change, including fever, diabetes mellitus, diabetes insipidus, portosystemic shunts, and diarrhea. Nonmedical causes can also occur. Minimal environmental stimuli, particularly in stalled horses, may result in learned polydipsia and/or oral playing in the water. Lack of other outlets for behavior may also result in animals, particularly horses, calves, and pigs, eating excessive amounts of salt, which then requires increased water intake to keep the appropriate hemodynamics. The sudden intake of large volumes of water can cause central nervous system signs as well as systemic signs of water intoxication (DeLahunta, 1983).

ALSO SEE: *Boredom, Drinking, Hyperthyroidism, Pollakidipsia, Polyuria*

Polydipsia Nervosa

Polydipsia nervosa is a variation of polydipsia related to a psychogenic increase in water consumption. It typically occurs in horses, where daily consumption is three to four times normal.

ALSO SEE: *Polydipsia*

Polygamy

Polygamy is a type of mating system in which individuals of one sex of a species mate with several individuals of the opposite sex. When one male has several females, the term polygyny is used. When one female has several males, the descriptive word is polyandry.

ALSO SEE: *Mating System, Monogamy, Polyandry, Polygyny, Promiscuity*

Polygyny

Polygyny is a type of polygamy in which individual males of a species have several females. In this type of mating system, care of the offspring is primarily a behavior of the female. This is the most common type of polygamy.

ALSO SEE: *Polyandry, Polygamy*

Polymorphism

Genotypic or phenotypic differences occur within a species. The two most widely recognized types of polymorphism are sexual dimorphism, in which males and females look different, and age dimorphism, in which there are physical differences between juveniles and adults.

ALSO SEE: *Age Dimorphism, Monomorphism, Sexual Dimorphism*

Polyphagia

The excessive desire for food, polyphagia, can be related to a number of factors. Certain medical conditions can be associated with this, such as diabetes mellitus and lesions of the hypothalamus. If the craving is for normal types of food that are accessible, severe obesity can result. When actual food is not available to certain affected individuals, anything can become food. This extreme behavior has been associated with hypothalamic tumors and with feline leukemia and can include the eating of literally anything chewable. Pica might then be the initial complaint.

It is often not possible to stop the problem because the causes are generally not treatable. An accurate diagnosis is desirable, however, to rule out those things that can be treated.

ALSO SEE: *Hyperthyroidism, Ingestive Behavior Problems, Obesity, Pica*

Polyuria

The passing of excessive volumes of urine is associated with polydipsia. Owners are generally more aware of an increase in urine output compared to water intake because of the inconvenience associated with large amounts of urine. Dogs ask to go out more frequently, or the stall bedding is soaked. When polyuria is identified as a problem, it is important to address the cause and the associated polydipsia. Diseases such as diabetes mellitus and renal failure can affect urine output, and so can conditions that affect the volume of intake.

ALSO SEE: *Hyperthyroidism, Pollakiuria, Polydipsia*

Population

A population of animals is the collection of the same species that live together in a relatively well-defined area.

ALSO SEE: *Animal Sociology*

Positive Attitude

As a specific behavior problem develops, the owner may begin to dislike the animal. Even though the behavior may have started as an accident or as the result of an unintended action, many owners come to feel that the animal may even be doing the behavior out of spite or to get even. Owners tend to carry grudges, which, of course, animals do not understand and can only interpret as a change in schedule or body language. A negative cycle develops that can eventually lead to the total destruction of the human-animal relationship. This attitude can develop to the point of being almost irreversible.

A positive attitude toward the animal will go a long way toward improving the relationship. One way to start this is to ask the animal to do anything that it can easily accomplish and to reward it positively for the success. The positive attitude is coupled with appropriate therapy for a successful outcome.

ALSO SEE: *Spite*

Positive Reinforcement

Positive reinforcement is a reward given for a behavior. The reward immediately follows the behavior and increases the likelihood that the behavior will be repeated. The type of reward that can be used will depend on the species and the individual. A primary reinforcer is associated with a survival need such as food, water, or shelter. Too much will decrease the effectiveness of its use during any particular session. A secondary reinforcer is one that through classical conditioning has come to be associated with a primary reinforcer. For most animals, food serves as a positive reinforcement. Praise coupled with food or social contact could become a secondary reinforcer and remain useful even after the primary reinforcer is stopped. Of the domestic animals, both the dog and horse will respond to praise and petting for training. Other species will accept it under certain conditions. The immediacy of the reward is important. The longer the interval between response and reinforcer, the less likely the animal is to connect the two and the longer it will take for the lesson to be learned.

ALSO SEE: *Classical Conditioning, Motivation, Negative Reinforcement, Praise, Punishment, Reinforcement Schedules, Reward*

Postcopulatory Behavior

Postcopulatory (post-mating) behavior occurs after ejaculation, including the dismount. The refractory period between matings may be included as part of the postcopulatory behavior or as a separate behavior. In domestic animals, there are a few variations. Dogs and tomcats usually self-groom, particularly their genitalia, soon after dismounting. A tom also quickly pulls away from a queen because of her aggressive reaction, probably a result of vaginal stimulation by the penile spines. A bull will draw his chin across the back of the cow as he dismounts. This behavior has been used to mark cows in estrus when teaser bulls are used for detection. In general, postcopulatory behaviors of stallions do not differ from those expected; however, an occasional stallion may faint when servicing his first few mares and cause a great deal of concern for the owners.

ALSO SEE: *Refractory Period*

Postures

Postures are signals given by different parts of the body as a form of communication.

ALSO SEE: *Ambivalent Postures, Distance-increasing Silent Communica-*

tion, Distance-reducing Silent Communication, Hard-to-Read Postures

Potential Danger

When dealing with aggressive behavior cases, one factor that should be considered is whether or not there is a real potential for danger to people. While some cases of aggression are potentially treatable, such as dominance aggression, the personality of the owner may not be strong enough to carry out the recommendations. The territorial protectiveness of a dog or cat may be too extreme, causing a potential threat to small children coming over to play.

Since public health has to be the first priority, removal of the animal from that environment might have to be the major recommendation. If the animal is only a threat to that particular person, as with a personality mismatch, the recommendation might be to find a new home for the animal. If, however, there is potential danger to the owner and/or others, euthanasia should be suggested.

ALSO SEE: *Aggression, Euthanasia*

Praise

Praise is a type of positive reinforcer given for a specific behavior. Most dogs respond to and learn with the use of praise by their owner, a technique that can be used to housetrain a puppy. Other species, such as horses, also respond to praise as a reward, although for most animals it is not a strong motivator.

ALSO SEE: *Housetraining, Motivation, Positive Reinforcement, Reward*

Precocial Animal

A precocial species is one in which the young are born in a relatively well-developed state and can follow their parents within a short period of time. Foals and calves are examples of precocial animals. In contrast, altricial animals are poorly developed at birth. Precocial bird chicks are called nidifugous nestlings.

ALSO SEE: *Altricial Animals, Nidifugous Nestlings*

Predation

Predatory behaviors are used by a number of species that depend on killing other animals for their own food. When a person thinks of predator animals, carnivores come to mind because of familiarity with the dog and cat and exposure to wildlife documentaries on the large cats. There are, however, a variety of other predator species, including birds of prey, spiders, and chimpanzees. Some species are solitary hunters, others hunt in groups, and still others wait for prey to come to them. Predation as it relates to veterinary medicine is important in dogs and cats. The evolution of this behavior in ancestors still influences the behaviors in domestic animals.

There are several stages of predatory behavior, each requiring slightly more motivation than the preceding one. Initiation of predation is independent of hunger, since the animal will spend a great deal of time searching before it can ever successfully kill. This situation occurs with the sight or sound of moving prey. For dogs, any movement away may be enough to trigger prey chasing. The first behavior of the series is the stalk. It is usually a crouched run or walk interspersed with pauses. Instead of moving forward, cats may shift their weight back and forth between their back feet (tread) and mouth a "silent meow."

The second phase is the catch. For cats this involves the pounce, where rear limbs remain on the ground to help guide the upper body if the mouse or rat makes a sudden turn. Dogs may pounce, but if going after large prey, they are more likely to grab at whatever part they can. The actual kill varies with the type of prey and the predator. Because cats kill animals smaller than themselves, they use the nape bite from the top of the neck to severe the spinal cord. Dogs (and the big cats) often catch prey at least as large as they are. The killing bite is also directed to the neck, but since it is coming from below, these animals have used suffocation of prey. For small prey, the dog may use a death shake. Following the kill, the prey may be taken to a quiet spot or to the young if necessary. Eating is the final phase.

Depending on the motivation, predation can stop at any phase, and that phase may be incomplete. Injured and dead prey are used to teach hunting skills and taste preferences to the young. Cats often bring dead or injured prey to the owner, perhaps as a modified form of maternal behavior.

Since predation is a normal behavior, it should not be punished. The only way to prevent these behaviors is to prevent access to prey. When predation is prevented, some animals may look for alternatives to meet their internal drive to perform these behaviors. Car chasing, cat chasing, and ankle attacks are examples of misdirected predation.

ALSO SEE: *Ambush Predator, Ankle Attacks, Car Chasing, Death Shake, Feast or Famine, Group Predation, Ingestive Behavior, Nape Bite, Predator Model, Predatory Aggression, Repeated Bites*

Predator Model

Any shape, image, or motion that represents a potential predator is considered to be a model. For many animals, the silhouette of a bird of prey can release a flight response. A ceiling fan can elicit an apparent fear in some domestic cats. Whether this response is innate has been questioned. It may be learned.

ALSO SEE: *Predation*

Predatory Aggression

This is a type of nonaffective aggression exhibited by predatory animals toward their prey. It involves one or more components of predation, usually the stalk, pounce, killing bite, and relocating to another spot to eat the food. If an animal does not hunt frequently, other things will trigger the instinct to chase moving objects. Chasing livestock, cars, bikes, joggers, ankles, balls, and other moving objects is internally rewarding. The animal feels good for having done it, so the behavior is reinforced and likely to occur again. A child that runs away from a dog can initiate prey chasing, and if caught could suffer severe wounds. For the dog, the longer the chase, the more aggressive the catch.

Stopping predatory aggression is difficult because of the internal reward with each success. The only sure way to prevent a recurrence of predatory aggression is to physically prevent the animal from chasing or having access to the initiating factor. Dogs that chase cars and are hit may go back to chasing cars when recovered. Thus, a negative experience may not stop all problems, but it is helpful for about half of the cases if diligently applied. Immediately at the start of each attack, a negative factor, such as a scare, long leash with raving owner, shock, or a jogger chasing back, must be applied. Livestock chasers have been made to drag rotting carcasses or to vomit from ingestion of an emetic, although neither technique has been particularly successful in stopping the problem.

ALSO SEE: *Ankle Attacks, Car Chasing, Chasing Cars, Chasing Livestock, Damming-up Theory, Hierarchy, Internal Reward, Livestock Chasing, Nonaffective Aggression, Repeated Bites, Separate, Shock Collars*

Preening

Preening is a type of oral grooming pattern in birds in which they use their bills (beaks) to clean and groom their feathers.

ALSO SEE: *Grooming Behavior, Habit Preening*

Preference Test

This is a form of behavior testing to determine preferences between various items or the ability to discriminate under specific conditions. In a feeding trial, the animal chooses between two or more flavors or textures of food. Farm animals have been given choices for light or no light, and radio on or off.

ALSO SEE: *Choice Test*

Preferred Associate

This is best described as a "friend." Animals can develop a special relationship with another, such that, even in a group, they spend more time with this individual than with others. Horses that are preferred associates tend to bed down together and show withers nibbling. One may step between its "friend" and an intruder. These animals are usually closely ranked in the group's social order.

Cats also can have a preferred associate, even though they are primarily asocial. They show mutual grooming behaviors and often sleep together. When one dies or leaves, owners often make the mistake of trying to replace the loss, often with a young cat.

ALSO SEE: *Additional Pets, Asocial, Mutual Grooming, Personal Distance, Withers Nibbling*

Prefrontal Lobotomy

Surgical treatments for aggression, specifically prefrontal lobotomies, have been reported to result in a placid personality. This procedure was more common several years ago when the specific diagnosis of the type of aggression was not made. With better understanding of causes and treatments for the various types of aggression, prefrontal lobotomies have lost their advocates.

ALSO SEE: *Aggression*

Pregnancy

Pregnancy is the physiological condition in females of having developing young within the uterus. The primary hormonal control during this time is progesterone, which has an antianxiety action, so the overall behavior change usually seen is a more relaxed female. The duration of pregnancy varies with species and is listed in Appendix B.

ALSO SEE: *Parturition, Pseudopregnancy, Appendix B*

Prenatal Learning

Prenatal learning is that which occurs before birth. This type of learning has been documented in birds, particularly relative to vocalization.

ALSO SEE: *Learning*

Presentation

Presentation is the special positioning of the body to encourage or allow another to interact. There is a wide variety of situations where presentation occurs. A bitch lies down so that her nipples are available to nursing puppies. The cat can use an arched back with piloerection as a defensive threat posture to warn off potential danger. The peacock displays his plumage to entice potential mates and warn other males away.

ALSO SEE: *Display, Epigamic Display, Epigamic Traits, Maternal Behavior, Nursing, Perceptive Behavior, Soliciting Behavior*

Prevent Access

Preventing access to certain areas or objects can be a successful way to treat certain behavior problems. When the history indicates the behavior happens in a certain location, merely blocking access to the area may be sufficient to eliminate the problem. A cat that urinates on the carpet in the spare bedroom usually stops housesoiling if the door is kept shut. A dog that gets on the sofa when the owner is gone stops when chairs and boxes block access to it.

Animals with oral behaviors like pica, prolonged sucking behaviors, cribbing, wind sucking, and destructive chewing tendencies can also be managed by preventing access to the items. This can be accomplished by blocking them from an area, removing the targeted object, or using a muzzle, if appropriate.

ALSO SEE: *Destructive Chewing, Muzzle, Pica, Prolonged Sucking*

Priming Stimulus

A priming stimulus is a particular stimulus that increases the motivation overtly. The presence of young can cause some individuals to show maternal behaviors even though they may not have any young of their own.

ALSO SEE: *Motivation, Spontaneous Behavior, Stimulus*

Proceptive Behavior

Proceptive behaviors are the presenting behaviors of females that are used to solicit sexual interaction from males. Genital presentation by baboons is an example.

ALSO SEE: *Female Behaviors, Presentation, Soliciting Behavior*

Progenesis

Progenesis is the more rapid onset of puberty and sexual maturation relative to physical development. Domestic livestock have been selectively bred for reproductive efficiency, and one result is that these animals show sexual behaviors at much younger ages than did their ancestors.

Progenesis is similar to neoteny, where physical development is slowed relative to puberty.

ALSO SEE: *Neoteny*

Progestins

Progestins are drugs that act like progesterone and are useful as drug therapy for certain medical and behavioral problems. Progestins decrease serum testosterone levels and thus are most successful when used on noncastrated males as a form of chemical castration. The second major effect of these drugs is that of an antianxiety tranquilizer, similar to that reported during the progesterone-related state of pregnancy. In behavior, the primary use of progestins has been in problems of male sexually dimorphic behaviors, including housesoiling by urine spraying. Since stress is a factor associated with many problem behaviors, the progestins have been moderately successful as a "shotgun" therapy. Unfortunately, in most stress-related behaviors, if the stressor is not removed it can eventually overpower the antianxiety tranquilizer effect. These drugs are also known to work for one or more repetitions of a problem and then not work. Reasons for this are speculative.

There is another behavior problem for which the progestins have been useful. One of the side effects of the drugs is appetite stimulation, particularly during the initial period of use. These drugs are indicated in prolonged cases of anorexia nervosa, particularly in cats, and for short-term appetite stimulation where owners are obsessively concerned about their pet not eating.

Additional side effects include endometritis/pyometra, spermatic aplasia, adrenocortical suppression, diabetes mellitus, mammary hyperplasia/neoplasia, and acromegaly. The rate of success is also variable with progestins, in part because of case selection, but also because of species variations. For any of the male sexually dimorphic behaviors in cats, the immediate and gradual successes in intact males approximate 85% to 90% (Hart and Barrett, 1973). In the dog, the best success rate, approximately 60%, is reduced with age and presumably learning. Thus, the older the dog and the more often the behavior has occurred, the less effective progestins are on male sexually dimorphic behaviors. The success rate for these drugs is much lower in neutered males and females, and it has not been determined for horses.

Because the side effects are potentially very serious, more suitable drugs or techniques should be used if possible, especially if long-term therapy is necessary. When progestins are used long term, owners should be advised of the side effects so they can weigh those against the consequences of not using the progestins.

ALSO SEE: *Drug Therapy, Sexually Dimorphic Behaviors, Appendix C*

Prolonged Sucking

Prolonged sucking is one form of the prolonged sucking syndrome usually seen in cats. This behavior is a continuation of nursinglike behavior, including both sucking and kneading with the forepaws, after weaning. In that context, the behavior has been equated with thumb sucking in children. The behavior occurs more often in orphaned and malnourished kittens and may be related to the practice of weaning kittens at 6 weeks instead of the 8 to 12 weeks that would occur naturally.

Prolonged sucking can be directed at many objects including the nipples of another cat, self-nursing, human skin, or areas of a companion dog. The behavior typically occurs when the cat is starting to relax, so soft purring may also occur. Over a long time, the nursing may gradually decrease but the kneading continues.

Prolonged sucking can also occur in other young, particularly calves, puppies, and piglets. It is most likely to continue in orphans or those separated early from the dam.

P

The behavior is self-rewarding, so a major effort is needed to stop it. The easiest method is to prevent access to the favorite object. Since this is not always possible, taste aversion can be tried if the behavior is particularly bothersome. Smell aversion, remote punishment, and direct punishment can also be used but are usually less successful.

ALSO SEE: *Internal Reward, Nursing, Prevent Access, Prolonged Sucking Syndrome, Remote Punishment, Retrojection, Smell Aversion, Taste Aversion, Wool Sucking*

Prolonged Sucking Syndrome

Certain cats continue to suck objects long after the time of normal weaning, and some begin the problem several months after weaning has occurred. There appear to be two primary types of this syndrome—one in which a kitten continues to suck objects (prolonged sucking) and one in which a Siamese or Siamese-cross cat begins sucking wool or other specific objects (wool sucking). The division between these two problems is not always clear, since young Siamese can suck nonwool objects, and some cats that have no obvious Siamese in their background go after wool objects. In addition, some of the cats chew or lick rather than suck, but this probably represents a variation of this syndrome.

Taste aversion, smell aversion, remote punishment, or direct punishment can be used for problem cats. Long-standing problems can be very difficult to stop because the behaviors are internally rewarding.

ALSO SEE: *Internal Reward, Prolonged Sucking, Remote Punishment, Smell Aversion, Taste Aversion, Wool Sucking*

Promiscuity

Promiscuity is a mating system in which there are no permanent pair bonds and an individual may mate with several individuals.

ALSO SEE: *Harem, Mating System, Polygamy*

Prompting and Fading

Prompting and fading is a training technique using a cue or prompt that is effective in eliciting a particular response. When the prompt/response pattern is learned, there is a lessening (fading) of the amount of the prompt while retaining the desired response. Once a horse has been taught to count using head nods as a cue, the deliberateness of the nod can be lessened to the point that it is barely perceptible to those watching.

ALSO SEE: *Learning*

Protean Behavior

Protean behavior is the use of erratic or sudden changes while attempting to flee from a predator. This could be sudden changes in direction while running or flying, or rapid changes in color or size.

ALSO SEE: *Escape Behaviors*

Protective Aggression

Protective aggression may be subdivided into territorial (protective) aggression, material (protective) aggression, and owner (protective) aggression. These involve guarding an area, a possession, or an owner from intrusion or attack.

ALSO SEE: *Affective Aggression, Material Protective Aggression, Owner Protective Aggression, Ritualized Fighting, Territorial Protective Aggression*

Pseudoconditioning

Pseudoconditioning is the increased likelihood that a neutral stimulus will elicit a specific response as a consequence of the repeated elicitation of that response by a stimulus with which it is already associated. Pseudoconditioning must be considered during classical conditioning.

ALSO SEE: *Classical Conditioning, Conditioning*

Pseudocopulation

Pseudocopulation is mating without ejaculation and can include mounting with or without intromission. The behavior may be shown by females and between individuals of the same sex.

ALSO SEE: *Homosexual Behavior, Mounting*

Pseudopregnancy

Pseudopregnancy is also called pseudocyesis and false pregnancy. It is a group of behaviors that can be shown by a nonpregnant bitch as the result of hormonal changes from corpora lutea of the last estrus. The corpora lutea in the dog normally regress approximately two months after estrus, which happens to be the time when parturition would occur as well. Affected bitches show behaviors typically associated with pregnancy, including nesting, adopting inanimate objects, and in extreme cases, restlessness and milk production. The behaviors can be subtle changes or of the same magnitude as actual parturition and nursing.

ALSO SEE: *Neutral Object, Substitute Object*

Psychogenic Constipation

Animals may continue to show constipation even after all usual causes have been eliminated or ruled out. Psychogenic constipation usually occurs when an extremely concerned owner continues to give a great deal of attention to the defecation and posturing behaviors of the animal. The problem animal is usually a dog, and the attention received seems to be important in the continuation of this condition. Decreased attention eliminates the problem.

ALSO SEE: *Attention Seeking, Exercise, Frustration, No Attention to Behavior, Psychogenic Problems, Schedule, Stress-related Behaviors*

Psychogenic Dermatoses

The manifestation of some psychogenic problems can be in the form of skin conditions. Flank sucking; lick granulomas; lesions of self-mutilation by horses, particularly stallions; hair pulling by primates; and excessive licking by cats are examples of how animals can react to stress and express it as a skin condition. In extreme, prolonged stress environments, immuno-deficient conditions may also develop.

Assuming food allergies and atopy have been ruled out, control of such a skin condition depends on eliminating those stresses that are bothering the animal. Treatment also includes a more rigid schedule and increased exercise.

ALSO SEE: *Antianxiety Tranquilizers, Excessive Grooming, Excessive Licking, Exercise, Flank Sucking, Frustration, Hair Pulling, Lick Granulomas, Psychogenic Problems, Schedule, Self-Mutilation, Stress-related Behaviors*

Psychogenic Diarrhea

Diagnosing psychogenic diarrhea can be extremely difficult because there are many medically related causes that are difficult to rule out. The psychogenic relationship with bouts of diarrhea should be suspected in high-strung personalities, particularly ones that are on low-exercise lifestyles, or in individuals that seem inwardly nervous, the type that would bite their nails if they were humans. Hospitalization, even without treatment, may clear up the problem, which then recurs when the animal gets home.

Treatment means minimizing the stresses that precipitate the bouts of diarrhea. Other helpful recommendations include adjusting the animal's lifestyle to a more rigid schedule and increasing exercise.

ALSO SEE: *Antianxiety Tranquilizers, Exercise, Frustration, Psychogenic Problems, Schedule, Stress-related Behaviors*

Psychogenic Pain

Animals may show pain that is very real to them, but for which no organic cause can be determined. In those cases it is important to evaluate the history for stress or excessive owner reaction. Treatment is similar to that for other psychogenic problems—minimize the stress.

ALSO SEE: *Antianxiety Tranquilizers, Attention Seeking, Exercise, Frustration, Psychogenic Problems, Schedule, Stress-related Behaviors, Sympathetic Lameness*

Psychogenic Problems

Stress to the point of distress can result in the development of behavior problems. Those problems that appear to have a medical basis but are a result of neurologic production are called psychogenic problems. These include psychogenic constipation, dermatoses, diarrhea, pain, seizures, shock, urinary incontinence, and vomiting.

The psychogenic component of these problems is often discovered accidently during the course of a more traditional medical treatment. The animal may be hospitalized and the problem stopped. It returns when the animal goes home. This cyclic response should be a diagnostic flag. Resolution of the problem will depend on identifying and eliminating the stress. Look particularly for things that may have changed in the animal's schedule, for insufficient exercise, or for excessive attention on the part of the owner. Antianxiety tranquilizers or progestins, with their antianxiety activity, may be helpful initially with psychogenic problems; however, they are not the cure. Drugs are only good for short-term management, so changing the environment becomes the ultimate key to success. A rigid schedule, increased exercise, and benign neglect are useful for many such problems.

ALSO SEE: *Antianxiety Tranquilizers, Exercise, No Attention to Behavior, Progestins, Psychogenic Constipation, Psychogenic Dermatoses, Psychogenic Diarrhea, Psychogenic Pain, Psychogenic Seizures, Psychogenic Shock, Psychogenic Urinary Incontinence, Psychogenic Vomiting, Psychological Well-being, Schedule, Separation Anxiety, Social Inhibition, Stress-related Behaviors*

Psychogenic Seizures

Seizures that are precipitated by apparently stressful events are known to occur in dogs. The manifestation is that of a classic seizure. Even such things as family arguments or intense staring at the animal can be seizureogenic. Control is achieved by removing the source of the stress.

ALSO SEE: *Antianxiety Tranquilizers, Exercise, Frustration, Psychogenic Problems, Schedule, Seizures, Stress-related Behaviors*

Psychogenic Shock

Among domestic animals, cats seem particularly prone to develop physiological shock from particularly stressful events. Some will go into a catatonic state; others become shocky. Cats have been reported to hide in dark corners, show depression, salivate, become anorexic, have dilated pupils, and have hyperesthesia. The shock syndrome may be a means of survival, since the lack of movement inhibits attacks by predators. In the extreme form, medical management of shock is necessary.

ALSO SEE: *Antianxiety Tranquilizers, Catatonic Reaction, Exercise, Frustration, Psychogenic Problems, Schedule, Stress-related Behaviors*

Psychogenic Urinary Incontinence

There are times when a physiologically and medically normal animal may show urinary incontinence. In dogs, the problem is most commonly associated with submissive urination, although it can be seen at other times. The mentally stressed, highly excited, or physically exhausted animal may lose the ability to hold urine, and the geriatric one may dribble urine in association with altered sensoria. Young dogs tend to outgrow the problem if handled properly, while old animals need a more guarded prognosis.

ALSO SEE: *Housesoiling—Submissive Urination, Hyperactivity, Hyperkinesis, Polyuria, Submissive Urination*

Psychogenic Vomiting

Psychogenic vomiting is a stress-related syndrome manifested as a medical problem. Diagnosis can be difficult because of the long list of differentials that must be considered, but psychogenic causes should be considered with nervous individuals. Hospitalization alone may clear up the problem until the animal returns home, because the owners are often busy people or overly protective.

Treatment includes adjusting the animal's lifestyle to a stricter schedule, increasing the exercise, and minimizing stresses.

ALSO SEE: *Antianxiety Tranquilizers, Exercise, Frustration, Psychogenic Problems, Schedule, Stress-related Behaviors*

Psychological Well-being

While the exact definition will be debated for a long time, psychological well-being generally refers to an emotional state resulting from minimal to no environmental stressors. This concept has come into vogue with the increased welfare concern for nonhuman primates in laboratory settings. The anthropomorphic equating of an active mind and a "happy" animal has lead to numerous studies in environmental enrichment.

ALSO SEE: *Environmental Enrichment, Frustration, Psychogenic Problems, Social Contact, Stress-related Behaviors*

Psychology

Psychology involves the study of mental processes and behavior. Learning is a major aspect of this discipline. Several subdivisions of psychology have been defined, including physiological, applied, social, educational, cognitive, and developmental. Comparative psychology looks at the similarities between humans and animals.

ALSO SEE: *Animal Psychology*

Psychomotor Agitation

Psychomotor agitation is excessive motor activity that is associated with stress. The activity is usually nonproductive and repetitious.

ALSO SEE: *Obsessive Compulsive Disorders, Stereotyped Behaviors*

Psychopharmacological Drugs

Psychopharmacological drugs are those that affect behavior through actions on the central nervous system.

ALSO SEE: *Drug Therapy, Appendix C*

Puerperal Aggression

Puerperal (maternal) aggression is that shown by a female shortly after parturition. It has a sudden onset, is very aggressive, and is temporary.

ALSO SEE: *Aggression, Maternal Aggression*

Pulling Back

Horses respond to frightening stimuli by trying to flee. If the animal is tied when the stimulus to flee occurs, it will pull back on the restraining device. If this device is not able to hold the weight pulling against it, the horse can escape. Thus, through trial and error, the horse can learn to pull back and break its halter or bridle if it wants to escape. It is important to use a strong halter and rope on animals learning how to stand tied. After several hard but unsuccessful struggles to get free, the horse will generally quit pulling back.

The problem horse that has mastered pulling back for escape must relearn the concept that escape is no longer going to happen. This can be accomplished successfully with a strong halter and rope. Some trainers will tie the rope to a rubber tire inner tube so that there is some stretch, and a quick snap when pressure is released. Punishment during the pulling phase may also be used judiciously. A second rope that is shorter than the halter rope can be used as a noose around the neck to cut off air (a hazardous technique that must be carefully applied) or it may be passed through the halter nose piece, between the front limbs and around the chest. Hitting the horse from behind with a broom while it is pulling also discourages pulling back without seriously injuring the animal. This technique associates punishment with a particular behavior to decrease the frequency of the pulling. For the horse that pulls back only at certain times, the single-leg horse hobble can teach it to allow saddling or other procedures.

ALSO SEE: *Escape Behaviors, Halter Breaking, Punishment, Trial and Error Learning*

Punishment

Punishment is the use of a negative factor (stimulus) with a behavior to decrease the frequency of the behavior. To be effective, the punishment must be properly timed and consistent. It must also be of enough significance to be meaningful to the individual.

Punishment of normal behaviors may be stressful to an animal, especially if appropriate alternatives are not provided. Cats do jump on things. They can be kept off objects such as counters if there are other high places they like, but they cannot be kept off all things. A horse gets mixed signals when it is punished with spurs and slaps of the reins, which say "go forward," and with pulling on the reins, which says "stop." The resulting frustration can lead to even more unacceptable behavior, such as rearing.

ALSO SEE: *Aggression and Telephones, Behavior Modification, Direct Punishment, Kicking, Motivation, Negative Reinforcement, Rearing, Remote Punishment*

Puppy Selection Test

There are a number of tests that can be given to puppies typically at the age of weaning to help choose certain types of personalities. They tend to point to active, nippy puppies (dominant) or those that are not (subordinate), and puppies that tend to be less social, more social, or independent. These are generally fun to administer; however, they have never been validated to actually correlate with adult personalities. Because environments can have a dramatic impact on genetic tendencies, a low reliability should be expected.

Purr

The cat's purr has been a sound of mystery for centuries. Purring is originated through a certain area of the brain (Gibbs and Gibbs, 1936) and actually occurs as air turbulence through a narrowed glottis. Intrinsic laryngeal muscles produce the partial glottal closure (Remmers and Gautier, 1972). Increased transglottal pressure causes the air turbulence and explains the inspiratory and expiratory phases of the sound. Purring can be loud to inaudible, depending on the cat and the situation. A popular theory, which still surfaces occasionally, held that the purr originated as blood turbulence in one of the great vessels, either the aorta or caudal vena cava, and was caused by an arched back during petting; however, electromyographic research techniques have localized it to the larynx.

Why cats purr will never be known with certainty, but it is easiest to equate the cat purr with a human smile. It usually occurs at times when we like to think the animal is happy, although it also is used when the act seems to be coaxing, proclaiming "aristocratic" status, or seeking acceptance.

An unusual purring situation veterinarians are likely to encounter involves a cat that has been chronically ill and is near death. Shortly before death, the cat may start purring. Some terminally ill human cancer patients experience a state of euphoria replacing pain and suffering. Possibly the cat is experiencing the same.

ALSO SEE: *Vocal Communication*

Puzzle Box

Puzzle box is a general term used for any boxlike apparatus used to study learning, memory, and other mental abilities. Examples include the Skinner box, maze, and finger puzzle.

ALSO SEE: *Learning, Skinner Box*

R

Rage Copulation

Rage copulation is mounting behavior directed toward an animal of the same sex and species during a display of aggressive dominance. It is common in dogs, territorial cats, and several other species. Contrary to the name, actual copulation is uncommon.

ALSO SEE: *Mounting*

Rage Syndrome

The rage syndrome is a general term that has been applied to unpredictable aggression in certain breeds of dogs. Most recently the problem has been associated with English springer spaniels; however, similar descriptions have been reported in Burmese mountain dogs, English cocker spaniels, and St. Bernards. Histories of affected dogs suggest that genetic factors are involved, although specifics are still being studied. In the rage syndrome, the episodes of aggression are usually unpredictable and severe. Physiological changes often indicate a high degree of arousal. These can include disorientation, trembling, urination, and/or defecation.

In some dogs, the aggression shown is actually dominance aggression. Other types of aggression have also been included under this generic term. In a few of the cases seen by the author, dogs that fit the parameters of the rage syndrome showed electroencephalographic changes characteristic of mental lapse aggression. It is important to diagnose as accurately as possible to determine if a treatment is possible; however, human safety must be the primary concern.

ALSO SEE: *Aggression, Genetic Problems, Mental Lapse Aggression Syndrome*

Rank Mimicry

Lower-ranking individuals can mimic certain behaviors of higher-ranking ones. The behavior is associated with attracting females.

ALSO SEE: *Male Behaviors*

Rank Order

This is another term that has been used to describe a social order or hierarchy.

SEE: *Social Order*

Reaction Norm

This is the normal pattern of behavior expected as a reaction to a stimulus, where the form of this movement remains independent of the particular stimulus. Shying in horses may be set off by many factors, ranging from a strange odor to a flapping flag.

ALSO SEE: *Shying, Stimulus, Stimulus-Response Relationship*

Reactive Anomalies

Behaviors that occur as a response to potential dangers are classified as reactive anomalies. They include behaviors of fight, flight, or immobility. Included in the specific types of reactions are mobile aggression, mobile alarm, hysteria, threatening, butting, biting, kicking, shying, striking, and tonic immobility.

ALSO SEE: *Biting, Butting, Hysteria, Kicking, Mobile Aggression, Mobile Alarm, Shying*

Reactive Distances

Reactive (or social) distances define the spacing of interactions of animals to herd mates, strangers, and area.

ALSO SEE: *Approach Distance, Critical Distance, Flight Distance, Group Distance, Home Range, Individual Distance, Perceptive Distance, Social Distance, Strike Distance, Submissive Distance, Territory, Withdrawal Distance*

Rearing

Rearing is a behavior in which the animal stands up on its hind limbs, waving its front limbs in the air. In species such as dogs and cats, it is a distance-reducing behavior. In horses it is a threat or aggressive posture. The behavior is also a common form of play aggression in yearling stallions.

ALSO SEE: *Distance-increasing Silent Communication, Distance-reducing Silent Communication, Escape Behaviors, Kicking, Striking*

Redirected Aggression

In redirected aggression, an animal redirects its emotional state toward an innocent bystander. The most common expression of this type of affective aggression is during a dog fight, where the person is bitten while trying to separate the dogs. Once worked up emotionally, an animal cannot instantly turn off that state if the cause suddenly goes away. In the time it takes the animal to calm down, it could redirect the excitement toward something else nearby. A horse excited by running horses in a nearby pasture may suddenly lash out at a pasture mate. A cat that is subjected to a bath may lash out at a nearby dog as soon as the owner releases it. The more worked up emotionally the animal is, the longer it takes to calm down and the longer it is subject to redirecting that emotional state aggressively.

In the wild, two responses commonly are used to inhibit a redirected attack. The first is to show extreme submission. The second is to show a posture that is totally unexpected for the situation, as if to give a visual "slap in the face." An aggressive attack might be countered with a mating posture or with mutual grooming.

ALSO SEE: *Affective Aggression, Aversion-induced Aggression, Avoid Excitement, Distance-reducing Silent Communication, Inhibition, Mutual Grooming, Neutral Object, Separate, Stress-related Behaviors*

Reestablish Dominance

In cases of dominance aggression where the dog treats the owner as a lower-ranking pack member, it may be necessary for the owner to establish or reestablish dominance. The relative difference in personalities between dog and owner can be important in determining whether this may even be possible and how difficult and how dangerous the process may be. Establishing owner dominance is not always possible.

If the dog assumed the position of leader by default, and the owner is able to give commands, the use of "No," a jerk correction on the collar, and obedience work can correct the problem. Dogs with dominant personalities need firm corrections. The owner must be able to enforce each command; direct eye contact with control, as with a halter or choke chain collar, can be used very effectively. The neck shake uses the canine lesson of throat control associated with victory in fighting to bring a point home without actual injury. Extremely dominant dogs and those that have been in control for a long time strongly resist efforts to control them, so the owner must be prepared, even with protective clothing if necessary. For these dogs, the Promise™ halter has proven to be very useful.

If the owner is physically or psychologically not strong enough to use force, a more indirect approach may be tried. The owner withholds all the dog's food and physical affection during the training period and avoids any action that is likely to evoke aggression. Periodically throughout the day, especially when the dog is seeking attention, the owner should give a command, such as "sit." For a correct response, the animal receives lots of attention and a small portion of food. As the dog learns this new routine, a gradual increase of the expected amount should begin. Over time, the owner feels more comfortable demanding a response and loses the fear of the dog responding with aggression.

ALSO SEE: *Dog Collars, Dominance Aggression, Neck Shake, No, Obedience Class*

Reflex

A reflex is an involuntary action resulting from a stimulus and, therefore, is under control of the nervous system. An example is the patellar reflex, in which a tap on the patellar tendon is transmitted to the spinal cord and connects to a motor nerve there which causes the quadriceps femoris muscle to contract and the lower limb to move. Reflexes are often part of a more complex behavior, such as the swallowing reflex at the end of food-seeking behavior. A reflex is present typically in several species of animals because it often is related to survival. Certain reflexes are present at birth and then disappear; an example is the rooting reflex, which causes neonatal puppies and kittens to orient toward warm, firm objects. Other reflexes develop under certain stimuli or conditions. Puppies and kittens develop self-initiated urination with time and maturation of the nervous system. Still other reflexes may develop and then disappear again. Until 4 days of age, a puppy suspended gently by its neck will curl into a ball (flexor dominance). From 5 to 18 days, the response is an arched back and extended legs (extensor dominance). After 18 days a normal puppy will simply hang limply when suspended.

ALSO SEE: *Fixed Action Pattern, Habit, Instinct, Reflex Rebound*

Reflex Rebound

When a behavior has not been used for a while, an appropriate stimulus may cause the excessive response of a reflex. When an animal has been in the dark for a long period of time, the eyes take longer than usual to adjust to a sudden, sustained bright light.

ALSO SEE: *Reflex*

Refractory Period

A refractory period is the time interval between the expressions of a behavior when the initiating stimulus remains present. The term describes the intervals between matings by a male when continuously presented with an estrous female. As a single male and female remain together, there is a gradual lengthening in the refractory period. In most species, the addition of a new estrous female, a novel stimulus, will shorten the male's refractory period. The interval between reactions to olfactory stimuli, such as catnip, is also called the refractory period.

ALSO SEE: *Catnip, Coolidge Effect, Male Behaviors, Motivational Energy*

Reinforcement Schedules

Once a desired behavior has been learned by positive reinforcement, the reward does not have to be given after each occurrence. Spacing of rewards can be varied by an interval schedule, a ratio schedule, or a combination of the two. Once the behavior has been learned, spacing of rewards has been shown to be more effective for retention of the lesson than continuous reinforcement.

Interval schedules reinforce the first response after a specific amount of time has elapsed. Fixed interval schedules reinforce the behavior after a set time has elapsed, such as every 20 minutes. Variable interval schedules reinforce the behavior after varying lengths of time, such as 5 minutes the first time, 30 minutes the second, and 20 minutes the third. The variable interval schedule reinforces the human gambling behavior of playing the slot machines.

Ratio schedules reinforce a certain response after the occurrence of a specified number of responses. Fixed ratio schedules reward the same response each time, such as after every third behavior. Variable ratio schedules reward a response at differing frequencies. The reward might be for the sixth, tenth, second, and fourteenth occurrence.

ALSO SEE: *Behavior Modification, Motivation, Positive Reinforcement*

Reintroduction

When an animal is separated from others it has been with, there can be problems with the reintroduction. In most species, if the separation is long enough, the void in the social order already has been filled when the individual returns. This could mean that the returning individual must establish a place within the group, necessitating the threats and possibility of aggression that go with that process. The problem is common in livestock species when certain individuals are shown in exhibitions. It also occurs occasionally in dogs when the dominant dog is hospitalized for surgery or a medical problem and returns with less strength than when it left.

A reintroduction should be carefully controlled to minimize problems. Reintroductions may be accomplished by keeping the individuals physically separate, but within sight of each other. In that way, visual threats can be used without the animals being able to fight. In territorial species, the actual physical reintroduction is safer in a neutral area, especially if the one removed is a higher ranking individual. For dogs, the normally submissive one may need to be removed temporarily until the dominant dog is back within the home, or the two dogs may need to be kept separate until the dominant one is strong enough to assert its dominance. Even then, a muzzle on the subordinate dog or on both dogs may be useful. Both could also be taken to a neutral area and walked past each other, making the subordinate dog show submissive signs, such as lying or sitting.

ALSO SEE: *Social Order*

Rejection of Neonate

Occasional females show aggression toward their newborns or actually desert them. For some, the aggression will decrease and stop after the young have suckled. Nourishment can be provided by hand feeding the rejected animal or by forcibly restraining the dam during nursing bouts. This problem is most common with the first parturition. Foal rejection is particularly troublesome because fostering seldom occurs, and foal care is a long commitment.

ALSO SEE: *Fostering, Maternal Behavior, Maternal Failure*

Releaser

A releaser is a communication, body posture, or behavior that stimulates a specific response. The word is generally interchangeable with "stimulus."

ALSO SEE: *Interspecific Releaser, Releasing Mechanism, Stimulus, Super Releaser*

Releasing Mechanism

The releasing mechanism is a combination of peripheral filters (senses) and releasers that result in a specific response. An innate releasing mechanism indicates a specific response to a stimulus even though the animal has not been previously exposed to that stimulus. For example, the distress vocalizations of a newborn kitten result in a specific reaction by all female cats in a certain hormonal state. An acquired releasing mechanism indicates a learning component. A dog's reaction to thunderstorms may become fearful over time. A third type of releasing mechanism is a modified innate releasing mechanism. Here, the instinctive component has been modified by experience.

ALSO SEE: *Peripheral Filters, Releaser*

Relict

A relict is an evolutionary vestige of an anatomical part or a behavior. The relict may be present only during embryological development, such as the vestigial gill slits in mammals, or it may be present in the adult as a relatively non-functional object, such as the human appendix, the canine dew claw, or the equine splint bones.

Remote Punishment

Remote punishment occurs when the animal connects the punishment with the behavior and location, not with the behavior and the owner. This type of punishment is most effective on behaviors in which an owner's presence may actually encourage the behavior, on problems that usually occur when the owner is out of the room, and on feline problems. Cats that jump on a table can learn not to if they are remotely punished with a spray of water or a blast from a remotely controlled hair dryer. A barking dog can be punished with a blast from a water hose with a sprayer attached. The owner's and veterinarian's imaginations are the only limit to the techniques that can be used. As with other forms of correction used for learning, timing is critical.

ALSO SEE: *Added Food Bowls, Aggression and Telephones, Climbing Curtains, Direct Punishment, Housesoiling—Defecation, Housesoiling—Spraying, Housesoiling—Urination, Indirect Punishment, Punishment, Shock Collars*

Remove the Stress

To treat any of the stress-related behavior problems successfully, it becomes important to reduce or minimize the effects of the stress on the animal. This can be accomplished temporarily in certain species with drugs. Many owners and veterinarians do not want the animal on drugs long term; the animal may become less responsive to the drug over time, or serious side effects may result from prolonged use. For any of these reasons, it may be considered more desirable to identify the source of the stress and remove or minimize it. General causes of problems include changes in the animal's schedule, especially relative to human interaction, or not enough exercise. Specific causes may include new cats roaming past a window, new activity next door, or a week with a heavy examination schedule for a student owner.

While it is not always possible to remove the specific stress, it may be possible to eliminate it from the animal's perspective. Roaming cats remain outside, but confining the resident cat away from a specific window, drawing the draperies, or pulling down a window shade (even on the outside of a window) can hide the visitors from view. Anticipation of a new stress, such as the birth of a baby, can allow for a gradual change in schedule so that the arrival will be less of a problem for the animal. Exercise can be increased for dogs by playing ball or chasing a frisbee. Permitting access to a pasture at night allows the show horse to keep its coat from sun bleaching, but increases the amount of exercise it gets.

ALSO SEE: *Drug Therapy, Exercise, New Baby, Schedule, Stress, Stress-related Behaviors, Appendix C.*

REM (Rapid Eye Movement) Sleep

Rapid eye movement sleep, also called fast wave sleep or paradoxical sleep, is one of two alternating major sleep periods. Neurologically it is an active time, with the electroencephalogram (EEG) showing low amplitude and fast activity, as in the awake state. In humans, dreams occur during REM sleep. This sleep phase is apparently important to renewing neurological functioning, because in sleep-deprived individuals the frequency and duration of REM sleep bouts increase for some time when sleep is again possible.

ALSO SEE: *Sleep, Slow-Wave Sleep*

Repeated Bites

Carnivores bite and shake their prey to kill it. After the kill they relax the grip and bite again, perhaps repeatedly. These subsequent bites are the repeated bites.

ALSO SEE: *Predation, Predatory Aggression*

Reproductive Behavior

Reproductive behavior includes a number of behaviors that ultimately lead to mating, pregnancy, and parturition. These behaviors are described in several ways. The sex of an animal is important in its behavior; male and female behaviors are described under the titles below. In addition, the reproductive behaviors include courtship, mating, postcopulatory, parturition, and maternal behaviors.

ALSO SEE: *Courtship, Female Behaviors, Genital Presentation, Harem, Long-Term Pair Bond, Male Behaviors, Maternal Behavior, Mating*

Behavior, Mating System, Monogamy, Multimate Group, Pair Bonding, Polygamy, Postcopulatory Behavior, Sex Advertisement, Sexual Selection

Resting Behaviors

There are two basic resting positions shown by animals—sitting and lying. In addition, horses have special anatomical features that allow them to rest while standing.

Sitting is a posture in which the animal's pelvic region contacts the ground, while the thorax is elevated. Although this posture is typically thought of with dogs and cats, other domestic animals use the posture as well. Horses may sit briefly, usually during a pause as they are getting up or between grooming bouts when they are rubbing their abdomen on the ground. Pigs use sitting as a common resting posture. Cattle that use the sitting position are usually heavy individuals of beef breeds.

Lying postures have ground contact at both the front and rear. This contact may be in sternal recumbency, where the ventral midline makes contact; lateral recumbency, where the ground contact is actually over the limbs on one side of the body; or a combination of sternal recumbency in front and lateral recumbency behind.

Horses have a specialized series of ligaments and bone formations, called the stay apparatus, that allows them to relax their muscles but remain standing. In this position, the horse can rest while standing.

Sleep, an obvious type of resting, occurs in two forms, described in more detail elsewhere. Slow-wave sleep can occur in any of the lying positions or in the standing position for the horse. REM sleep apparently must occur in a lateral recumbency.

ALSO SEE: *Dog-Sitting, REM Sleep, Slow-Wave Sleep, Stretching*

Retrain to Eliminate

Long-standing problems with canine or feline housesoiling may mean the animal never was appropriately housetrained or that it unlearned the accepted behavior, learning instead to eliminate in an unacceptable location or on an unacceptable surface. For these animals, it may be necessary to retrain them to eliminate where the owner wishes. This procedure takes the owner's time and effort, so he or she must be committed to the project.

For dogs, retraining to eliminate usually means teaching the housesoiling dog to go outside. This is done most easily in many cases by using the same timing and techniques as if housetraining a puppy.

For cats that do not use the litter box, retraining may be helpful. Confinement to a noncarpeted room with food, water, a bed, and a litter box may be sufficient to remind the cat of its early training. After a long period of time, a gradual reintroduction to more areas of the house is allowed. It is important initially to give the cat access to a variety of litter types to allow the cat to choose which

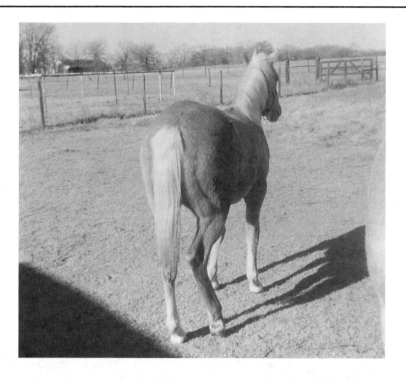

Resting Behaviors. While horses can rest in a standing position, most will show the relaxation of one rear foot, as is seen in this figure.

it prefers. In extreme cases of long-term housesoiling, after the more routine procedures have failed, it may be necessary to try a more drastic retraining procedure if the cat owner does not want to consider making the cat an indoor-outdoor animal. For this technique the cat is again confined to a small room with its provisions. In addition to a litter box, litter is sprinkled lightly over the entire floor so that the animal must eliminate on litter. After several weeks, litter is swept so that a fourth of the floor is bare. If the cat uses the bare floor, recover the area with litter. If the cat uses the litter-covered part, keep that arrangement for several more weeks and then try half bare floor and half litter-covered floor. Repeat the process, gradually reducing the litter-covered floor area until only the litter box remains. After several weeks with it, the cat can be gradually reintroduced into the rest of the house.

ALSO SEE: *Housesoiling, Housetraining, Indoor-Outdoor*

Retrojection

Retrojection describes an animal's use of its own body part(s). A common example is associated with self-sucking seen in orphaned or early weaned young, as in prolonged sucking in cats.

ALSO SEE: *Prolonged Sucking*

Returning to Old Home

A complaint of cat owners who move is that their pet keeps returning to its old home or runs off in an apparent attempt to do so. The problem is more common when the move is only a short distance. The cat's strong attachment to a territory and its general sense of direction are the apparent drawing forces. The problem of the cat returning to an old territory usually can be prevented with careful planning. Confinement of the pet inside the home, a garage, or a shed for several days to weeks helps the animal establish a new small territory and decreases the tendency to leave.

Other species occasionally return to an old home, but the attraction is usually social. Dogs have been identified by collar tags at their former home. Horses, too, have crawled under or jumped fences to return to a pasture from which they had recently been moved.

ALSO SEE: *Confinement*

Reward

A reward is a reinforcer that follows a behavior. It can be positive or negative in its interpretation by an animal and tends to encourage repetition of the behavior. The type of reward can also be internal, promoting a good feeling, or it can be external, such as food or praise.

ALSO SEE: *Internal Reward, Motivation, Negative Reinforcement, Positive Reinforcement*

Ritualized Fighting

Fighting between members of the same species where the objective seems to be to intimidate rather than to do physical damage is called ritualized fighting. A specific behavior pattern is followed, and if fighting actually occurs, it usually comes after intense threats. Ritualized fighting is most often associated with rivals for territory, mates, food, or social rank.

ALSO SEE: *Aggression, Dominance Aggression, Protective Aggression, Territorial Protective Aggression*

Roaming

Roaming is the tendency of an animal to stray occasionally from its territory. This characteristic is a male sexually dimorphic behavior and thus is controllable to a certain degree by the reduction of testosterone.

ALSO SEE: *Castration, Drug Therapy, Sexually Dimorphic Behaviors*

Rocking

Rocking is a stereotyped behavior exhibited by primates. The animal sits and moves its body forward and back. While the behavior is generally regarded as abnormal, it does occur occasionally in the wild. It is most typically seen in caged laboratory primates and may be related to the lack of other forms of exercise or mental stimulation. Since the behavior is self-rewarding, it can quickly develop into a habit and become very difficult to eliminate. It is a coping behavior that provides exercise, so it may not always be desirable to eliminate it.

ALSO SEE: *Stereotyped Behaviors*

Roles of Domesticated Animals

Domesticated animal species have provided a number of diverse services for humans. The roles can be divided into 12 categories as described below.

Clothing—One of the earliest contributions made by animals, both wild and domestic, was that of clothing. The hides furnished leather articles, and the hair and wool added fibers that could be made into items of apparel.

Food—Even before domestication, animals were a source of meat for the hunter and the extended family. After domestication, milk, and in some cultures, blood, also became important.

Transportation—A number of species have served as a primary means of transportation, carrying humans on their backs or pulling them in wagons or other vehicles. Horses have been a major part of many cultures, with burros, cattle, reindeer, camels, and dogs contributing also.

Extension of human senses—The limits of human senses have been extended through the capabilities of animal senses. While guide dogs for the blind are the most obvious example, hearing-ear dogs, tracking dogs, and drug- and bomb-detection dogs have filled needs in other areas.

Protection—Animal skins and pelts have provided shelters. Dung is a source of warmth. Dogs have protected owners against intruders and assisted the police and military in their duties. Even canaries have protected miners by serving as an early warning against poison gas in the mine.

Research—Laboratory animals have made major contributions to the knowledge of certain diseases, the development of treatments for these conditions, the understanding of all disciplines of human and veterinary medicine, and the development of products that are safe for consumers. In recent years, the search for alternative methods to study the extensions of these areas has decreased the number of animals used by researchers and increased the contributions of individual research projects.

Physical health—Human health has been protected through animal contributions. Numerous species have been involved in the growth of vaccines, although recombinant DNA techniques are dramatically changing this need. The exercise provided by horses has helped the physically normal person maintain health. The handicapped rider benefits from the muscle exercise of hippotherapy, a relatively new technique that is being added to rehabilitation programs. Even the physical exercise associated with walking a dog can be included.

Occupations—A number of people depend on animals for their direct livelihood. Obvious inclusions are animal trainers and veterinarians.

Educator—The animal raised with a child often becomes an educator. The openness of reproduction provides lessons of sex. Companionship teaches aspects of discipline with love, and death teaches about bereavement.

Mental health—Many animals have had an association with religion, whether as religious figures or as favored species within a religion. A more direct contribution to mental health comes from the companionship provided by the animals. Recreation, whether by hunting, riding, racing, or other similar events, is also important for humans. Events such as bull fighting, dog fighting, and chicken fighting also provide recreation, although they tend to be more controversial within Western cultures. Animals also can serve as status symbols for the owners. Registered breeds and unusual appearances reflect the owners' images of themselves.

Manufacturing—Maintaining a large number of animals in close confinement for maximum production within a unit is commonly called "factory farming." It is common in egg and broiler chicken production and in hog production units. In addition, the waste products of animals are used to supply fertilizer, heat, methane gas, and animal feed.

Communication—While animals have carried messengers for military and civilian needs, such as the pony express, they also have been the primary message carriers. Trench dogs used in World War I carried messages across the battlefield. Carrier pigeons continue as occasional messengers even today.

Rolling

Animals groom their coats in a number of ways, including by rolling on the ground from side to side and while on one side. This action is often in loose dirt and helps bring dust into the coat. Rolling usually is followed by the animal shaking the dirt free again. Rolling may also be done in mud or in loose dirt after the animal is wet. The mud on the coat is allowed to dry and probably serves as natural protection against insects. Less agile animals may decrease the amount of action and wallow instead.

An additional type of rolling occurs in dogs and occasional other species. Dogs are famous for rolling in manure and decomposing matter. While the exact reason for the behavior is not known, the author proposes two theories. The first theory says that this behavior is the animal's way of taking on a specific scent. It should be remembered that the animal's aesthetic values and likes and dislikes are different than those of the human. Under this theory, the behavior is analogous to putting on cologne or perfume. The second theory holds that rolling on smelly things allows the dog to scent-mark larger areas with its own body odors, being another form of marking behavior.

ALSO SEE: *Grooming Behavior, Marking, Self-Marking, Shaking, Wallow*

Rolling Skin Syndrome

The rolling skin syndrome is another term for the feline hyperesthesia syndrome.

SEE: *Feline Hyperesthesia Syndrome*

Running Away

Fleeing is a natural escape mechanism for some species of animals. For horses and others that evolved on the open plains, running is a logical defense strategy. Since domestication, that escape mechanism can get the animal into trouble. Fences and gates become real dangers during an instinctive reaction. Bolting from a handler is another example.

Running away has a second connotation. Dogs and cats occasionally will leave what has been a longtime home. The amount of time they are gone can vary from a few hours for the dog that escaped from the backyard to the animal that never comes back. Dogs that escape from a fenced yard, whether by digging out or climbing over a fence, may spend time running through the neighborhood. Other dogs keep running away from an approaching owner or pay no attention to being called. For some dogs, much energy and/or not enough social interaction can cause the dog to run and seek out peers. Both behaviors are self-rewarding. The dog can also be taught to run away by being punished each time the owner approaches. Cats tend to run away from an established home if there are social changes in the territory. A pariah may leave and generally not return if the social stress is too great.

ALSO SEE: *Bolting, Climbing, Digging—Outdoors, Escape Behaviors, Fence Jumping, Flight Distance, Flightiness, Internal Reward, Pariah, Returning to Old Home, Stress-related Behaviors*

Satellite Male

Satellite or peripheral males live along the edges of a social group. In some species, they are part of the group; in others, they just happen to be around. The individuals are usually young adult males that have not yet established their own social group. Satellite males may have occasional opportunities to mate with one or more group females.

ALSO SEE: *Animal Sociology*

Scent Marking

Scent marking is the use of an odor to mark a particular territory, individual, or self. The odor may be associated with saliva, glandular secretions, urine, or feces. These scents are a form of olfactory communication used mainly by macrosomatic animals.

ALSO SEE: *Macrosomatic Animals, Pheromone, Self-Marking, Urine Spraying*

Schedule

One factor associated with many problem behaviors is a change in schedule for the animal. Owners seldom realize how important a schedule is to their animal or just what routine is already established.

Dogs and cats are attuned to times when they interact with their owners, even to times when they are petted while the family watches television. Their stares on weekend mornings make sleeping late impossible. When one person is home all day, the animal may get used to attention on demand.

Changes in the daily schedule can be stressful to the animal. Little changes such as a late arrival or missing a snack, or bigger ones such as a new baby, different work times, a vacation, or house guests can be very disruptive. The exact reaction varies. It may be simply a more intense greeting, but it also can include destructive behaviors, stereotypies, or aggression. When a problem starts, the tendency is to make additional changes to contain the problem instead of returning to the previous situation. Occasionally it is not possible to return to the old schedule, such as when a new baby arrives. If the event can be anticipated, gradual change minimizes the impact of the event. Another technique is to make the new schedule very firm so that the animal can determine what occurs when and change faster.

Recommendations for problems associated with stress often include a firm schedule for the animal.

ALSO SEE: *Attention Seeking, Climbing, Destructive Behaviors, Destructive Chewing, Digging—Indoors, Digging—Outdoors, Excessive Grooming, Excessive Licking, Excessive Vocalization—Howling, Fear of Change, Frustration, Fun in Location, Gradual Introduction, Hot Spots, New Baby, Psychogenic Problems, Self-Mutilation, Spite, Stereotyped Behaviors, Stress-related Behaviors*

Scratching

Scratching is a behavior of chickens in which they scratch the ground with one leg and then the other. It is usually associated with eating.

Mammals may show a similar scraping or scratching of the ground with either front or hind feet. Pawing can be associated with aggression, marking, or apparent impatience.

ALSO SEE: *Marking, Pawing*

Searching Automatism

Searching automatism is the side-to-side movements of a neonate's head that occur spontaneously and in association with tactile stimulation. These movements stop when the neonate finds a mammary teat to suckle. The behavior, common in kittens and puppies, decreases as the infant gets older and can search for a teat using vision and smell.

ALSO SEE: *Nursing*

Sebacide

Sebacide, a type of infanticide, is usually called fratricide.

SEE: *Fratricide*

Seizures

Epilepsy and seizures due to other causes can have a major behavioral component. They are best recognized in dogs, but probably occur in other species too. The condition can be expressed as a behavior change only—tail chasing, star gazing, aggression, fly snapping, limb flicking, and the feline hyperesthesia syndrome. Histories are important in establishing a diagnosis and will conform to those of the more classic forms of seizures. The animal is usually a young adult; the onset is gradual with increasing frequency and severity. There may be a triggering event such as excitement, and owners may be aware of a pre- or post-seizure phase. A blank stare and unawareness of the surroundings is common. The dog may try to be close or to hide after the brief seizure.

Treatment may be initiated if the frequency, duration, or intensity is severe. Antiepileptics are the standard drugs used. While new drugs are slowly finding their way to veterinary medicine, the old standbys are the most commonly used, even with their side effects. The drugs, doses, and clinical evaluations for follow-up are the same as for the more typical types of seizures.

ALSO SEE: *Brain Disorders, Drug Therapy, Epileptic Aggression, Feline Hyperesthesia Syndrome, Feline Ischemic Encephalopathic Aggression, Fly Snapping, History Taking, Limb Flicking, Psychogenic Seizures, Tail Chasing*

Selective Breeding

Selective breeding occurs when the choice of reproductive partners is made by humans choosing certain traits they hope will be passed on to the offspring. This process is critical to domestication in the first place, and then becomes important to the establishment of breeds or the enhancement of physical or behavioral features.

ALSO SEE: *Domestication*

Self-Licking

Self-licking can refer to the normal form of self-grooming with the tongue, or it can also be applied to excessive licking.

ALSO SEE: *Excessive Licking, Grooming*

Self-Marking

Self-marking is a form of scent marking involving the application of an odorous substance to one's own body. Rolling in smelly material and urinating on the rear limbs are examples. The apparent function is for scent communication.

ALSO SEE: *Rolling, Scent Marking*

Self-Mutilation

Self-mutilation is damage that an animal causes to itself, usually in response to excessive environmental stress. While any species is susceptible to the behavior, it is most common in dogs, cats, horses, and primates. The behavior usually takes the form of psychogenic dermatoses and responds to the routines of schedule and exercise along with reduced environmental stresses. There is apparently some form of internal reward, because normally painful behaviors continue without intervention.

ALSO SEE: *Avoid Situations, Destructive Chewing, Excessive Licking, Exercise, Feline Hyperesthesia Syndrome, Frustration, Hair Pulling, Lick*

Granulomas, Over-Grooming, Psychogenic Dermatoses, Schedule, Stereo-typed Behaviors, Stress-related Behaviors, Tail Chewing

Semisocial

The term semisocial is used to describe certain insect species, including some primitive bees (including bumblebees) and wasps, where all members of the colony are of the same generation.

More advanced insect colonies are described as eusocial.

ALSO SEE: *Eusocial*

Senile Aggression

Senile changes have not been proven to occur in animals; however, there are some bouts of aggression that may be related to such changes. Aggression has been associated with aging of Type A personalities in humans, so the possibility of an animal model does exist. Tumors could also play a role in causing this syndrome.

Behaviorialists working at separate colonies of geriatric beagles report instances in which dogs that had been housed together for a long period of time would kill and partially eat one of the penmates. There is evidence that the dog killed may have been caught in the pen fencing. It has not been determined whether the dogs simply turned on a defenseless dog or whether distress cries triggered aggression to destroy the noise so as not to make the pack "vulnerable." There are case histories of older dogs that have become uncontrollably mean-tempered toward all people, including their owners. Additional behavioral study is necessary to clarify this type of aggression.

ALSO SEE: *Cannibalism, Irritable Aggression, Mental Confusion, Pack Response Aggression*

Sensitive Period

Sensitive periods are limited times within an animal's life when the individual is particularly sensitive to certain types of learning, such as imprinting. The term "critical period" is often used interchangeably, although "sensitive period" implies a less well-defined beginning and end.

ALSO SEE: *Critical Periods, Imprint Learning*

Separate

Certain types of aggression cannot be stopped as long as environmental factors do not change. There are also situations in which the animal, owner, or another animal is in potential danger. These are times when continuous separation may be the only workable solution. Intermale aggression requires a constant separation of dogs showing the trait, or fighting will occur. Prey chasing by dogs is prevented best by keeping the dog separate from cats, livestock, and cars if there is any tendency for chasing. Dominance aggression toward a person or redirected aggression toward a small conspecific may also require continuous separation.

ALSO SEE: *Dominance Aggression, Fight It Out, Intrasexual Aggression, Predatory Aggression, Redirected Aggression*

Separation Anxiety

Separation anxiety is used to describe behaviors that occur when the animal, usually a dog, is left alone. Historically the problem usually happens as the person is leaving or immediately thereafter, so the owners comment that it does not matter if they are gone five minutes or five hours. The specific behaviors vary depending on the location and the dog but commonly include destructive chewing, excessive vocalizing, digging, garbage eating, urination, defecation, aggression as the owner leaves, or psychogenic problems.

Management of these problems can be difficult because it takes both time and effort, and the more severe the problem, the more difficult the solution. Since the dog's concern is over the owner's absence, it must gradually be accustomed to that absence. The owner should go through all the motions of getting ready but not actually leave. When the excitement is triggered by a specific event, such as the jiggling of car keys, the specific anxiety-eliciting behavior can be performed to accustom the dog to it. Additional components should be added to distract the dog. A favorite food or toy can be presented, and the owner should leave briefly as soon as the dog's attention is focused on the item. Changes in length of time absent are also helpful; for example, walking out and coming immediately back in and then walking out and returning after 30 seconds. The absence is gradually increased and made more random. The dog should not be punished for the inappropriate behavior. Ideally while the retraining is going on, the owner should be gone just under the length of time the dog can tolerate. Crating the severe cases usually is not helpful, since many of these dogs injure themselves as they attempt to get out. Antianxiety tranquilizers may be necessary in the more severe cases.

The owner should not reward the behavior by returning while the dog is showing the behavior. Walking in when the dog is barking translates to the dog that barking will eventually bring the owner. Use a noise as a distraction if necessary so that the door opens when the dog is not showing the behavior.

ALSO SEE: *Aggression, Avoid Situations, Cloth with Odor, Destructive Chewing, Digging, Drug Therapy, Emotional Come and Go, Excessive Vocalization, Excessive Vocalization—Barking, Excessive Vocalization— Howling, Garbage Eating, Psychogenic Problems, Social Contact, Stress-related Behaviors*

Separation Syndrome

Separation syndrome is the collection of problems that can occur if an infant is separated from its mother after the bond has been formed. Common sequelae include stereotypies, self-mutilation, and the inability to later form appropriate social bonds. The separation syndrome is a type of deprivation syndrome.

ALSO SEE: *Deprivation Syndrome, Self-Mutilation, Stereotyped Behaviors*

Sex Advertisement

Sex advertisement is a term generally used to describe any behavior or physical feature that helps in the establishment of a pair bond. It can include special coloring, vocalizations, courtship dances, and contacts.

ALSO SEE: *Reproductive Behavior*

Sex Attractant

A sex attractant is a pheromone that functions to attract and/or guide individuals together to ensure successful reproduction.

ALSO SEE: *Pheromone*

Sex-related Aggression

Sex-related aggression, a type of nonaffective aggression, is generally regarded as a normal behavior under hormonal and neurologic control. The nape bite is shown primarily by dogs, toms, and stallions when mounting. This grip is considered an inhibited bite, since its apparent purpose is not to leave a wound. In other forms of sex-related aggression, anestrous females may react aggressively toward attempts to mount, and the estrous queen will strike at a tom as he dismounts after mating. An occasional complaint may indicate that an individual male is too rough or that the owner does not understand what is normal for the species. Owners can be educated, but little can be done to modify an individual animal's style.

ALSO SEE: *Mutual Grooming, Nonaffective Aggression*

Sexual Behavior

Sexual behavior is reproductive behavior.

SEE: *Reproductive Behavior*

Sexual Dimorphism

When differences occur between individuals within a species, it is called dimorphism. When the differences between the sexes occur relative to the

appearance and behavior, the term sexual dimorphism is appropriate.
ALSO SEE: *Dimorphism, Monomorphism, Sexually Dimorphic Behaviors*

Sexually Dimorphic Behaviors

Maleness and femaleness are not absolute traits. They represent a graded scale of physical and behavioral features usually associated with a particular sex, but which overlap considerably. Male behaviors generally include marking, roaming, intermale aggression, mounts, and pelvic thrusts. Female behaviors are typically those associated with sexual and maternal behaviors.

Determination of general dimorphic characteristics occurs around the time of birth. That is when a testosterone surge masculinizes the brain to be responsive to testosterone at puberty. Without the perinatal testosterone, the brain retains feminine behaviors. If this hormone surge occurs prior to birth, a female twin or adjacent fetuses may be partially affected.
ALSO SEE: *Castration, Female Behaviors, Intrasexual Aggressions, Male Behaviors, Roaming*

Sexual Selection

Sexual selection describes the various types of competition that eventually leads to successful reproduction. Intrasexual selection describes the interactions between members of the same sex to achieve access to the opposite sex. The aggressive interactions of males during a breeding season are examples. Intersexual selection is the choice of a specific partner.
ALSO SEE: *Advertising Dress, Dissociation, Reproductive Behavior*

Shaking

Shaking is a side-to-side rapid rotational motion used as a grooming behavior. It probably functions to rid the coat of excessive amounts of dirt or water and is used by horses, dogs, and cats, particularly after rolling.

The death shake associated with prey killing by carnivores has also been called shaking.
ALSO SEE: *Death Shake, Grooming Behavior, Rolling*

Shaping

Positive reinforcement is used to reinforce a series of behaviors that progress toward a desired behavior. Paper training puppies starts with papers covering the entire floor and praising the puppy for eliminating; gradually the size of the paper-covered area is decreased, and the puppy is still praised for eliminating on the paper. Eventually the size of the area covered by paper is quite small, but the puppy continues to use it. Teaching a dog or cat to ride in a car or a horse to ride in a trailer employs the same principle. The animal is rewarded for coming close to the vehicle, and then for putting its head in. The next reward comes for getting in and then for being shut in for a brief period of time. Eventually the animal is taken for a short ride and gradually for longer ones.

ALSO SEE: *Positive Reinforcement, Punishment, Skinner Box*

Sheep

Sheep, *Ovis aries*, were domesticated from *Ovis orientalis*, the Asiatic mouflon, or wild sheep, approximately 9000 years ago (Clutton-Brock, 1981). As with modern sheep, the mouflon was a grazing animal, and it came from the mountain areas of Asia Minor. Early association with humans was probably for the food and clothing the animals could provide.

ALSO SEE: *Domestication, Appendix B*

Shelter-seeking Behavior

Behaviors that help protect an animal from weather or insects can be termed shelter-seeking. Such behaviors include seeking protection in buildings or under trees (dangerous in lightning storms), crowding for warmth or protection (dangerous for domestic poultry), mutual fly chasing by standing so another's tail protects the face, and standing in deep water to ward off biting insects.

ALSO SEE: *Grooming Behavior*

Shock Collars

Shock collars are electrically activated shocking devices attached to a collarlike strap. There are two basic designs. One has an attached sensing device that activates the shock when the dog barks. This type of collar has no external control, so the barking of a second dog or other sharp noise may activate the shock, or a dog that reacted by yelping may continuously activate the shocker.

The second type of shock collar has a remote control device so that a person must push a button to activate the shock. As with any type of punishment, timing of the shock is important. Some types also use a weighted dummy collar so that the animal will not learn to be on its best behavior only when the collar is worn. This type of collar can be useful on some individuals for certain types of behavior problems for which remote punishment is desirable. These collars are commonly used in training bird dogs.

There are, however, problems with the use of shock collars. For some horses or dogs, the amount of the shock may cause them to show another undesirable reaction, such as panic running or extreme submission. The amount of shock delivered each time may be inconsistent, so the degree of punishment varies independently from the problem behavior. Physical variations, such as the amount of hair or degree of wetness, can also vary the shock received. Appropriate use with careful monitoring of the entire application and response can produce successful results. Inappropriate use can cause more problems than the animal had originally. In each case it is necessary to evaluate all contributing factors because one problem behavior may be replaced by another if the initiating factors are not changed.

ALSO SEE: *Remote Punishment*

Shying

Shying is a flight reaction most commonly seen when a horse is startled by an object. Because horses evolved to flee potential danger, their reaction to unknowns often involves flight. Things which are startling are often those that move so rapidly that the horse cannot focus on them, such as a bird flying up from underfoot or plastic flapping on a fence. Objects perceived as being out of place can also cause reaction.

Experience generally tempers the severity of the shying. A gentle introduction to trail riding by traveling with a calm, older horse and by patient introduction to things that are frightening help the young horse develop into a dependable trail horse. Intangibles such as an individual's personality and mood can also affect the animal's tendency to react to a given situation.

ALSO SEE: *Vision*

Siblicide

Siblicide is another term used to describe fratricide.

SEE: *Fratricide*

Sibling Rivalry

While sibling rivalry in its truest form refers to fights among offspring of the same parents, the term is also used to describe the confrontations between dogs or cats sharing the same living space. Rivalry is most often associated with food. Whether this means squabbles over preferred resources or over a particular food item, the differences are usually settled by the relative positions within the social order. With animals kept as pets, humans may side with a lower-ranking animal and compound the difficulty in settling the disagreement.

ALSO SEE: *Dominance Aggression, Social Order*

Silent Heat

Certain females show no or very low levels of behavioral estrus even when there is a physiologically normal estrus. Silent heats are usually associated with

S

cows, but occur in mares, bitches, and probably other species as well.

ALSO SEE: *Female Behaviors*

Skinner Box

The Skinner box is a type of puzzle box used to study operant conditioning. An animal, originally a bird, was rewarded for a random behavior, such as turning its head toward a lever. Gradually the behavior was shaped so that the head not only turned, but it touched, and later pushed, the lever for its reward.

The apparatus is named after B.F. Skinner, who popularized its use in psychology.

ALSO SEE: *Puzzle Box, Shaping, Skinnerian Shaping of Behavior*

Skinnerian Shaping of Behavior

B.F. Skinner defined operant conditioning for the study of learning by dividing it into three primary components. The first was a stimulus situation, or cue, in which the response occurs. The second component was the response itself, and the third was the reinforcing consequence, or reinforcer. Using this combination in a series of more demanding tasks, he could shape a behavior from one that barely resembled a desired result to one that was relatively complex.

Getting a rat to push a lever when a light comes on is the goal. The sequence starts by rewarding the animal with food if it turns its head toward the lever when the light first comes on. Eventually it must turn its body, then approach, then touch, and finally push the lever in order to get the food. Getting a monkey to pull a rope for food starts by getting it to touch a rope. Including food within a braided rope can accomplish this. Then just touching a plain rope brings a reward. Then the rope must be pulled. Eventually the rope can be pulled from one area of the cage, and the reward can be received in another. This type of shaping is valuable for behavioral enrichment for zoo and laboratory animals.

ALSO SEE: *Kicking, Learning, Negative Reinforcement, Operant Conditioning, Positive Reinforcement, Skinner Box*

Sleep

Sleep is an unconscious state of resting that is believed to be necessary for most mammals. The two phases of sleep alternate between slow-wave and fast-wave (REM) electroencephalographic activity during a sleep session.

With the exception of fish, all vertebrates are believed to sleep. It is believed that fish must continuously swim to breathe and therefore cannot go into a deep sleep. Sharks that inhabit a unique oxygen-rich environment off the Mexican coast are the only known fish exception.

ALSO SEE: *REM Sleep, Resting Behaviors, Sleeping Position, Slow-Wave Sleep*

Sleeping Position

A wide variety of positions are used by animals for sleeping. For mammals, the typical postures are lateral recumbency, sternal recumbency, or a combination of cranial-sternal and caudal-lateral. Lateral recumbency is the typical posture for REM sleep. Occasional individuals, usually dogs or cats, sleep on their backs. Horses use their reciprocal apparatus to be able to rest in a standing position, with one rear limb resting on the toe. Birds may stand on one leg with the head tucked under a wing. Bats sleep hanging upside down.

ALSO SEE: *Resting Behaviors, Sleep*

Slow-Wave Sleep

Slow-wave sleep is the first of two types of sleep an animal enters during a sleep period. The electroencephalogram (EEG) is synchronized and has a regular pattern of high-amplitude slow waves. This pattern alternates with REM sleep several times during a sleep period. If the duration of slow-wave sleep increases, the length of sleep increases.

ALSO SEE: *REM Sleep, Sleep*

Smell

The sense of smell in humans is rudimentary compared to that of domestic animals, especially the dog. Because of this, we have a great deal of trouble designing tests that accurately measure olfaction.

To put canine smell in perspective, compare the olfactory bulbs of a human to those of a large dog. The human has approximately 2×10^7 olfactory cells, and the bulbs have a surface area of about 500 mm^2. The dog has about 2.8×10^8 cells and 7000 mm^2 area. The comparative difference is significant. A dog can smell a dilution of 1 part of alpha-ionone in 10^7 parts dilutant (Moulton, 1972). For comparison, this means being able to detect 1 drop of odor diluted in 10^7 drops of water (Fuller and Fox in Hafez, 1969), or roughly 1 drop in 25 barrels of water. This, however, is probably not the limit of sensitivity of the dog's nose. A plant odor was detected at a dilution of 10^{13} parts (Dan Craig, personal communication). If that is compared to 1-drop equivalents, a single drop of the odor could be detected in a 24.8 million barrel dilution. The possibilities for drug detection, bomb detection, and scent tracking are almost limitless. One molecule could easily alert a trained detection dog, and field experience indicates how well these animals can do.

The sense of smell of cats is probably between that of dogs and humans. Cats use saliva, urine, and sebaceous gland secretions to mark certain objects, so messages are communicated through olfaction. The cat olfactory area has approximately 6.7×10^7 cells (Beadle, 1977). This species also reacts behaviorally to a number of plant odors, with catnip most well known.

Olfaction in horses has not been well studied, but experience indicates it is superior to that of humans. Stallions smell feces and urine in social encounters, indicating that smell is important behaviorally. Horses can detect odors from dead poisonous snakes, decaying carcasses, and fires that are much too weak for human noses.

Pigs apparently have an exceptional sense of smell. Behaviorally, scents from the preputial pouch, saliva, and carpal glands are important, indicating that smell plays an important role. Pigs that find the musty odor of truffles underground rely on their noses and are easily trained.

ALSO SEE: *Catnip, Cloth with Odor, Flehmen, Marking, Sniffing Humans, Vomeronasal Organ*

Smell Aversion

Smell aversion is the use of odor as a deterrent. In one technique, a "stinky" aerosol spray is selected, and the animal allowed to smell the nozzle. Then the owner holds the can in front of the animal so that the spray will come out at 90° from the animal's face, not directly at it. While the can is sprayed for one to two seconds, it is moved rapidly toward the animal's face in a threatening manner. The animal should react by trying to get away, and cats, in particular, can scratch or bite. The goal is to have the animal associate the smell with the hissing, threatening experience. With the animal out of the room, the object being chewed is sprayed and the fumes allowed to settle before the animal has access to it.

The odor used for the spray should not be one typically found in the home. The exception would be for the wool-sucking cat that targets the underarm areas of dirty shirts or human skin. In this case, a deodorant spray would be an appropriate choice.

ALSO SEE: *Aversive Conditioning, Destructive Chewing, Direct Punishment, Taste Aversion, Wool Sucking*

Snapping

In foals, snapping is another term to describe jaw chomping. The term also describes an abbreviated biting behavior by dogs, usually used as a warning.

ALSO SEE: *Distance-increasing Silent Communication, Jaw Chomping, Warning Behavior*

Sniffing Humans

Many large dogs show the unacceptable behavior of putting their nose in a person's crotch and sniffing. Women usually receive this attention. Dogs live in a scent-oriented world because of their keen sense of smell, and scents are their primary means of identifying individuals. The vaginal secretions of women make the smell of the crotch area attractive to the dog.

Since the behavior is normal but unacceptable, punishment is not appropriate. Instead, it is best to divert the dog's attention or ask for an alternate behavior.

ALSO SEE: *Divert Attention, Smell, Substitute a Behavior*

Sniff-Yawn

The sniff-yawn is a behavior of bovine females after they encounter their just-born young. The female licks the placental fluids, raises its head, licks its nose, and yawns. During the yawn the eyes are usually closed and the tongue rolled upward. Within a few seconds, the yawn stops. The exact purpose of the behavior is unknown, but it has been speculated that it is similar to flehmen, introducing fetal odors into the vomeronasal organ.

ALSO SEE: *Flehmen, Maternal Behavior, Vomeronasal Organ*

Snout Rubbing

Snout rubbing is a porcine variation of nose rubbing, which is usually associated with crowding. Thus, it probably represents a stereotyped behavior. The incidence of snout rubbing tends to increase as tail docking is used to decrease the incidence of tail biting. Snout rubbing also can be associated with anal massage and ingestion of feces in some pigs.

Pasturing, lower stocking rates, and environmental enrichment with things to root and move around have been useful for managing this problem.

ALSO SEE: *Environmental Enrichment, Nose Rubbing, Tail Chewing*

Social Behavior

Social behavior describes the types of interactions between members of the same species. It can also include symbiotic interspecies relationships. These interactions vary depending on the type of group and the environmental situation. Social behaviors include sexual behaviors, mutual grooming, social orders, maternal behavior, communication, and socialization. Most social interactions are allelomimetic, but a few are agonistic. Dominance allows minor disagreements to be settled with only a mild threat, preserving life, limb, and group benefits. With the exception of the cat, domestic animals are social, group animals. These interpersonal activities are extremely important, and forced isolation causes problems: dogs will escape to find social contracts and horses will run through fences.

Dogs spend up to 85% of their time in close proximity with pack members (Fuller and Fox in Hafez, 1969). That equates to more than 20 hours a day. Owners must recognize what prolonged absences mean to their dog. While it is not practical to spend 20 hours each day with the animal, a dog owner can maximize the benefits of time together with a schedule. People who are absent for long periods need to consider seriously whether they should have a dog or whether a second dog may be an appropriate social companion. Dogs that protect pack members, an instinctive social behavior, are considered heros.

Feral horses live in harem groups or small herds when stallions and mares are present. Domestication and castration complicate this social arrangement and can result in large herds. Even within groups, individual friendships can develop, and such friends are called preferred associates.

Cattle can live in larger herds than horses, but within the herd there are subgroups. Individual cows often belong to several of these subgroups with a place in the social order of each. As group members, cows are active followers of a few leaders so that the herd moves in relatively parallel patterns. This cohesive tendency is weakest in individuals recently introduced to the herd. Sheep also have active followership in their flock structure.

Pigs are extremely flexible in their group size. Feral animals live in female herds of 4 to more than 20 individuals, with boars joining them during breeding season (Hafez and Signoret in Hafez, 1969). Groups approaching 80 individuals can occur. Domestic pigs accept a wide variety of social densities; however, crowding can be stressful. Body contact is an important social behavior and is maintained during resting, even in hot weather.

ALSO SEE: *Agonistic Behavior, Allelomimetic Behavior, Antisocial, Asocial, Bachelor Groups, Communication Behaviors, Greeting Behaviors, Grooming Behavior, Harem, Hero, Maternal Behavior, Preferred Associate, Reproductive Behavior, Schedule, Social Contact, Social Groups, Socialization, Social Order*

Social Contact

Animals that normally live in groups spend a certain portion of each day in close proximity to other members of that group. There are many benefits to this contact, including protection, mutual grooming, cooperative food gathering, and assistance in raising the young. There also may be intangible benefits of being with conspecifics, because prolonged periods of separation can be associated with behaviors of separation anxiety, stress, stereotypes, and psychogenic components. The amounts and timing of social contact needed by the various species are not well studied, but this area is receiving a great deal of attention relative to the general welfare of laboratory animals.

ALSO SEE: *Animal Welfare, Psychogenic Problems, Separation Anxiety, Stereotyped Behaviors, Stress-related Behaviors*

Social Distance

The social (reactive) distance is a broad category defining the spacing of interactions of animals to herdmates, strangers, and area. Variations in social distances can occur due to a number of influences, including the environmental context (such as crowded vs. not crowded), physiological state (such as sex hormone fluctuations), "mood," selective breeding (such as production breeds of poultry), intensity of stimulation (such as a rapid or slow approach), and learning (particularly from early experience).

A second definition of social distance is a subcategory of the broad one defined above. It represents the space between the individual distance, which is limited to preferred associates, and the distance at which an animal that is moving away from its group will turn around and go back to the group. A young horse being ridden from the barn for the first time will start acting up when it reaches the outer limit of the social distance.

ALSO SEE: *Individual Distance, Preferred Associates*

Social Facilitation

Social facilitation is a phenomenon in which the behavior of an individual has an additive or reciprocally stimulating effect on others. An alarm or flight reaction by a few individuals in a group can result in the flight of all members of that group. Social facilitation can affect other behaviors as well, including reproduction, ingestion, and elimination (Fox, 1986).

ALSO SEE: *Sympathetic Induction of Mood*

Social Grooming

Social (mutual) grooming occurs when one individual grooms another. The site groomed is often one that the individual would have a difficult time taking care of alone, such as the neck, shoulders, or back. In addition to a grooming function, these interactions probably help intensify social bonds and minimize tensions within a group.

ALSO SEE: *Grooming Behavior, Mutual Grooming, Withers Nibbling*

Social Groups

Animals live together in many types of groups, generally defined as social groups, from loose congregations to tight-knit interdependence.

ALSO SEE: *Aggregation, Animal Sociology, Anonymous Group, Association, Colony, Group Cohesion, Harem, Individualized Group, Population, Satellite Male, Society*

Social Inhibition

Social inhibition is the suppression of a specific behavior because of the influence of another. The presence of a high-ranking group member can minimize salivary flow and interest in eating. It can also minimize interest in an estrous female. Appeasement displays can minimize or stop an aggressive display. Psychogenic problems are extremes of social inhibition.

ALSO SEE: *Appeasement Behavior, Psychogenic Problems*

Socialization

Socialization is a special learning process during which an individual learns to accept close proximity to various species or to conspecifics of its own group. This may be as narrow as imprinting on a dam or neonate (imprinting), or as broad as learning to tolerate a multispecies environment. For the most part, socialization is restricted to a specific time period. That is certainly true for maternal/infant imprinting. The actual limits of socialization are best understood in dogs, although some general principles apply. The socialization period begins shortly after the senses are functional and continues until the animal begins to show strong interest in its environment.

In dogs, the socialization period extends from 3 weeks to approximately 12 weeks. It can be argued that these few weeks are the single most important time in the life of the dog (Scott and Fuller, 1965). This is when it must learn its own species, as well as cats, horses, sheep, and other animals. It is also the time it must be around humans, both adults and small children. Since the lessons of socialization are visually oriented and most dogs (and especially puppies) have poor visual distinction, the form of an adult human is perceived as different in proportions to that of a child. This is especially true if the child is under approximately 7 years of age; it still has the juvenile proportions, including a larger head, and diapers really distort proportion. The child's movements are also more jerky and swaying.

During the socialization period for puppies, many changes occur just because of physical and neurologic maturation. In addition, the puppy's interest in other living beings peaks between 5 and 7 weeks during the peak approach period. It can be altered drastically by negative experiences at the start of stable learning (week 8) and is set for the rest of the animal's life by the start of the peak avoidance period (week 12) (Fox, 1965). The lessons of socialization must be reinforced occasionally in the weeks and months to come and may be lost or altered by traumatic occurrences.

Once socialized, a dog may actually crowd closer to an owner or social peer if punished or abused because it feels safer by being close than by leaving. For example, a dog follows the family child going for a bike ride but is not supposed to. The child stops and yells and hits at the dog to make it go home. Instead of leaving, the dog crouches into a submissive posture and crawls closer to the child. Passive attention also has a strong attraction for the socialized dog and explains why dogs reliably go to the person who does not like dogs. The actual amount of time or exposure needed for socialization is probably not great compared to total time of the period (Scott and Fuller, 1965). Overnight isolation during the peak approach period might actually speed the process of socialization (Fox, 1965).

Socialization is important for species identification in cats, but their asocial nature makes characterization more difficult. The socialization period begins around 3 weeks, when kittens are physically able to interact with their world. It probably ends at about 9 weeks, as they become much less interested in social beings and much more engaged in environmental exploration (Beaver, 1992).

Foals and calves are born with eyes and ears open, and they are aware of things around them almost immediately. For them, socialization may end within a few hours. A foal knows its dam in 3 hours and knows it is a horse even if it is orphaned within hours of birth and raised by a nurse goat. Human interaction with newborn foals can result in easier handling as the horse gets older (Miller, 1991). Calves take a little longer, since an orphan can imprint on other species. Baby piglets are intermediates in the physical and sensory development of neonates. Their socialization period probably begins around the start of the second week of age.

Improper socialization in dogs can become a major problem. It hinders the dog's ability to relate to people. In any animal species, poor socialization can affect the choice of reproductive partners and thus the probability of reproductive success.

ALSO SEE: *Exploratory Behavior, Fear of People, Improper Socialization, Improper Socialization Aggression, Imprint Learning, Isolated Syndrome, Kennelosis, Peak Approach Period, Peak Avoidance Period, Place Imprinting, Rank Order*

Social Order

A social order is the arrangement of dominance within a group. The general description of a social order (dominance order, pecking order) is linear. That is, animal **A** is dominant to animal **B**, which is over **C**, which is over **D**. This relationship can be pictured as:

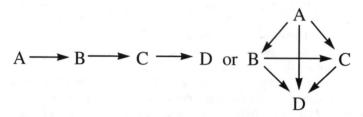

Linear-tending groups share some positions. When animals share one position, any situation in which a subtle threat normally settles the matter results in a more aggressive confrontation. Children or dogs raised as equals bicker frequently, and at least for dogs, measures to establish a definite position should be taken. This minimizes competitive aggression. A linear-tending relationship with a shared position could be pictured as :

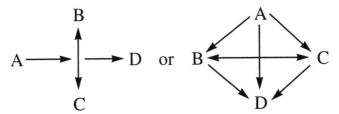

Another type of linear-tending group would have a position shared by a group with their own internal relationship.

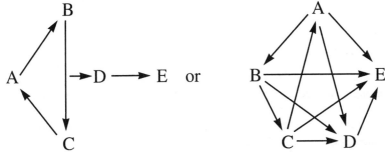

Complex groups have unique relationships between and among individuals and are common in cattle and sheep. Within a herd or flock there can be several smaller social groups that have a few members in common with other groups. Thus individuals may be ranked in two or three different groups.

A dog pack is variable in size depending on a number of conditions, but is linear to linear-tending in social arrangement.

The feral horse herd as a whole is quite stable and consists of a dominant stallion, a few mares, and their offspring up to three years of age. Bachelor groups of young stallions have a strong linear social order with only the highest ranking acting as a top stallion. Leadership in an action or movement is not necessarily related to the social ranking, and group social order is linear-tending. In a harem group, leadership is taken by the dominant stallion approximately 75% of the time (Waring, 1983).

Cattle and sheep have a cohesive bond that allows them to form large complex groups. They have an active followership so that all members tend to go where those in the front go. This is the reason that grazing cattle tend to be oriented in the same direction. Leadership is distinct from followership in cattle. In voluntary movement, the front few cows tend to be high-ranking, while in a forced movement, low-ranking cows are in front.

Swine social orders are complex and consist primarily of females with young. Boars normally join only during the mating season. Feral herds are generally of less than 20 individuals, although this species is extremely adaptable so that large groups can exist.

ALSO SEE: *Asocial, Bachelor Groups, Competitive Aggression, Dominance, Dominance Aggression, Establish Dominance, Central Hierarchy, Hierarchy, Hyporexia, Peck Order, Rank Order, Sibling Rivalry, Social Behavior, Status Signal*

Society

A society is a social group living together that shows a division of labor and regulation of activity. Parental care is generally well advanced. After humans and other primates, insects are the most commonly mentioned societies.

ALSO SEE: *Animal Sociology, Social Behavior*

Sociobiology

Sociobiology studies the biological basis for social behavior, primarily by examining how a gene pool can most successfully be passed on to succeeding populations.

ALSO SEE: *Adaptation, Behavioral Ecology, Kin Selection, Parental Investment, Parent-Offspring Conflict*

Soil Eating

The eating of soil or other foreign matter is a behavior problem seen most often in horses, cattle, dogs, and cats. Kittens typically eat litter a few days before starting litter box usage. A form of pica, soil eating is frequently related to mineral deficiencies, so diets must be carefully evaluated. Phosphorus, iron, and salt deficiencies are most common. Management systems should also be evaluated, since horses often respond to increased exercise.

ALSO SEE: *Exercise, Pica*

Soliciting Behavior

Soliciting behavior is the female behavior used to encourage copulation by a male. It is a part of the courtship behaviors.

ALSO SEE: *Courtship, Presentation, Perceptive Behavior*

Solitary

Solitary describes the lifestyle of individuals that live alone except to mate. Most felids are solitary, as are orangutans. These individuals are also called asocial or antisocial.

ALSO SEE: *Antisocial, Asocial*

Somnolent Impotence

Somnolent impotence is a condition in bulls that orient correctly behind an estrous cow, but adopt an inactive, sleeplike state. The head may be laid on the female's back. This condition may be an expression of narcolepsy.

ALSO SEE: *Male Behaviors, Narcolepsy*

Song

A song is a complex series of vocalizations. Functions vary with the species and the situation. The difference between a song and a call is poorly defined, although the latter tends to be much shorter, with less variations in it. Mammals, including whales, dolphins, and primates, have been studied for their song production. Birds are the best understood at this time and various patterns have been determined. Some of the patterns are species-specific, while others are a local dialect learned during specific developmental stages.

ALSO SEE: *Communication Behaviors, Vocal Communication, Vocalization*

Spay

A common expression used to describe an ovariohysterectomy or an ovariectomy.

ALSO SEE: *Ovariectomy, Testosterone-induced Aggression in Mares*

Species-Specific

A species-specific behavior is one that is characteristic of a particular species. The meaning if strictly interpreted refers to behaviors found only in that species. The more general definition includes behaviors that are found in all members of the specific species, regardless of whether the behaviors do or do not occur in other species. The hissing response of the cat is a species-specific behavior. So is the rumination of cattle (and other ruminants).

Spite

Owners often think a behavior problem is directed toward them—a spiteful reaction to something they have done. "Spite" in an animal can never be proven since the animal cannot talk about its reasons for doing something. Most behaviors happen for a specific reason; however, once the problem starts the owner may develop a negative attitude toward the animal. This results in less attention or increasingly harsh treatment, and then the animal may direct the problem behavior toward a specific individual. This directional behavior may be an attempt to get attention, since negative attention can be better than none at all. Dogs and cats typically show housesoiling or destructive behavior. For horses and some cats, the behavior may be irritable aggression.

Correction of the problem depends on building a positive interaction at the same time that schedules and primary problems are addressed.

ALSO SEE: *Destructive Chewing, Housesoiling—Spraying, Housesoiling— Urine Marking, Housesoiling—Urination, Irritable Aggression, Positive Attitude, Temper Tantrum*

Spontaneous Behavior

Spontaneous behavior has no obvious outside stimulus or control. The initiation of a spontaneous behavior and its control are under influences of the central nervous system. These behaviors can be motor or vocal.

If a behavior normally is dependent on an external stimulus, but appears to occur spontaneously, it is called a vacuum activity. Careful observation may be necessary to determine whether there is a stimulus or not, since priming stimuli can be difficult to detect.

ALSO SEE: *Priming Stimulus, Vacuum Activity*

Springer Rage Syndrome

This is a form of the rage syndrome seen in English springer spaniels.

SEE: *Rage Syndrome*

Stall Kicking

Horses that cannot get rid of excessive energy through exercise will find other ways to vent the energy. Stalled animals develop vices such as stall kicking. The behavior develops gradually and eventually becomes a habit, as if the horse likes the sound or feel of the kicking; the behavior has become internally rewarding even though it can cause physical injury. Stopping a stall kicker can be as difficult as stopping any habit. The appropriate approach to control is to make the behavior cause punishment and to provide an acceptable outlet for the excess energy. Kick chain (chains attached to leather leg straps) are commonly used. These cause a chain to whirl and hit the kicking leg. Shock-absorbing and sound-dampening padding will discourage other horses. Individual solutions using ingenuity are appropriate. With any solution, exercise or pasturing should be incorporated.

ALSO SEE: *Habit, Internal Reward, Kicking, Vices*

Stall Weaving

Stall weaving is stereotyped weaving.

SEE: *Stereotyped Weaving*

Star Gazing

Animals may be reported to "stare at the stars" or "into space." Periods of the behavior are usually brief. The occurrence is probably more frequent than recognized, and it is most commonly recognized in dogs. The primary differential diagnosis is a seizure; however, the mildness of the condition seldom requires drug therapy. Star gazing as a form of seizure may be one of at least two behavioral patterns associated with the condition. Environmental conditions such as undetected odors or sounds could produce a similar temporary response.

ALSO SEE: *Seizures*

Status Signal

A status signal is a display that indicates the age, experience, or position in a social order. The silver back on an older male gorilla is one example of such a signal. Status signals may reduce the amount of aggression within the group.

ALSO SEE: *Social Order*

Stereotyped Behaviors

A stereotyped behavior is an intentional, repetitive behavior that is nonfunctional. Many of the behaviors are performed in a rhythmic manner. They usually develop in an effort to cope with environmental stress such as isolation, little exercise, or no schedules. Stalled horses and laboratory primates are particularly vulnerable; however, these behaviors are seen in several species. There is considerable debate about whether stereotyped behaviors are totally bad for the animal, in that they do help it to cope, but there is no argument that it is better that they not develop at all. The behaviors are believed to have an internal reward and thus may continue as a favored activity even over eating or social interactions. Narcotic antagonists have been used on affected animals to stop the behavior temporarily. This indicates that brain chemistry may also be altered during the behavior. The development of long-acting narcotic antagonists should prove helpful in treating these behaviors, but they can only be considered as part of the answer.

ALSO SEE: *Appetitive Behavior, Boredom, Drug Therapy, Excessive Licking, Frustration, Habit, Head Nodding, Head Rubbing, Head Shaking, Ingestive Behavior, Internal Reward, Obsessive Compulsive Disorders, Psychomotor Agitation, Rocking, Schedule, Snout Rubbing, Social Contact, Stereotyped Pacing, Stereotyped Weaving, Stress-related Behaviors, Tail Chasing, Tongue Dragging, Tongue Play, Tongue Rolling, Vices*

Stereotyped Pacing

Stereotyped pacing is an adaptive pattern used by animals confined in a small area for long periods of time. It is an effort to use excessive energy and perhaps to overcome the lack of environmental stimuli. Evidence suggests that the behavior may release endorphins to help decrease stress. Stereotyped pacing is usually a walking or trotting gait along a specific path in a fixed pattern. This could be in a circle or back and forth in a straight line. A head toss may occur at each end of the line. Expression of this pacing is seen most typically in kenneled dogs, stalled horses, caged large carnivores, and caged nonhuman primates. As with any habit, once the pattern is established, the behavior is difficult to eliminate. It is important to correct the environment and encourage nonstereotypic activity. Punishing the behavior at each occurrence may also be used with the other measures. Prevention of the development of the behavior is much better than having to eliminate it. However, since it is a coping behavior that does provide exercise, eliminating it may not always be desirable.

ALSO SEE: *Stereotyped Behaviors, Stereotyped Weaving*

Stereotyped Weaving

Stereotyped weaving is a rhythmic lateral rocking motion in which an animal shifts its weight between its forelimbs. The rear limbs often move also, with the resulting rhythm being that of a walking gait. This behavior most commonly develops in individuals that are confined to small areas for long periods. It may be an attempt to get rid of excess energy or to cope with a bland environment. Once the behavior pattern has been established, it can be difficult to eliminate. For horses that show stereotyped weaving in a trailer, hobbles on the forelimbs can prevent the horse from getting the limbs far enough apart to weave. Since this can also affect their ability to brace during cornering, care must be used.

ALSO SEE: *Stereotyped Behaviors, Stereotyped Pacing, Trailer Rocking*

Stimulus

A stimulus is a condition that triggers a certain response by an animal or plant. The response can be physiological or behavioral, and the stimulus can be external or internal. Overt stimuli are priming stimuli and are not obvious to an observer.

ALSO SEE: *Priming Stimulus, Reaction Norm, Releaser, Stimulus Filtering, Stimulus Model, Stimulus-Response Relationship, Stimulus Summation, Threshold*

Stimulus Filtering

Selection of specific stimuli from an environment is dependent on central and peripheral filters. Although the environment contains a vast assortment of potential stimuli, only those that are recognized and passed along to the brain can be acted on centrally. Even then, action also depends on other factors of the filtering systems.

ALSO SEE: *Central Filters, Filters, Peripheral Filters, Stimulus*

Stimulus Model

A stimulus model is an alternate object that can elicit the same response as the item it models. A mounting dummy is used as a stimulus model to collect stallion semen for artificial breeding. A tape of distress vocalizations of a mouse can initiate hunting in a cat. Odors or appearances can also be mimicked to stimulate a specific response.

ALSO SEE: *Mimicry, Stimulus*

Stimulus-Response Relationship

The stimulus-response relationship is a quantitative relationship between the amount of stimulus it takes to produce an appropriate response and the degree of that response. In habituation learning, there is an inverse relationship between the amount of stimulus and the degree of response over time.

ALSO SEE: *Habituation Learning, Reaction Norm, Stimulus*

Stimulus Summation

The combined effect of several stimuli may elicit a stronger response than the response to a single stimulus. When this is true, the total of the stimuli is the stimulus summation. A single mosquito may bite a horse almost without visible reaction by the horse; however, as the number of mosquitoes increases, the horse's reaction also changes, even to running.

ALSO SEE: *Stimulus*

Stool Eating

Stool eating is another term used for coprophagy.

SEE: *Coprophagia*

Stool Eating—Another Species

Eating the feces of another species is most commonly done by dogs. It is important to understand that the aesthetic values of this animal are much different than those of humans. Dogs eat cat feces probably because of the smell and protein in it. Feces of cattle and horses are eaten for the content of predigested vegetable matter.

ALSO SEE: *Coprophagia, Grass Eating*

Stotting

Stotting is a jumping behavior in which all four legs are kept stiff. It is usually associated with excitement, fright, or play in certain gazelles and antelope.

ALSO SEE: *Locomotion*

Stress

Stress is a pressure or strain placed on a system. In animals, there is always a certain degree of stress to find food or water, avoid predators, and avoid agonistic behaviors. If the amount of pressure is great enough, the body's endocrine system, particularly the adrenal gland, will interact. The immediate reaction is from the adrenal medulla, and longer interaction is with the adrenal cortex. Continued stimuli can become distressful, and more extensive body changes result.

Several behaviors are associated with stress and the animal's attempt to minimize the distress.

ALSO SEE: *Cronism, Remove Stress, Stress-related Behaviors*

Stress-related Behaviors

Stress-related behaviors fill one major subdivision of behavior problems. These are expressed in an animal's attempts to cope with stress or distress. To stop these problem behaviors, it is important to eliminate the primary cause. Because the precipitating factors can be difficult to find, it may be necessary for the owners to keep a diary related to the problem and events preceding it. In addition to working on the specific stressor, it is often helpful to increase the amount of exercise the animal gets and to keep it on a rigid schedule. Antianxiety tranquilizers may also be helpful in the short term. Laboratory and zoo animals are being helped with efforts to provide enriched environments instead of barren cages.

ALSO SEE: *Anorexia Nervosa, Attention Seeking, Boredom, Buller Steer Syndrome, Catatonic Reaction, Climbing, Cronism, Destructive Behaviors, Diary, Digging, Displacement Activity, Drug Therapy, Environmental Enrichment, Excessive Grooming, Excessive Licking, Excessive Vocalization—Barking, Exercise, Feline Hyperesthesia Syndrome, Flank Sucking, Frustration, Frustration-induced Aggression, Ground Pecking, Ground Rutting, Hair Pulling, Improper Socialization Aggression, Organizing Behavioral Histories, Psychogenic Problems, Psychological Well-being, Redirected Aggression, Remove Stress, Running Away, Schedule, Self-Mutilation, Separation Anxiety, Social Contact, Stereotyped Behaviors, Stress*

Stretching

Stretching is a behavior, usually associated with resting, in which the animal briefly extends its limbs in a specific way. Animals that move on four limbs alternately stretch the front by extending the limbs far forward, or the rear pair by moving forward to extend the hips. Birds extend limbs on the same side at any time so that they can balance on the opposite foot, or they can stretch by extending both wings and rear limbs using gentle flapping to briefly hold the stretch. There may be a tendency for several members of a group to stretch at the same time (pandiculation).

ALSO SEE: *Pandiculation, Resting Behaviors*

Strike Distance

The strike distance is that distance an animal will reach or go to during an attack by an approaching intruder. For a horse, this represents the reach of the forelimbs or hind limbs. For a dog that is tied, it could represent the length of the chain.

ALSO SEE: *Critical Distance, Reactive Distances, Social Distance*

Striking

Striking, a distance-increasing behavior, is a sudden, forceful forward movement of one or both front feet, usually in an apparent attempt to hit something in front. The target of a horse could be a rival stallion or a stallion advancing toward an anestrous mare. A horse that gets too close, a dog, a cat, or an insect around the nose can also elicit striking. People can also be targets of an aggressive act, especially if they are inflicting pain. For this reason, it is best to avoid standing directly in front of a horse.

ALSO SEE: *Distance-increasing Silent Communication, Kicking, Rearing*

Submissive Behavior

Submissive behavior is the performance of distance-reducing silent and/or vocal communications by the least dominant animal to minimize or prevent an aggressive encounter. This definition may include or exclude appeasement behaviors.

ALSO SEE: *Active Submission, Appeasement Behavior, Cut Off, Distance-reducing Silent Communication, Passive Submission*

Submissive Distance

The social (reactive) distance at which an animal begins to show distance-reducing silent communication (submissive) postures to an approacher is called the submissive distance.

ALSO SEE: *Distance-reducing Silent Communication, Reactive Distances, Social Distance*

Submissive Inertia

Submissive inertia, tonic dyskinesia, hypotonia, and tonic immobility are other terms for catatonic reactions.

SEE: *Catatonic Reaction*

Submissive Tricks

To help owners establish and maintain the dominant position over their dog, the pet can be taught certain tricks that actually have a submissive meaning. "Shaking hands" uses the raised paw greeting position that a subordinate shows to a pack leader. "Sit" and "down" are passive submission postures, as is "roll over." These behaviors are difficult to teach to a dominant dog because it does not want to show submissive signs. If one family member can make the dog respond appropriately, that person can enforce an appropriate response if the dog does not want to respond to another family member's command. A dominant dog may not learn these tricks initially, and other methods to establish the dominance of the owner may be needed.

ALSO SEE: *Dominance Aggression, Establish Dominance, Passive Submission*

Submissive Urination

Submissive urination is a behavior of passive submission used by dogs. Young dogs show the behavior to people more frequently than older dogs, as if they position themselves low in the social order compared to their owners. Most dogs outgrow submissive urination by the time they reach sexual maturity, although an extreme threat in their minds may still elicit the behavior occasionally. Owners sometimes interpret submissive urination as housesoiling; however, the causes of the two are quite different. Punishment makes submissive urination worse, since the dog is already showing submission. The person should show body postures that are not threatening and gradually let the dog increase its confidence in social situations. It might also be helpful for owners to make the first contact with the animal outside the house. While this does not lessen the degree of submissive urination, it reduces the perception of the problem.

The drug phenylpropanolamine may be helpful in some cases of submissive urination by young dogs because of its action to tighten the urinary sphincter.

ALSO SEE: *Avoid Excitement, Decrease Body Threat, Housesoiling—Submissive Urination, Increase Pet's Confidence, Passive Submission, Psychogenic Urinary Incontinence, Appendix C*

Substitute a Behavior

When an animal is showing an unacceptable behavior, one technique to get it to stop is to ask for and reward a substitute behavior. When a dog tracks in mud because it dashes into the house without waiting for its feet to be wiped, making it sit as it enters the house stops it from tracking mud throughout. A dog that jumps on people can sit to be petted instead. Because the animal can only perform one behavior, choose one that is opposite to the one the animal chooses, and reward the desired response.

S

ALSO SEE: *Aggression and Doorbells, Aggression and Telephones, Dashing through Doors, Jumping on People, Offensive Threat, Sniffing Humans*

Substitute Object

A behavior may be directed toward an otherwise neutral object because the appropriate one is not available. Bitches often "mother" stuffed toys, the substitute objects, while going through a false pregnancy.

ALSO SEE: *Pseudopregnancy*

Suckling Order

In certain animals there is a defined order of the young relative to each other during nursing. This is another name for teat order.

SEE: *Teat Order*

Super Releaser (Supranormal Releaser)

A super releaser is a stimulus that releases a particular behavior pattern more easily than the normal stimulus. A bird that will roll its own egg out of the way of a larger egg is one example. The cuckoo chick's coloration is more attractive to its host parent so that it receives preferential treatment to the bird's own chick.

ALSO SEE: *Releaser*

Swine

The wild boar is the animal from which modern pigs, *Sus scrofa*, were derived as subspecies, and it can still be found in its wild form in Europe, Asia, and North Africa (Clutton-Brock, 1981). Domestication probably began about 7000 B.C. with pigs used for meat. The domesticated European subspecies make up most of the familiar meat-producing breeds. Pigs of Asia tend to have shorter legs and an extreme fat-bellied appearance.

Old World fossil evidence traces pig ancestry to *Propalcaeochoerus* of the Oligocene Period (30 million years ago). This was a small, four-toed animal with well-developed canine teeth.

ALSO SEE: *Domestication, Appendix B*

Sympathetic Induction of Mood

In certain situations, the mood or emotional state of one animal is transferable to other group members. One important type of reaction that can be transferred is related to group preservation. Deer or horses that perceive potential danger will stamp a foot or snort a warning and then flee if necessary. Herdmates typically react by increasing their alertness, snorting, and reacting as if danger is nearby. Territorial protective aggression by one pack member may initiate the same defense in other pack members, resulting in a show of unity.

ALSO SEE: *Avoid Excitement, Learned Excitement, Mood Induction, Territorial Protective Aggression*

Sympathetic Lameness

Lameness can be used as an attention-seeking behavior. An animal may limp for a true medical condition, usually mild, but continues to limp after all conditions indicate it should be recovered. The animal has learned that by limping it will be rewarded whether by a rider dismounting or by attention being given to the leg. The overly concerned owner is quick to fall into this situation. Occasionally the animal limps on the wrong limb or alternates with periods of normal walking, making the diagnosis easier. When attention is no longer given, the lameness disappears.

ALSO SEE: *Attention Seeking, No Attention to Behavior, Trial and Error Learning*

Sympathomimetic Intoxication

Occasionally an animal shows an unexpected reaction to a sympathomimetic substance. The types of reactions include aggression, hypervigilance, psychomotor disturbances, tachycardia, pupillary dilation, and vomiting. Sympathomimetic intoxication can occur in response to drugs used in treating hyperactivity and hyperkinesis.

ALSO SEE: *Drug Therapy, Hyperactivity, Hyperkinesis*

Synchronization

Synchronization involves the development of similar timing relative to behaviors or physiological events. Many times synchronization occurs because of stages of the moon or the length of daylight. Reproductive states can be synchronized in sows by dramatic management changes. For example, all nonpregnant females that are hauled in a trailer will show estrus in four to six days. Certain hormones are also capable of synchronization of estrus, a helpful technique in multiple ovulation–surrogate mothering in cattle.

Syndrome

A syndrome is a group of symptoms that occur together and that constitutes a recognizable condition.

T

Tail Chasing

Tail chasing is a behavior problem in which dogs and some cats run in tight circles, as if chasing their tails. Some do get the tail and do physical damage to themselves, but most only go through the actions of the chase. The causes of the behavior are numerous. In some breeds, such as bull terriers, there is strong evidence of a genetic predisposition and a relationship to hydrocephalus (Dodman, 1992). In others, the timing, duration, and response to medications indicate tail chasing is a seizure. Many dogs have learned the behavior, probably as a response to little physical activity. The chasing behavior helps get rid of excessive energy, and that probably serves as its own internal reward. Over time it can become stereotyped.

Therapies depend on cause. A substitute behavior, such as "sit," can be asked for to break the pattern of running. This must also be coupled with greatly increased amounts of exercise and environmental stimulation. Narcotic antagonists are gaining favor in the treatment of stereotypies. Treatment for hydrocephalus may be tried in appropriate individuals. Antiepileptics work reasonably well on true seizuring tail chasers. Tail chasing can be very difficult to get to respond. Severely affected individuals have been euthanized, but for less severe forms, it may be necessary to accept the behavior, at least partially.

ALSO SEE: *Boredom, Drug Therapy, Exercise, Genetic Problems, Hydrocephalus, Internal Reward, Stereotyped Behaviors, Substitute a Behavior, Tail Chewing*

Tail Chewing (Tail Biting)

Biting the tail of a conspecific is a problem for swine and horses. Some horses chew tails as part of environmental exploration, with weanlings and yearlings tending to mouth objects. Protein deficiencies can also produce tail chewing.

For pigs, tail biting has led to a great deal of concern over husbandry practices because there is an apparent connection with environmental stress. While specifics vary in individual operations, the incidence of tail chewing seems to increase with crowding and adverse environmental factors. The distal half of the tail is apparently less sensitive because pigs that tolerate chewing on it do not usually tolerate chewing on the proximal stub. Amputation of at least half the tail is a common practice to control the problem. Less crowding; behavioral enrichment with straw, balls, or pasture; or housing the offending pigs together also decreases the incidence.

Tail biting in dogs is usually self-directed and classified as a self-mutilation behavior, often associated with tail chasing. In cats, the behavior is usually part of the feline hyperesthesia syndrome.

ALSO SEE: *Feline Hyperesthesia Syndrome, Pica, Self-Mutilation, Tail Chasing*

Tail Rubbing

Tail rubbing can be a problem in horses. The etiology is not well understood, but parasitism must be ruled out.

Tail Switching (Flagging)

The deliberate back-and-forth movement of the tail as a distance-increasing sign is called switching or flagging. It can be very fast or a slow motion. In dogs, the tail posture is vertical or over the back, and the motion is fast. Tail switching is easily confused with tail wagging, which has a nonaggressive meaning. Horses clamp the tail tightly against the body and slowly move it from side to side. Horses also give a quick swish or hold the tail tightly in as a response to something unpleasant, such as a spur poke. Calves rapidly switch their tails while butting the cow for more milk.

ALSO SEE: *Distance-increasing Silent Communication, Tail Wagging*

Tail Wagging

Tail wagging is a back-and-forth movement of an animal's tail associated with distance-reducing postures. It is a free movement, without the indication of stress associated with tail switching.

ALSO SEE: *Distance-reducing Silent Communication, Passive Submission*

Tame Animal

A tame animal is an individual (wild, domesticated, or feral) that allows a human in close proximity, within its personal distance. The flight distance toward humans has been reduced to zero.

ALSO SEE: *Domestication, Feral Animal, Flight Distance, Personal Distance, Wild Animal*

Taste

The sense of taste is not well studied in animals. In general most respond well to chemicals associated with salt, sour, and bitter, with minimal response to sweetness. Considering natural diets, it is not surprising that sweetness is not a major part of the taste spectrum. Individuals can, however, develop a strong liking for foods with high sugar content. All the other taste components are self-limiting in the normal animal. Since sweet is minimal in the natural diet, animals never developed a mechanism to limit its consumption.

Most taste studies in farm species have centered around taste and texture preferences, since feeding has become such a major factor in commercial operations.

ALSO SEE: *Ingestive Behavior*

Taste Aversion

Most destructive oral behavior problems can be treated with taste aversion, perhaps in addition to other treatments. Taste aversion works on the principle that a bad association with a particular taste results in that taste becoming repulsive. Any bad-tasting product may be used, including hot pepper sauce, bitter apple flavor, creosote, chloramphenicol, or a number of commercial products. The problem animal is allowed to smell the product, and then several milliliters of solution are squirted into the mouth. The desired reaction is salivation and repulsion. The product is used to cover the problem area or item so that when the animal gets a small smell or taste, it is reminded of the bad experience. The events are similar to what happens to people who get sick after eating a particular food. They do not want it again for a long time.

ALSO SEE: *Aversive Conditioning, Destructive Chewing, Direct Punishment, Excessive Licking, Inappropriate Licking, Psychogenic Dermatoses, Self-Mutilation*

Teat Order

A teat order is the use of a specific teat each time a neonate nurses. It has specific implications in the domestic cat and pig. For kittens, there are usually more teats than kittens, and over the first week, an individual's nursing becomes localized to one or two specific teats. For piglets, the choice is more restricted, since their number and the number of nipples is fairly close. By the end of the second week of nursing, piglets show a preference for a specific teat. The largest piglets tend to chose the front nipples, which also supply the most milk and are the most protected. The caudal teats have the least milk and increase the likelihood of the piglet being stepped on and injured. The slowest weight gains also occur here, thus maximizing the size differential in the piglets. The hierarchy established in this way carries over to social situations later.

ALSO SEE: *Fostering, Nursing, Social Order, Transitional Phase*

Teeth Clapping

This is another term used to describe jaw chomping in foals.
SEE: *Jaw Chomping*

Temperament

An animal's temperament is the general consistency with which it behaves. This does not include abnormal learned behavior such as stereotypies. The consistency of the behaviors usually takes time to develop and is not adultlike until some time after sexual maturity. In cats, the most noticeable change occurs around the time of sexual maturity, when the social behavior of kittenhood is traded for the asocial behavior of adulthood. Behavioral maturation into adulthood occurs in dogs at approximately twice the age of sexual maturity. In livestock species, the stabilization of temperament also occurs at approximately twice the age of puberty. For horses, it may take three to four years, and in cattle, the time is about two and a half years.

Environment versus genetic influences on adult temperament is very controversial. The work of Scott and Fuller (1965) in dogs showed there are a number of genetic components to behavior in a controlled environment. The genetic influence of a sire or dam on temperament has also been debated. For most animals, environmental influences have an undetermined effect, although their value should not be underestimated. The impact of a mare, cow, or other mother on its offspring may be greater because of their environmental influence as well as the genetic contribution.

Human personalities have been rated popularly as Type A and Type B. Animals, particularly cattle, have been divided into several other groups based on the Pavlovian concept of temperament. This gave rise to four subdivisions (Hafez, Schein and Ewbank in Hafez, 1969): (1) Strong, balanced, sanguine, and lively; (2) Strong, balanced, phlegmatic, and quiet; (3) Strong, nonbalanced, choleric, and noninhibited; and (4) Weak, melancholic.

Temper Tantrum

While animals do not throw the classic temper tantrum as seen in humans, by doing or not doing things at times individuals can show strong elements of their personality that correspond to the human behavior. It is important to analyze the situation because the uniqueness of an animal's senses allows it to perceive something that we would have trouble identifying. A horse that has loaded many times may suddenly refuse. A cat may react aggressively to not getting its usual treat at a specific time. It can be argued that urine marking can also be done "to get even." A dominant dog may physically fight the restraint of a halter.

Treatments for such animals involves tenacity. The animal should never be allowed to get its way unless the behavior is totally uncharacteristic. It may take some detective work to really understand what is upsetting the animal, but always follow through with a command. If the animal is successful, the behavior is likely to be repeated, and the eventual elimination becomes more difficult. By determining why the cat or dog is marking, adjustments can be made to minimize the environmental factors that cause the marking.

ALSO SEE: *Aggression, Dog Collars, Housesoiling—Spraying, Housesoiling—Urine Marking, Spite, Trailer Loading, Trial and Error Learning*

Territorial Behavior

Any behavior used to advertise or defend a territory is called a territorial behavior. Aggression is commonly used to defend the borders; however, the behaviors can also include threatening, marking, and vocalizing.

ALSO SEE: *Territorial Protective Aggression*

Territorial Protective Aggression

Territorial protective aggression, or territorial aggression, is a form of affective aggression in which an animal defends an area from invasion or reacts in certain ways to individuals already within the area. (It is also a type of mobile aggression.)

While the establishment of territories is common in wild animals, in domesticated animals it is shown only by cats and certain dogs. It is important for dog owners to differentiate between territorial and owner protective aggressions. Many dogs allow intruders into their territory—more commonly thought of as guests in the home—but are very protective of their owner. Other dogs have been trained to show aggression at the door but are not really territorial. A cat may jump on an intruder or burglar as an expression of territorial protection and be recognized as a hero. A few owners have complained about the cat that attacks guests in their home. For those cats, it is best simply to confine them in a room until the guests have gone.

Territorial defense is strongest at the center of a territory and in a small territory such as a car. As the edges are reached, the aggression is reduced to a threat, and the voice tone qualities change to reflect this. Once outside the territory, the pet is much less aggressive. Territorial protective aggression is difficult to modify because the behavior itself is rewarding to the animal.

When an animal is already within a territory, a second type of territorial aggression may be seen. This is a common behavior expressed by cats. A territorial tomcat can mount and nape bite any other cat within its territory, male or female. The mounted animal responds by vocalizing aggressively and by assuming a crouched posture until it can escape. If the tom leaves his territory, he could become the cat being mounted. In a pet situation, the territorial cat does not have to be an intact tomcat; females and neutered males can also control a territory.

ALSO SEE: *Affective Aggression, Aggression and Mail Carriers, Hero, Inter-*

nal Reward, Mobile Aggression, Mounting, Mutual Grooming, Owner Protective Aggression, Protective Aggression, Ritualized Fighting, Territorial Behavior, Territory, Unconsciously Learned Aggression

Territory

A territory is the social (reactive) distance within a home range that is actively defended. Wild species may have more than one type of territory, such as one for eating and one for reproduction or resting. Territorial defense is strongest toward the center and in smaller spaces. Of the domestic animals, only cats and some dogs, especially terriers, are very territorial. Cats often continue to return to an old territory, if not physically prevented. Certain dogs are very protective of their territory and may need to be introduced to others only away from their space. Fences can limit a dog's territory, making it identical to the home range.

ALSO SEE: *Home Range, Reactive Distances, Returning to Old Home, Social Distance, Territorial Protective Aggression*

Testosterone-induced Aggression in Mares

Some mares show aggression to other horses and to people that is excessive in regard to other conditions. These mares tend to have dominant personalities, may show stallion behaviors, and have muscle tone and condition better than expected. High testosterone levels have been associated with this aggressive condition (Beaver and Amoss, 1982). An ovarian tumor can be the source of the testosterone. In other cases, the adrenal or pituitary may be abnormal.

ALSO SEE: *Aggression, Dominant Personality, Hormone Imbalance Aggression, Ovariectomy*

Thanatosis

Thanatosis is playing dead. The opossum uses this as a means of defense and protection, as do several other species. The catatonic state is another example of this behavior.

ALSO SEE: *Catatonic Reaction*

Thinking

Thinking is the use of reason or logic to come to some conclusion. It implies the ability to project into the future as well as to draw from the past. Thinking is also known as insight learning.

ALSO SEE: *Insight Learning, Intelligence*

Threat Behavior

Threat behaviors are vocal or positional patterns used to repel another for the prevention of aggressive interactions. These are also called threat displays.

ALSO SEE: *Canine-Tooth Threat, Distance-increasing Silent Communication, Threat Displays, Threat Yawn*

Threat Displays

Threat displays involve the use of one or more types of distance-increasing body postures. These can be used as a show of reactive anomaly.

ALSO SEE: *Canine-Tooth Threat, Distance-increasing Silent Communication, Genital Presentation, Reactive Anomalies, Threat Behavior, Threat Yawn*

Threat Yawn

The threat yawn is a yawnlike, open-mouth behavior used as a threat. The behavior is shown by several species of primates and by the hippopotamus.

ALSO SEE: *Threat Behavior, Threat Displays*

Threshold

The threshold is the minimum amount of stimulus needed to elicit a response. The threshold level may vary with the frequency of a specific behavior. If that behavior has not occurred recently, the amount of stimulus needed may decrease. This decrease may be lowered to such a degree that the behavior appears spontaneously as a vacuum activity.

ALSO SEE: *Stimulus, Vacuum Activity*

Thunderphobia

Thunderphobia and brontophobia are terms used to describe the fear of thunder.

ALSO SEE: *Fear of Thunder*

Time-Out

Time-out is a behavioral technique used to punish a dog briefly by depriving it of the social attention that initiated the problem. A dog responds to the doorbell by running and barking or by jumping on visitors. In both cases, it may be seeking attention of the owners or the guests. Putting the dog in a room by itself for 5 to 10 minutes deprives it of the social contact it seeks. This technique should be coupled with a behavior modification program for successful resolution. The dog can be asked to sit at the door and is then sent to the room only when it disobeys. Long periods of isolation are counterproductive and may actually aggravate the initial problem. Several short sessions of "time-out" interspersed with a reintroduction to the scene until the unacceptable behavior no longer occurs is much better than a long isolation.

ALSO SEE: *Aggression and Doorbells, Confinement, Jumping on People*

Time Synchronizer

A time synchronizer is an external stimulus that affects the physiological rhythms of an animal over a period of time. The amounts of sunlight and moon phases are the most common.

ALSO SEE: *Biological Rhythms*

Timid Personality

Personalities in any species can be inherited as well as transformed by an environment. Timidity or the tendency for it can be a heritable trait. Careful analysis of a pedigree should be made before a genetic connection is made. Scott and Fuller's (1965) work with shelties, beagles, fox terriers, cocker spaniels, and basenjis showed a breed difference in their dogs as well as an individual difference.

Traumatic experience can also result in a timid personality. While we are most familiar with these events in dogs, individuals in other species are also susceptible.

ALSO SEE: *Aggressive Personality, Decrease Body Threat, Dominant Personality, Fear of People, Fear Biting*

Tongue Dragging

Tongue dragging is a behavioral pattern shown by horses in which the tongue is allowed to hang out of the mouth. It is often folded longitudinally on itself, and it may or may not be sucked. Lack of environmental stimuli is generally listed as a contributing factor to the development of the behavior as a habit.

The protrusion of the tongue is particularly distracting in the show arena. In halter classes, handlers have used pain, such as pricking with a thumbtack, to discourage the behavior; in performance classes, the tongue can be restrained with a net or spoon bit. While tongue amputation has been used, it is not recommended.

ALSO SEE: *Boredom, Stereotyped Behaviors, Tongue Play*

Tongue Play

Tongue play is most common in horses and cattle that are confined for long periods of time. If allowed to continue, usually without an increase in exercise or change in the environment, tongue play can become a stereotypic problem behavior.

Sucking on littermates or herd mates is also a play behavior usually associated with orphans or early weaned young. It, too, can become a problem if allowed to continue.

ALSO SEE: *Licking, Play Behaviors, Prolonged Sucking, Stereotyped Behaviors, Tongue Dragging, Tongue Rolling*

Tongue Rolling

Cattle may show a behavior of rolling their tongues in irregular ways. Typically the tongue is extended out of the mouth and then rolled back into the mouth or toward the nostril in an exaggeration of normal grooming. Swallowing or gulping air may also occur. Tongue rolling is probably the bovine equivalent of tongue dragging in horses. Evidence suggests the behavior can be learned by watching other problem animals and that there might be a genetic predisposition in some individuals.

Successful elimination of tongue rolling is difficult, and the longer the habit is established, the more difficult the solution. Free movement, forced exercise, equine wind-sucking straps, and a metal ring in the frenulum of the tongue have been used to manage the problem.

ALSO SEE: *Genetic Problems, Licking, Stereotyped Behaviors, Tongue Dragging*

Tonic Dyskinesia

Tonic dyskinesia, tonic immobility, hypotonia, and submissive inertia are other terms for catatonic reactions.

SEE: *Catatonic Reaction*

Tonic Immobility

Tonic immobility, tonic dyskinesia, hypotonia, and submissive inertia are other terms for catatonic reactions.

SEE: *Catatonic Reaction*

Trailer Kicking

Some horses develop the habit of kicking trailer doors or pawing while they are being hauled. After a long trip, a horse may show this behavior if the vehicle slows down or stops, or it can become restless when needing to urinate but unable to assume the appropriate posture. Other horses fight the confinement of the trailer because of negative experiences in the past. The obvious concerns for the owner are injury to the horse and damage to the trailer. A common approach to this problem is the use of hobbles, although properly timed punishment for the behavior can also curtail it.

ALSO SEE: *Hobbles, Kicking, Trailer Rocking*

Trailer Loading

Loading large animals into a trailer or truck can become a very frustrating experience if behavioral principles are not used. For each species, there are little things that can make a big difference. With the exception of horses, most animals experience only one or two trailer rides and so are not able to learn a system or a specific trailer. The experience is strange and so are the smells. For all animals, it is generally helpful if the inside of the vehicle is intensely lighted and no shadows occur on the path or ramp.

Horse trailering is often a repeated event, so it is particularly important that the first several experiences are good ones. Owners should not wait for the first lesson to be the day of a show or race. Loading can be practiced long before. Patience is critical. Only gentle pressure to keep the head in position and to lead should be used; pulling on the head is not acceptable. Many horses are easier to load if another horse is in front or beside it, so an experienced horse should be loaded first. The person working the halter rope should not stand immediately in front of the horse, particularly in a narrow trailer, since horses try to avoid running into a person, and the narrow trailer stall could give the perception of having to hit the person. A long lead rope through an escape door keeps the handler out of the way. Encouragement should come from behind. Since the goal is to have the horse move forward, forward motion should be rewarded. Standing or backward motion becomes less desirable, and punishment of the head must be avoided. Vocal or physical encouragement from the rear is then used. Pauses may be necessary so the horse can investigate before it continues. Once inside, a reward should be given, and food is generally well-accepted. Initial trips should be short and slow, with particular attention given to starts, stops, and cornering.

Cattle can easily be driven along high, close-sided, curved chutes, following the animal in front. Lighting and lack of shadows are particularly important. It is best not to let the animals see distractions to the side, including people who are too close. Electric cattle prods, whips, and ropes are used to move and load cattle; however, these are generally not necessary if proper attention is given to the environment.

Since sheep are followers, goats are used to lead the sheep, waiting until the last one is loaded before quickly ducking out as the gate is shut. Sheep will also go to a sheep temporarily tied in the front of a trailer.

ALSO SEE: *Decrease Body Threat, Flight Distances, Temper Tantrum*

Trailer Problems

Horses can make trailering a difficult experience. Some kick, stall weave, rear to get front feet in the manger, scramble when cornering, or simply will not load. Most problems start during a bad hauling experience, such as when a driver corners too fast or when a trailer is too small for the horse. The horse may also become uncomfortably hot, thirsty, or bothered by insects. When stall partitions run all the way to the floor, the horse may not have enough room to spread its feet for balance in the turns. It may then become panicky and lean to one side while climbing on the wall or partition—scrambling. Partial partitions are generally better.

Once a trailering problem has started, it may be easier to manage than to eliminate. Many horses do well if hauled in a stock trailer or conventional two-horse trailer with the center partition removed or swung over. Other horses do well in slant-load trailers or in the kind in which they face backward.

Retraining can be done, particularly if the problem has not become extremely severe. Antianxiety tranquilizers may be useful initially in this program. Desensitization occurs by a gradual process of slowly reintroducing the horse to the trailer with lots of positive reinforcement, short sessions, and patience. It is also important to make sure that the factors related to initiating the problem are eliminated.

ALSO SEE: *Drug Therapy, Trailer Kicking, Trailer Loading,Trailer Rocking*

Trailer Rocking

Horses can cause trailers to rock as they shift their weight back and forth. The most common cause of mild side-to-side rocking is the horse shifting its weight. Severe side-to-side rocking often is caused by a horse that performs stereotyped weaving when it is hauled. Hobbling the horse is helpful, although care must be used while hauling because the horse's ability to maintain balance will have been compromised. A full-length partition in a side-by-side trailer may also be helpful, or it may be useful to haul the horse at an angle, as in a slant-load trailer, or to haul it facing the rear of the trailer. Back-and-forth jerking movements of the trailer occur when horses kick at the trailer tailgate and when an animal rears back and manages to get its frontlimbs into the trailer manger. Horses that somehow fall and are unable to get back on their feet and horses that are trying to escape, as when frightened by a piece of paper that blows into the back of an open trailer, can also cause severe rocking of a trailer.

ALSO SEE: *Stereotyped Weaving, Trailer Kicking*

Trained Aggression

Trained aggression uses an animal's instinctive reactions to protect or to guard something. It is most common in dogs such as the German shepherd, Doberman, Rottweiler, and more recently the pitbull dog, which learn to serve as guard, sentry, patrol, and attack dogs. In some methods of training, the aggression is directed at everyone but the trainer (the classic "junkyard dog"), while in others there are varying degrees of control, from the cue to start an attack to the most demanding cue—to halt an attack. Aggression is seldom a complaint by the owners of these dogs, and veterinary treatment is generally not a problem if they are trained for cues, since the owners will handle the dog in an appropriate manner.

ALSO SEE: *Affective Aggression, Learned Aggression*

Training

Training is a broad term used to describe the learning of lessons that are controlled by a human.

SEE: *Learning*

Transitional Phase

In animal species in which the young suckle, there is a transitional phase when the infants start eating adult foods but continue to nurse. The specific time period varies not only among species but also within a species. In puppies, the transitional phase begins about 3 weeks of age and continues until weaning at approximately 6 weeks. Kittens also begin this phase at approximately 3 weeks. Weaning will normally be completed at between 8 and 12 weeks, although single kittens may continue nursing as long as a year. Foals begin trying to reach grass and to eat grain by a few weeks of age. This increases gradually over the next several weeks. The environment has a lot to do with the time of weaning. In areas where grass is minimal, mares tend to wean foals at a younger age. When grazing is good or supplements are provided, natural weaning may not occur for over a year. The usual age of weaning is generally between 4 to 6 months.

Calves begin ingesting grass and grains in limited amounts after a few weeks, with forced weaning around 4 months. There is a great deal of variation in the cattle industry in regard to taking calves off the dam, especially in dairy operations and commercial beef ranches. Rumination begins at about 3 weeks and reaches adult levels between 6 and 8 months.

Piglets nurse until weaned at approximately 6 to 8 weeks. For them, the ingestion of solid food can begin around 1 week.

ALSO SEE: *Food Preferences, Ingestive Behavior*

Transport of Young

Transport of the young is used to describe any method of moving the juveniles by either parent. They may ride on the parent's back, in a pouch, clutching the fur, or in the mouth. They may also be carried temporarily by the mother from place to place, as is common with kittens and puppies.

ALSO SEE: *Carrying In*

Trial and Error Learning

In trial and error learning, learning is associated with the reward of a natural, spontaneous act. The behavior continues to be rewarded, resulting in a decreased interval between occurrences. A cat jumps on a kitchen table and finds food. This increases the likelihood that it will jump on the table again. Each time it finds food, the tendency is stronger to repeat the behavior. A horse plays with a latch using its lip and opens the door to its stall. The escape is likely to be tried again. Rowdy behavior, like biting at pants legs, can increase the attention a dog gets, rewarding the behavior. Substituting no reinforcement or a punishment instead of a reinforcer decreases the tendency for the behavior to occur again.

ALSO SEE: *Learning, Local Enhancement, Operant Conditioning, Temper Tantrum*

Trichophagia

Trichophagia is another term for hair eating.

SEE: *Hair Eating*

Unconsciously Learned Aggression

Unconsciously learned aggression involves an animal gradually learning to show aggression because of subtle behaviors by the owner. When owners fear the environment, they often get a dog "for protection." Then without realizing it they use trial and error rewards for barking or growling when the doorbell rings. The dog responds and soon becomes aggressive to all visitors, including friends. When told the behavior can be changed, the owners will respond, "But will my dog protect me?" They have confused learned aggression with owner protective aggression.

To eliminate the behavior, a number of techniques in behavior modification can be used. Extinction is one technique most successful if the problem is not long standing. Habituation to the doorbell ringing without being answered is another useful technique, particularly when the dog is also asked to sit. Any inappropriate response is immediately corrected with a "no" and "sit," time-out, or punishment, as with a water sprayer.

Other animals can show unconsciously learned aggression. Horses that rear in play because they have been stalled too long and are feeling good can learn that the behavior causes the person to back away. The horse then learns to control a situation with aggression. In this case, what started out as play changed to learned aggression without the conscious effort of the owner or trainer.

ALSO SEE: *Affective Aggression, Behavior Modification, Competitive Aggression, Extinction, Learned Aggression, No, Time-Out, Trial and Error Learning*

Urination

Urination, physiologically, is the process of expelling urine from the body. Behaviorally, the process has a number of facets.

Neonates may not be able to urinate unless they receive anogenital stimulation from the dam's licking. The anogenital reflex is present in species in which the young must stay in a single location for a prolonged period of time. It ensures that the dam is there to clean up the urine so the den or nest smell does not attract predators. This reflex is present in puppies, kittens, fawns, and others. While calves can eliminate on their own, they also can be stimulated to do so.

In dogs, the puppy gradually begins to urinate on its own from a squatting or forward-leaning position, a posture similar to that used by adult females. As the male dog approaches puberty, the squatting posture changes to a posture where one rear limb is elevated and abducted. Small amounts of urine are squirted, usually directed toward certain objects. Thus, males will use urine to mark territory or objects and to leave information. Limb elevation is hormonally controlled and is dependent on neonatal masculinization of the brain by testosterone, with another surge of the hormone at puberty.

While there are several things that typically result in urination in dogs, behavioral stimuli tend to be specific odors. The odor of urine from another dog and excreta from other animals (dogs often urinate directly on horse urine and bird droppings) are common stimuli. Frequency of urination varies considerably, depending on sex and environmental factors.

Feline urinary patterns are initially associated with the anogenital reflex. A few days before they eliminate on their own, kittens can be seen playing in loose dirt or litter. The typical cat urination pattern is to dig a small hole in soft dirt or litter, assume a deep squatting posture over the hole, urinate, turn and smell the contents of the hole, and earth rake the dirt to cover the urine. Studies have shown that the earth raking behavior is instinctive, triggered by smell. Cats show the raking behavior motions even on a hard surface like linoleum (Beaver, 1992).

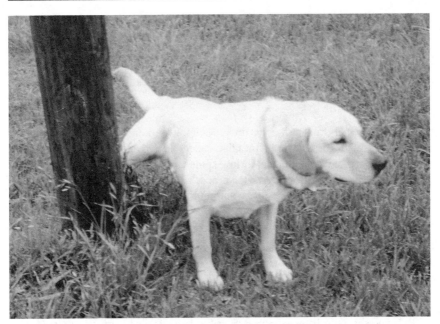

Urination. Male dogs start lifting their leg during urination, as seen here, when testosterone levels increase at puberty.

The covering behavior is learned, usually from the queen. Adult cats urinate 2 to 3 times daily.

Adult cats have a second method to expel urine—spraying. This behavior is associated with territorial marking and can be a response to environmental stress. The posture used for spraying is a standing posture, a vertically held tail that quivers as urine is expressed, and a position backed up almost to the vertical object to be sprayed. Urine is forcefully expelled in short bursts. The standing orientation puts the scent at nose level for other cats that might pass by.

Horses have sex-based posture differences. A mare spreads her rear limbs apart, arches her back, and tips her pelvis so that urine can fall almost straight down. Geldings and stallions move their forelimbs forward, spread their rear limbs somewhat, and slightly arch their backs, at least initially. Many horses, especially males, try to urinate on surfaces that do not have a tendency to let urine splash. Thus, areas preferred tend to be grassy or deeply bedded. They may avoid urinating in horse trailers unless it is necessary.

Typically horses urinate 5 to 10 times each day; however, they can develop patterns of urinating, usually associated with times or events, such as after a race or before eating.

Cattle also have gender-based urinary postures. Cows assume a posture similar to that of the mares, usually with a greater arch to the back. Bulls and steers are in a typical standing posture. Urination for them is almost passive. Cattle normally urinate about 8 times each day.

Swine are variable in their urinary behaviors, but they tend to eliminate near their water source, especially in confinement.

ALSO SEE: *Defecation, Elimination Behavior, Housetraining, Marking, Sexually Dimorphic Behaviors, Urine Spraying*

Urine Drinking

Animals that drink urine are most commonly found in dairy herds that are closely confined during winter months, especially when the cows are kept on concrete flooring. Urine collects in low spots and becomes available. The problem disappears when these cows have access to pasture and when there is an evenly distributed access to fresh water and salt. The behavior occurs in other animals as well. Dogs may slowly lick urine from other species, as if sampling it. The behavior probably serves to introduce the associated odors into the incisive ducts.

ALSO SEE: *Drinking, Flehmen, Vomeronasal Organ*

Urine Spraying

Urine spraying is a sexually dimorphic behavior, primarily associated with felids and used to scent mark territorial boundaries and certain things within a territory. A cat will stand, backed up against the vertical object it chooses to mark. The tail is held up and often quivers. Pulsing bursts of urine hit the object to leave an olfactory mark at the level of the cat nose. This is a normal behavior, which, if it occurs within a home, becomes objectionable.

ALSO SEE: *Housesoiling—Spraying, Intention Spraying, Marking, Scent Marking, Sexually Dimorphic Behaviors, Urination, Warning Behavior*

Vacuous Chewing

Vacuous chewing is an atypical oral behavior in pigs. The individual shows chewing movements even though nothing is in the mouth. It is probably similar to bar biting, with a relationship to poor environmental stimuli, since provision of straw, bedding, corn cobs, and other novel stimuli can reduce the incidence of this problem.

ALSO SEE: *Bar Biting, Boredom, Jaw Chomping*

Vacuum Activity

A vacuum activity is the expression of an instinctive behavior without an apparent external stimulus. The action may actually represent a lowered stimulus threshold, as described in the damming-up theory, or it may be truly spontaneous. Examples could include birds that sing when not defending a territory, attracting mates, or warning rivals, or it could include mating behaviors shown at inappropriate times or targets by animals that have not been allowed to mate.

ALSO SEE: *Damming-up Theory, Instinct, Spontaneous Behavior, Threshold*

Vices

A vice is a potentially dangerous behavior shown by an animal. It includes the various forms of aggression. A broader, second definition is any type of problem behavior, particularly the stereotyped behaviors of horses.

ALSO SEE: *Aggression, Stereotyped Behaviors*

Vigilance

Vigilance describes the alert state of an animal, usually relative to observation for predators. This can be shown by an individual for its own protection, by peripheral members of a group, or by specially positioned "guards."

ALSO SEE: *Warning Behavior*

Vision

The senses of animals can differ markedly from those of humans, so their interpretation of surroundings will be quite different. In general, predators are more dependent on motion to find food, since camouflage and environment hide the prey. Animals of prey are also dependent on movement to serve as an early warning against predators. For these animals, detailed vision, such as that of humans, is less important.

Dogs and cats, which are predators, have relatively wide areas in their visual fields for binocular vision and wide blind angles behind their heads. The dog has a visual field of 97° binocular vision, 88° additional monocular vision with each eye, and 87° blind area. The visual field for the cat is 120° binocular vision, 80° additional monocular fields for each eye, and 80° blind area (Beaver, 1992). Since pouncing on small prey is important in predation, binocular vision is relatively important to both species. The Siamese visual field and neurologic connections differ from those of cats in general. These cats, whether cross-eyed or not, have little binocular vision (Guillery, 1974). It is as if each eye cannot see past the median plane. Thus, their field of vision is 140° monocular vision for each eye and an 80° blind area.

Horses and cattle are prey for carnivores, so their visual systems are quite similar to each other. Survival depends on a wide field of vision rather than on binocular focusing. For horses the visual field is 65° binocular vision, 146° monocular vision for each eye. The blind area is approximately 3° (Schmidt-Morand, 1992). As with all animals, these angles of vision are dependent on the shape of the head and the placement of the eyes. Because of its nose, the horse has another blind spot under its head, in front of its feet. To see objects in the approximately 4-foot blind area, the animal must lower its head and pull its nose caudally. The concept of a blind area immediately in front of the feet is important for a horse working logs in a trail course or walking through areas with unsure footing.

Another unique feature of the horse eye and probably that of cattle has to do with the animal's ability to focus on objects. Focus is usually taken care of by the lens with the attachment of the ciliary muscles. In the horse, the lens does not have the elasticity typical of other animals, so focusing must be accomplished by another method—head movement. There are two theories about how this occurs. The first is called the ramped retina theory. According to this theory, the lower part of the retina is closer to the lens than the upper part, thus giving a sloped line to the posterior globe. Light from distant objects would focus on the lower retina while that from closer objects would enter the bottom of the eye to reach the upper retina. The second theory is based on the anatomy of the retina. The area centralis, the area of sharpest vision, is a strip along the ventral half of the retina. Sharpest focus would occur for light entering the top of the eye. The net effect of either theory is the same. In order to focus on an object, the horse would need to be able to move its head up and down to focus. Any fast movement, such as a bird flying up from the ground, would only appear as a blur because the horse could not get the object in focus and keep it in focus fast enough. The instinctive tendency to flee would trigger the response to shy away from the blur. Head position and the limited binocular scope for the horse is critical for its ability to judge distances for jumping and running. Vertical jumps are easier to gauge, while horizontal jumps usually call for more dependence on the rider.

Vision for pigs is dependent on the position of the eyes relative to the skull. Since the pig is an omnivore, it would be expected to have a visual system unlike strict predators or prey species. The approximate visual field is 40° binocular vision and 115° additional monocular vision for each eye; a 90° blind field reflects this uniqueness.

All the domestic animals except the pig normally have a tapetum. By acting as a biologic mirror, this reflective area helps magnify the amount of light that enters the eye. This adaptation increases available light for better night vision; however, it tends to decrease the acuity of vision to some degree when a single light source activates several spots on the retina.

The ability to see matures as the nervous system matures, especially for animals that are born with their eyes sealed. Early experiences train the brain about certain types of images. Experimentally, visual deprivation of neonates can result in behavioral blindness. Forms, outlines, and movement are critical to both the visual learning and social development of puppies and kittens.

ALSO SEE: *Color Vision, Shying, Socialization, Fear of Falling*

Vocal Communication

Humans are vocally oriented and have a tendency to place undue emphasis on animal vocal communication. While sounds are important for certain species to prevent direct interactions between groups, vocal communication tends to relay emotional states rather than specific messages. Vocal patterns are well studied in certain species and not in others.

Dogs—Vocalization can occur by birth. While patterns will change over time, the general vocabulary changes only slightly. Nonprotest sounds of puppies have a mewing and clicking quality. They peak in frequency by approximately 7 days and disappear at 4 to 5 weeks. Protest sounds in puppies also peak at about 7 days. The whimpers disappear at about the same time as nonprotest sounds, but the yelps continue to be associated with pain, and whining develops for mentally or physically "unpleasant" situations, including submissive ones. Barking and howling generally serve as a threat or warning and are discussed elsewhere. Growl vocalizations typically are associated with aggression. The deep tone usually indicates strong intention and no fear. A louder, higher pitch is more of a threat display. Growls can occur as a play vocalization. Other sounds with a sneeze, yawn, or squeal are anticipatory. An "inverted sneeze" typical of brachycephalic breeds occurs most commonly during excitement. Sighs usually are associated with resting. During typical pack communication, there are combinations of several sounds giving indications of numerous emotional states.

Cats—Cat patterns have been well studied and have been divided phonetically into 17 different ones (Moelk, 1944). Most, like the growl, are associated with aggression, and the heat cry, sex call, and hiss are common with reproduction and territory. The "silent meow" is used at times when noise would be a disadvantage, as when watching birds. Soft clicking can also be heard when a cat is watching birds or is otherwise excited. The purr is discussed separately.

Horses—Spectrographic recordings of many equine vocalizations have been described in the context of their associated behaviors (Waring, 1983). Blowing is a vocal communication that carries for a great distance and signals a warning. The snort is associated with restlessness, especially when the horse is constrained by a barrier. Whinnies also carry for distances. These can communicate a stallion's challenge, or distress of separation as when a foal has been separated from the mare. A nicker is a softer, low-pitch sound, associated with a number of situations. It is usually used when begging, as for food; however, some horses whinny instead. Mares nicker at foals when there is potential danger. Stallions nicker in sexual behavior when approaching a mare. Mares welcome foals back, and stalled horses welcome food. Squeals are associated with aggressive encounters between horses, especially in sexual behavior when stallions meet mares and full acceptance has yet to occur. Vocalizations of a groan and snore are usually associated with resting.

Cattle—Vocalizations in cattle have been characterized phonetically and according to the situation by Kiley (Houpt, 1991). The soft "mm" is a reassurance between cow and calf or a vocalization while waiting to be milked or fed. The louder "mm(h)" is given in tense situations as when isolated, while the "(M)enh" is the roar made by bulls. A hungry calf may use the "menh" call.

Swine—A. Grauvogl has described more than 20 different sounds emitted by pigs (Hafez and Signoret in Hafez, 1969), but few other individuals can identify that many. The general grunting noises have several, ill-defined meanings. Some, such as the "mating song" have been timed and well-characterized, but most are not yet recognized as unique. Barking sounds serve as a warning, usually bringing a quick retreat. Squeals are associated with distress, as when a baby pig is picked up.

ALSO SEE: *Barking, Communal Song, Distress Call, Excessive Vocalization, Excessive Vocalization—Barking, Excessive Vocalization—Howling, Excessive Vocalization—Whining, Howling, Purr, Song*

Vocalization

Vocalization is the sound produced by the interaction of air, vocal folds or syrinx, and vibrations within the respiratory tract. The sound is usually associated with communications.

ALSO SEE: *Sniff-Yawn, Song, Vocal Communication*

Vomeronasal Organ

Just above the hard palate, the nasal mucosa covers a secondary organ of olfaction, the vomeronasal organ. This paired, cigar-shaped structure receives odors, probably in the form of volatile fatty acids, through an opening in each nasal cavity and/or through the incisive ducts in the mouth. The incisive ducts open on both sides of the incisive papilla, immediately behind the central incisor teeth. The behavior called flehmen helps odors get into the incisive ducts by opening the mouth and at least partially obstructing the nostrils. In horses, the incisive ducts are closed, so odors must enter through the nostrils instead. This unique equine feature apparently developed in parallel with the alar cartilages, which keep the nostrils open during flehmen. The activated sensory cells of the vomeronasal organ transmit electrical messages via the vomeronasal nerves to specific areas of the brain.

The vomeronasal organ, formerly called Jacobson's organ, is apparently triggered by odors associated with sexual behavior and perhaps social behavior.

ALSO SEE: *Flehmen*

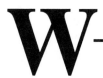

Wallow

Wallowing is a grooming behavior in which an animal spends time rolling and lying in mud or muddy water. It serves as a means of keeping cool and of covering the coat and skin with mud for protection against insects. In domestic animals, the behavior generally is associated with swine, although other species wallow to a lesser extent. Animals in dry locations may also create a wallow by urinating in a dust area and then rolling there.

ALSO SEE: *Grooming Behavior, Rolling*

Warning Behavior

A warning behavior is one that alerts others in the group of possible danger and/or the intruder that it should not approach closer. These behaviors may be vocalizations, such as a bark or growl. Other noises, such as snorts, foot stomping, and antler thrashing have similar meanings. The animal also may warn by using body language, such as the defensive threat in cats or flattened ears in horses. Pheromones or urine marking can produce olfactory warnings.

ALSO SEE: *Distance-increasing Silent Communication, Housesoiling— Urine Marking, Pheromone, Vigilance, Vocal Communication*

Weaning

Weaning is the process of stopping the infant's dependence on its mother, especially for milk. For young that nurse, there is a gradual change to solid food (transitional stage) before nursing stops completely. Weaning is normally completed by 6 weeks in puppies, 12 weeks in kittens, and 6 months in foals. For single kittens and for foals of well-fed, nonpregnant mares, weaning may not take place until much later. Calves and piglets vary in times of weaning because of management systems.

ALSO SEE: *Ingestive Behavior, Nursing, Transitional Phase*

Weaving

Weaving is a behavior problem also known as stereotyped weaving.

SEE: *Stereotyped Weaving*

Wild Animal

A wild animal is a member of a species that has evolved to its present form without any major human influence.

ALSO SEE: *Domestication, Feral Animal, Tame Animal*

Wind Sucking

Wind sucking is a serious behavior problem in horses that can result in medical problems. This behavior usually develops in a horse that had been a cribber when little was done to control that problem or its causes. Long-term confinement with minimal exercise or mental stimulation may eventually produce the problem. This behavior is exemplified by a horse that bites firmly onto a board or pipe, tenses the muscles in its neck, sucks in, and swallows air. Some horses would rather wind suck than eat, and most lose body condition because of the problem.

The behavior becomes its own reward, so treatments are not very successful. A wind-sucker strap usually is tried first to stop the problem. This is placed tightly around the cranial neck and apparently causes discomfort when the behavior is attempted. Many horses learn to ignore the strap. Surgical myotomies only make it more difficult for the horse to bite an object and tense its neck. The result is usually cosmetically unpleasant and seldom successful. Behavioral therapy, if intensive, can be more successful. The key is long-term therapy with several components. A muzzle can prevent the horse from getting a hold on a board or pipe. In addition, greatly increasing the amount of exercise the horse gets will measurably improve the chances. For a few horses, just being in a pasture may be enough; others will simply spend their pasture time wind sucking on a fence. Shock collars have been used successfully with a few horses. Recent studies with narcotic antagonists indicate that eventually there may be a group of drugs that can help extinguish internally rewarded behaviors such as wind sucking.

ALSO SEE: *Cribbing, Drug Therapy, Internal Reward, Muzzle, Shock Collars, Taste Aversion*

Withdrawal Distance

Once an animal begins to flee from an intruder, it will run for a limited distance, the withdrawal distance, if it is not being pursued. If the animal were to continue fleeing for great distances when not in danger, it would use more energy than needed and could possibly run into another source of danger. For domestic animals and captive wild animals, the distance may be artificially limited by fences.

Horses evolved on the plains, with running as their instinct for survival. If a threat is perceived, the instinct to run the full withdrawal distance often causes a horse to injure itself on a fence or other object. Since these limitations did not exist when the instinct evolved, the horse never developed adaptive protective mechanisms.

ALSO SEE: *Reactive Distance, Social Distance*

Withers Nibbling

Horses that are preferred associates will commonly start grooming each other after a period of separation. Using the teeth and upper lip, they stroke and bite each other's withers, neck, and back areas. This withers nibbling behavior helps groom areas that are difficult to self-groom, and it probably serves as a greeting and reassurance between individuals.

ALSO SEE: *Grooming Behavior, Mutual Grooming, Preferred Associate, Social Grooming*

Wood Chewing

It is common to find horses that chew and eat wood in stalls and paddocks. There can be a nutritional relation to inadequate amounts of salt or roughage. Studies have shown severe wood chewing can occur if hay levels are less than one pound per hundredweight. When nutrients are not deficient, a lack of environmental stimuli and exercise predisposes horses to this condition.

The addition of sawdust to concentrated diets has been advocated. Muzzles and taste aversion can be combined with access to pasture and increased exercise to eliminate or minimize the problem.

ALSO SEE: *Boredom, Exercise, Muzzle, Taste Aversion*

Wool Pulling

Wool pulling is a variation of hair pulling seen in sheep. Animals that are confined and on high-concentrate diets seem to be affected most.

ALSO SEE: *Hair Pulling*

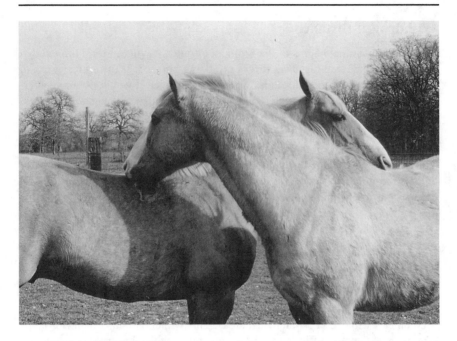

Withers Nibbling. Two pasture mates demonstrate withers nibbling.

Wool Sucking

Wool sucking is a variation of the prolonged sucking syndrome, and it apparently has a genetic basis. The affected cats usually are Siamese or Siamese crosses. For some of these animals, the sucking apparently begins at the time of weaning, although it will commonly begin in a completely weaned cat before six months of age, and the behavior often includes chewing not just sucking. The targeted object usually is made of wool or is fluffy in texture. Other objects that pick up sebaceous secretions, such as the underarm areas of dirty tee shirts, may also be sucked or chewed. The cat may stay with a specific object or damage several items.

The behavior probably is internally rewarding, because it is extremely difficult to eliminate. Often the cat's access will have to be limited; if it can be limited to just one item, that may be a desirable outcome. Taste aversion is the most effective technique for eliminating the problem. Smell aversion and remote or direct punishment can be used, but the results are not as good.

ALSO SEE: *Genetic Problems, Internal Reward, Prevent Access, Prolonged Sucking, Prolonged Sucking Syndrome, Remote Punishment, Smell Aversion, Taste Aversion*

Z

Zoomorphism

Zoomorphism is attributing animal characteristics to humans. This occurs most often when rationalizing human behavior in terms of that shown in animals.

Zoomorphism is the opposite of anthropomorphism.

ALSO SEE: *Anthropomorphism*

BEHAVIOR PROBLEM HISTORY FORM

Date:
Owner:
    Name:
    Address:
    Phone:
Signalment:
    Age:
    Sex:
    Species:
    Breed:
    Name:
Background Information:
    Other pets:

Name	Age	Sex	Species	Breed

    Family members:
        Number of adults:
        Number and ages of children:

    Observation of the problem:
        Has the owner seen the animal show the behavior?
    Source of the animal:

Animal shelter	Got as a gift
Auction	Newspaper ad
Breeder	Pet store
Former owner	Raised it
Found as a stray	Relative or friend

    Age of the animal when obtained:
    Medical history:

What exactly is the problem?
When did the problem begin?
    Duration:
    Progress of the problem:
        Getting progressively worse
        Has stayed at the same severity
        Is gradually getting better
        Has periods when it does not occur
        Has only happened once or twice
    Other events that occurred about the time the problem started:

When does the problem happen?
  Frequency:
    Several times daily
    Daily
    Every other day
    Every few days
    Weekly

    Every other week
    Monthly
    Irregularly

    Other (describe)

Timing of occurrences:
    Morning
    Afternoon
    Evening
    Daytime
    Late night

    Only when people are present
    Only when no one is present
    People can be present or absent
    People are nearby but not close

Where does the problem occur?
  In the house:
    Basement
    Breakfast area
    Child's bedroom
    Closet
    Den, TV, family room
    Dining room
    Entryway to house
    Guest bedroom
    Hallway
    Kitchen

    Laundry (utility) room
    Living room
    Master bathroom
    Master bedroom
    Recreation room
    Second bathroom
    Stairway
    Upstairs
    Near the litter box
    Other (describe)

  In the garage:
  Outdoors:
    In a fenced backyard:
      Center of the yard
      Near a fence
      In a flower bed
      In the garden

      Near a gate
      Near the house
      In a shady area

    In an unfenced backyard:
    In a fenced front yard:
    In an unfenced front yard:
  In other locations:
    In the car:
    In a stall:
    In a shed:
    In a paddock:
    In a pasture:
    Other (describe):

Specific items or people targeted:
  Specific items:
    Bed
    Blanket
    Cabinets
    Carpet

    Furniture (which piece)
    Houseplants
    Manger
    Shoes

Clothes (whose)   Stall
   Clean   Telephone
   Dirty   Trailer
Curtains/Blinds   Trailer door
Door   Wall
Doorbell   Window
Fence   Window or door sill
Floor   Other (describe)
Specific individuals:
   Animal itself
   Particular person
General Information:
  Location of the animal when the owners are gone:

On a chain	In a paddock
In a crate	In a pasture
In a fenced yard	In a stall
Anywhere in the house	
In a kennel	Other (describe)
Confined to a bathroom	
Confined to the kitchen	
Confined to the utility room	
Anywhere outside	
In a specific room (which one)	

  Location of the animal when the owners are home:

On a chain	In a paddock
In a crate	In a pasture
In a fenced yard	In a stall
Anywhere in the house	
In a kennel	Other (describe)
Confined to a bathroom	
Confined to the kitchen	
Confined to the utility room	
Anywhere outside	
In a specific room (which one)	

  Location where the animal usually sleeps:

In the area of its chain	In a specific room (which one)
In a crate	In the fenced yard
Anywhere in the house	Anywhere outside
In a dog kennel	In the barn
In the kitchen	In a paddock
In the master bedroom	In a pasture
In a child's bedroom	In a stall
On the bed	Other (describe)

  Type of food the animal gets:

Canned (brand name)	Grain
Dry (brand name)	Hay
Semi-moist (brand name)	Pasture
Table scraps	Prepared feeds

Home prepared meals (describe)
Frequency and time of feeding:
    Once each day at
    Twice each day at
    Three times daily at
    Four times daily at
    Other (describe)
Formal Training:
    Obedience training:
        Owner took dog to obedience class
        Owner taught dog a few commands (which)
        Dog was sent to a trainer
            Attack training
            Guard dog training
            Obedience training
            Amount of time owner worked with dog and the trainer
        General amount of success with obedience lessons
    Professional horse trainer:
        Length of time with the trainer
        Amount of time owner worked with horse and trainer
    No formal training
Does the animal show a "guilty" look associated with the problem?
Are there any recent changes in the family or the animal's environment?

Additional history for cases of aggression:
    Targets of the aggression:
        Humans:

Adult owners	Child in the immediate family
Adults the animal knows	Children the animal knows
Adult strangers	Child strangers
Men only	
Women only	Ages of the children

        Animals:
            Same species
                Same sex as the problem animal
                Different sex from the problem animal
            Another species (describe)

        Itself directed
            Flank area
            Forelimb
            Side of the body
            Tail
Associated behaviors:
    Can the owner predict when the animal will show the behavior?
        What are the signs?

What does the animal do immediately after the problem behavior?

Additional history for cases of housesoiling:
    For problem dogs:
        Normal patterns:
            Location of normal elimination:
                Anywhere in the house
                On carpet in the house
                On paper in the house
                Within a fenced yard
                Anywhere outside
                Other (describe)
            Frequency of normal elimination if dog goes outside:

Outside all day	Afternoon
Outside all night	Early evening
Uses dog door	Late evening
Early morning	On demand
Late morning	After bedtime
Noon	Other (describe)

            Posture for urination:
                Lifted leg
                Standing
                Squatting
    For problem cats:
        Litter box use:
            Has the cat ever used the litter box?
            Does the cat use the litter box currently?
                Always for feces
                Occasionally for feces
                Never for feces
                Always for urine
                Occasionally for urine
                Never for urine
        Litter box management:
            Number of litter boxes:
            Number of cats using the litter boxes:
            Location of the litter box(es):

Closet in a bedroom	Laundry (utility) room
Closet in a hall	Master bathroom
Garage	Master bedroom
Guest bedroom	Second bathroom
Kitchen	Other (describe)

            Brand of litter used:
                Any recent changes in brands of litter?
            Frequency with which feces are removed:
            Frequency of complete litter dumping:
            Frequency of washing the litter box:
    Other information:
        Products used to clean up soiled areas in the house:

APPENDIX B

GENERAL SPECIES INFORMATION

	Dogs	Cats	Horses	Cattle	Swine	Sheep	M
Scientific name	Canus familiaris	Felis catus	Equus caballus	Bos taurus / Bos indicus	Sus scrofa	Ovis aries	Capra hircus
Intact, adult male	Dog	Tomcat	Stallion	Bull	Boar	Ram, buck	Billy, buck
Neutered male			Gelding	Steer	Barrow	Wether	Mutton
Young male			Colt				
Intact, adult female	Bitch	Queen	Mare	Cow	Sow	Ewe	Doe, nanny goat
Young female			Filly	Heifer	Gilt		
Young animal either sex	Puppy	Kitten	Foal	Calf	Piglet	Lamb	Kid
Group name	Pack		Herd	Herd	Herd	Flock	Flock
Social behavior	Linear dominance	Territorial	Linear dominance	Complex dominance	Complex dominance	Active fellowship	Complex dominance
Male Puberty	6-9 months	9-12 months	16-20 months	10 months	5-8 months	5-7 months	8 months
Female puberty	6-8 months	3-12 months	10-24 months	9-12 months	6-8 months	6-16 months	4-12 months
Average		5-7 months	18 months		7 months		5-7 months
Estrus period	7-10 days			9-28 hours	40-80 hours	24-48 hours	36-48 hours
If mated		4-6 days					
If not mated		10-14 days					
Average			5 days	18 hours	40-44 hours	36 hours	40 hours
Estrus Cycle	4-12 months	21-29 days	19-23 days	13-23 days	18-28 days	14-19 days	12-24 days
Average	6 months	Seasonal	21 days; Seasonal	21 days	21 days	16 days; Seasonal	21 days; Seasonal
Gestation	63 days	63-65 days	322-344 days	281-290 days	113-116 days	144-152 days	135-160 days; 151 days
Average delivery time	3 hours	1-2 hours	10-30 minutes	30-60 minutes	1-4 hours	30-90 minutes	
Delivery intervals	20-60 minutes	1-50 minutes			10-35 minutes		
Average number young	4	3	1	1	9	1-2	1-2
Added time for placenta			2 hours		12 hours	5 hours	
Name for birthing	Whelping	Queening	Foaling	Calving	Farrowing	Lambing	Kidding
Time to estrus after parturition		Seasonal	4-14 days	32-86 days / Affected by nursing	1-3 days		
Average	4 months		9 days	60 days	2 days		
Placenta type	Zonary	Zonary	Diffuse	Cotyledonary	Diffuse	Cotyledonary	Cotyledonary
Time of fetal implantation	13-15 days	11-12 days	40 days	30 days	11 days	18 days	
Ejaculate volume	7-10 cc		50-125 cc	2-10 cc	200-300 cc	0.8-1.25 cc	
Sperm count	5-20×10^8 cc		6-30×10^7 cc	8-12×10^8 cc	1-4×10^8 cc	1-3.5×10^9 cc	

APPENDIX **C**

DOSES OF DRUGS USED IN BEHAVIOR THERAPY

The following listing of drugs is not intended to be complete because many conditions, such as hypothryoid aggression, are treated by conventional therapy. It does, however, include most of the drugs that are currently used. The doses suggested are compiled from a number of sources and represent the range recommendations currently being used. The reader is directed to in-depth books, formularies, and articles (Allen, Pringle, Smith, et al., 1993; Brander, Pugh, Bywater, et al., 1991; Dodman, Shuster, Court, et al., 1987; Dodman, Shuster, White, et al., 1988; Hart, Eckstein, Powell et al, 1993; Overall, 1992; Plumb, 1991; Texas A&M University, 1990; Upson, 1985; Voith and Marder in Morgan, 1992; White, 1990) dealing with pharmacology and psychopharmacology to learn more about indications and contraindications for the use of any particular drug.

Acepromazine maleate (Acepromazine™)
Behavior use: decrease spontaneous activity, decrease response to stimuli, sedation
Action: phenothiazine tranquilizer
Dogs: 0.22-1.1 mg/kg PO; 0.11-1.1 mg/kg IM/SQ/IV; 0.55-1.1 mg/kg PO; 0.055-0.11 mg/kg IM/SQ/IV
Cats: 0.55-2.2 mg/kg PO; 0.22-2.2 mg/kg IM/SQ; 1.1-2.2 mg/kg PO; 0.11-0.22 mg/kg IM/SQ/IV
Horses: 0.04-0.08 mg/kg IM/SQ/IV

Alprazolam (Xanax™)
Behavior use: fears
Action: benzodiazepine tranquilizer
Cats: 0.125-0.25 mg/kg PO q12h; 0.125-0.25 mg/cat PO q12h

Amitriptyline hydrochloride (Elavil™)
Behavior use: generalized and separation anxiety, excessive grooming, urine spraying
Action: tricyclic antidepressant, tertiary amine
Dogs: 1-2 mg/kg/day PO q24h or divided; 2.2-4.4 mg/kg PO q12h
Cats: 5-10 mg/cat/day

Azaperone (Stresnil™, Suicalm™)
Behavior use: control aggression and fighting, decrease excitement
Action: butyrephone neuroleptic
Pigs: 2.2mg/kg IM

Buspirone hydrochloride (Buspar™)
Behavior use: urine spraying, stereotypies, obsessive compulsive disorders, fear of thunder, various phobias

Action: anxiolytic, partial serotonin agonist
Dogs: 2.5-10 mg PO q8-12h
Cats: 2.5-5 mg PO q8-12h; 5-7.5 mg PO q12h

Chlordiazepoxide
Behavior use: antianxiety affect, urine spraying
Action: benzodiazepine tranquilizer
Dogs: 2-20 mg PO as needed
Cats: 2-5 mg PO

Chlorpheniramine maleate (Chlor-Trimeton™)
Behavior use: mild sedation for apprehension, travel by car
Action: antihistamine
Dogs: 4-8 mg PO q12h
Cats: 2 mg PO q12h

Chlorpromazine hydrochloride (Thorazine™)
Behavior use: decrease spontaneous activity, decrease response to stimuli, sedation
Action: phenothiazine tranquilizer
Dogs: 1 mg/kg PO q12h
Cats: 1 mg/kg PO q12h
Pigs: 1.1 mg/kg IM

Clomipramine hydrochloride (Anafranil™)
Behavior use: generalized and separation anxiety, obsessive compulsive disorders,
     excessive grooming, lick granulomas
Action: tricyclic antidepressant, tertiary amine
Dogs: 1-3 mg/kg/day PO; 1-3 mg/kg PO q12h x 4-5 wk

Clorazepate dipotassium (Tranxene™)
Behavior use: antianxiety affect, fear of thunder
Action: benzodiazepine tranquilizer
Dogs: 0.55-2.2 mg/kg PO; 11.25-22.5 mg PO q8-12h; 5.6 mg/small dog PO q24h;
     11.25mg/medium dog PO q24h; 22.5 mg/large dog PO q24h; 11.25-22.5 mg
     PO q12-24h
Cats: 0.55 - 2.2 mg/kg PO; 0.5 - 1.0 mg/kg q12-24h

Dextroamphetamine
Behavior use: narcolepsy and hyperkinesis in dogs, mainly for diagnosis
Action: short-acting stimulant
Dogs: 0.5-1 mg/kg PO; 0.2-1.3 mg/kg PO as needed

Diazepam (Valium™)
Behavior use: antianxiety affect, stop grand mal seizures, appetite stimulant, urine
     spraying, fear of thunder
Action: benzodiazepine tranquilizer
Other: gradual withdrawal is recommended
Dogs: 2-20 mg IV/PO as needed; 0.55-2.2 mg/kg PO as needed

Cats: 2-5 mg IV/PO as needed; 1 mg IV with food; 1-2 mg PO q12h; 1-3 mg PO q12-24h

Horses: 0.1-0.3 mg/kg IV as needed

Diphenhydramine hydrochloride (Hydramine™)
Behavior use: mild sedation for apprehension, travel by car
Action: antihistamine
Dogs: 4 mg/kg PO q12h
Cats: 4 mg/kg PO q12h

Doxepin hydrochloride (Sinequan™)
Behavior use: excessive grooming
Action: tricyclic antidepressant, tertiary amine, with antipruritic action
Dogs: 5-10 mg/kg PO q12h; 0.5-1.0 mg/kg PO q12h; 0.5-1.0 mg/kg PO

Ethylisobutrazine hydrochloride (Diquel™)
Behavior use: control intractable dogs, reduce self-mutilation
Action: phenothiazine
Dogs: 2.2-4.4 mg/kg IV to effect; 4.4-11.1 mg/kg IM for profound tranquilization

Fluoxetine (Prozac™)
Behavior use: depression, obsessive compulsive disorder
Action: antidepressant, serotoninergic agent
Other: onset and withdrawal take 3-6 weeks
Dogs: 1 mg/kg/day PO

Imipramine hydrochloride (Tofranil™)
Behavior use: generalized and separation anxiety, mild narcolepsy
Action: tricyclic antidepressant, tertiary amine
Dogs: 2.2-4.4 mg/kg PO q12-24h

Medroxyprogesterone acetate (Depo Provera™)
Behavior use: antianxiety tranquilizing effect, decreases serum testosterone and resulting male behaviors, increases appetite
Action: injectable, long-acting progestin
Dogs: 8-10 mg/kg IM; 5-10 mg/kg SQ/IM; 11 mg/kg SQ/IM
Cats: 100 mg/cat IM; 10-20 mg/kg SQ/IM; 50 mg females, 100 mg males SQ 3x/year; 5-10 mg/kg SQ/IM; 11mg/kg SQ/IM

Megestrol Acetate (Ovaban™, Megace™, Ovarid™)
Behavior use: antianxiety tranquilizing effect, decreases serum testosterone, increases appetite
Action: oral progestin
Dogs: 2.2 mg/kg/day PO for days 1-7, 1.1 mg/kg/day (or 2.2 mg/kg, every second day) PO for days 8-14, if positive results, the maintenance dose level should be as low and infrequent as possible; 2.2-4.4 mg/kg/day PO for 2 weeks, then 1/2 dose for 2 weeks; 1.1-2.2 mg/kg/day for 2 weeks decreasing by 1/2 every 2 weeks

Cats: 5 mg/day PO for days 1-7, and 2.5 mg/day (or 5 mg every second day) PO for days 8-14, if positive results, maintenance dose should be as low and infrequent as possible; 2.5-5.0 mg/day PO for 7 days, 2.5-5.0 mg/week; 5-10 mg/day PO for 1 week then decreasing every 2 weeks to minimum effective dose

Horses: 65-85 mg/500 kg PO q24h

Methylphenidate hydrochloride (Ritalin™)
Behavior use: hyperkinesis, narcolepsy
Action: time released stimulant
Dogs: 5mg/small dog PO q12; 10 mg/medium dog PO q12h; 20 mg/large dog PO q12h; 5+ mg/day PO; 20-40 mg/dog

Naloxone hydrochloride (Narcan™)
Behavior use: obsessive compulsive behaviors and stereotypies diagnosis
Action: narcotic antagonist
Dogs: 11-22 micrograms/kg SQ/IM/IV

Naltrexone (Trexan™)
Behavior use: obsessive compulsive behaviors and stereotypies diagnosis
Action: narcotic antagonist
Dogs: 2.2 mg/kg PO q24h; 2.2 mg/kg PO q12-24h
Cats: 25-50 mg PO q24h

Phenobarbital
Behavior use: anticonvulsant, tranquilization (particularly in cats), feline excessive vocalization
Action: barbiturate
Dogs: 2-4 mg/kg PO q12h; 2-3 mg/kg PO/IM/IV as needed; 2.2 mg/kg PO/IM/IV q12h
Cats: 2-4 mg/kg PO q12h; 2-3 mg/kg PO/IM/IV as needed

Phenylpropanolamine hydrochloride (Dexatrim™, Ornade™)
Behavior use: submissive urination
Action: sympathetic agonist
Dogs: 12.5-50 mg PO q8-12h; 1.1-4.4 mg/kg PO q8-12h; 1-2 mg/kg PO (25 mg maximum)

Phenytoin sodium (Dilantin™)
Behavior use: anticonvulsant
Action: anticonvulsant
Dogs: 5-30 mg/kg PO q8h; 15-35 mg/kg PO q8-12h

Primidone (Mysoline™)
Behavior use: anticonvulsant
Action: anticonvulsant
Dogs: 55.5 mg/kg PO q12h; 25-30 mg/kg PO q12h

Promazine hydrochloride (Sparine™)
Behavior use: decrease spontaneous activity, decrease response to stimuli, sedation

Action: phenothiazine tranquilizer
Dogs: 2.22-4.44 mg/kg IM/IV; 1-4 mg/kg PO/IM as needed
Cats: 2.22-4.44 mg/kg IM/IV; 2-4 mg/kg PO/IM as needed
Horses: 0.44-1.11 mg/kg IM/IV; 1.1 mg/kg IV; 0.4-1.0 mg/kg IV
Pigs: 0.44-1.0 mg/kg IV/IM

Propranolol hydrochloride (Inderal™)
Behavior use: reduce sympathetic activity, mild fear of thunder
Action: Beta adrenergic blocking agent
Dogs: 5+mg/small dog PO q8h; 10-20 mg/large dog PO q8h; 5-20 mg PO q8h; 5-40mg PO q8h

Trimeprazine tartrate (Temaril™)
Behavior use: decrease spontaneous activity, decrease response to stimuli, sedation, antipruritic
Action: phenothiazine tranquilizer with antipruritic, antiitussive, and antiinflammatory properties
Dogs: 1.1-4.4 mg/kg PO q6h; 2.5mg/10 lbs up to 40 lbs, 15 mg if over 40 lbs PO q12h, reduce dose by 1/2 after 4 days

References and Additional Reading

Allen, D. G., Pringle, J. K, Smith, D. A., Conlon, P. D., and Burgmann, P. M. 1993. Handbook of Veterinary Drugs. Philadelphia, J. B. Lippincott Company, p. 678.

American Psychiatric Association. 1987. Diagnostic and Statistical Manual of Mental Disorders, 3rd ed. Washington, DC, American Psychiatric Association, p. 494.

Anderson, R. K., and Foster, R. E. 1987. Promote Good Manners with Gentle Leader™. Minneapolis, Alpha-M Inc.

Antelyes, J. 1973. The patient's name: a clinical bonus. Small Anim. Clinician 68:232-235.

Beadle, M. 1977. The Cat: History, Biology, and Behavior. New York, Simon and Schuster.

Beaver, B. V. 1980. Veterinary Aspects of Feline Behavior. St. Louis, C. V. Mosby, p. 217.

Beaver, B. V. 1989. Environmental enrichment for laboratory animals. ILAR News 31 (2):5-11.

Beaver, B. V. 1989. Feline behavior problems other than housesoiling. J. Am. Anim. Hosp. Assoc. 25 (4):465-469.

Beaver, B. V. 1989. Housesoiling by cats: a retrospective study of 120 cases. J. Am. Anim. Hosp. Assoc. 25 (6):631-637.

Beaver, B. V. 1992. Feline Behavior: A Guide for Veterinarians. Philadelphia, W.B. Saunders Company, p. 276.

Beaver, B. V. 1993. Profiles of dogs presented for aggression. J. Am. Anim. Hosp. Assoc. 29 (6):564-569.

Beaver, B. V., and Amoss, M. S., Jr. 1982. Aggressive behavior associated with naturally elevated serum testosterone in mares. Applied Anim. Ethology 8:425-428.

Beaver, B. V., Fischer, M., and Atkinson, C. E. 1992. Determination of favorite components of garbage by dogs. Appl. Anim. Behav. Sci. 34:129-136.

Bennett, M., Houpt, K. A., and Erb, H. N. 1988. Effects of declawing on feline behavior. Companion Anim. Pract. 2:7.

Berger, J. 1986. Wild Horses of the Great Basin: Social Competition and Population Size. Chicago, The University of Chicago Press, p. 326.

Brander, G. C., Pugh, D. M., Bywater, R. J., and Jenkins, W. L. 1991. Veterinary Applied Pharmacology & Therapeutics, 5th ed. Philadelphia, Bailliere Tindall, p. 624.

Brown, S. A., Crowell-Davis, S., Malcolm, T., and Edwards, P. 1987. Naloxone-responsive compulsive tail chasing in a dog. J. Am. Vet. Med. Assoc. 190 (7):884-886.

Clutton-Brock, J. 1981. Domesticated Animals from Early Times. Austin, University of Texas Press, p. 208.

Craig, J. V. 1981. Domestic Animal Behavior: Causes and Implications for Animal Care and Management. Englewood Cliffs, NJ, Prentice-Hall, Inc., p. 364.

Crowell-Davis, S. L., and Houpt, K. A. 1985. Coprophagy by foals: effect of age and possible functions. Equine Vet. J. 17:17-19.

Crowell-Davis, S. L., and Houpt, K. A., eds. 1986. Behavior. Vet. Clin. of North Am.: Equine Pract. 2 (3):465-671.

DeLahunta, A. 1983. Veterinary Neuroanatomy and Clinical Neurology, 2nd ed. Philadelphia, W.B. Saunders Company, p. 471.

Diagnosis: Barbering, or hair-pulling. Lab. Anim. 20 (3):18, 1991.

Dodman, N. H. 1992. Tail chasing in a bull terrier. Presentation at the Am. Vet. Soc. Anim. Beh., August 3, 1992, Boston, MA.

Dodman, N. H., Shuster, L., Court, M. H., and Dixon, R. 1987. Investigation into the use of narcotic antagonists in the treatment of a stereotypic behavior pattern (crib-biting) in the horse. Am. J. Vet. Res. 48 (2):311-319.

Dodman, N. H., Shuster, L., White, S. D., Court, M. H., Parker, D., and Dixon, R. 1988. Use of narcotic antagonists to modify stereotypic self-licking, self-chewing, and scratching behavior in dogs. J. Am. Vet. Med. Assoc. 193 (7):815-819.

Edwards, A. J. 1988. Answers to some questions about buller steers. Kansas Vet. Med. Assoc. Newsletter:5-7.

Fagen, R. 1981. Animal Play Behavior. New York, Oxford University Press, p. 684.

Fenner, W. R. 1982. Quick Reference To Veterinary Medicine. Philadelphia, J. B. Lippincott Company, p. 592.

Fox, M. W. 1965. Canine Behavior. Springfield, IL, Charles C. Thomas, p. 137.

Fox, M. W. 1966. Canine Pediatrics: Development, Neonatal and Congenital Diseases. Springfield, IL, Charles C. Thomas, p. 148.

Fox, M. W. 1971. Psychopathology in man and lower animals. J. Am. Vet. Med. Assoc. 159 (1):66-77.

Fox, M. W. 1986. Laboratory Animal Husbandry: Ethology, Welfare and Experimental Variables. Albany, State University Press of New York, p. 267.

Fraser, A. F. 1992. The Behaviour of the Horse. Wallingford, Oxon, UK, C•A•B International, p. 288.

Fraser, A. F., and Broom, D. M. 1990. Farm Animal Behaviour and Welfare, 3rd ed. Philadelphia, Bailliere Tindall, p. 437.

Gambaryan, P. P. 1974. How Mammals Run. New York, John Wiley and Sons, p. 367.

Ganz, L., and Fitch, M. 1968. The effects of visual deprivation on perceptual behavior. Exp. Neurol. 22:638-660.

Gibbs, E. L., and Gibbs, F. A. 1936. A purring center in the brain of the cat. J. Comp. Neurol. 64:209-211.

Goodall, J. 1976. The Chimpanzees of Gombe: Patterns of Behavior. Cambridge, MA, Belknap Press, p. 673.

Guillery, R. W. 1974. Visual pathways in albinos. Sci. Am. 230:44-54.

Hafez, E. S. E., ed. 1969. The Behaviour of Domestic Animals, 2nd ed. Baltimore, The William and Wilkins Company, p. 647.

Hafez, E. S. E., ed. 1975. The Behaviour of Domestic Animals, 3rd ed. Baltimore, The William and Wilkins Company, p. 532.

Hart, B. L. 1981. Olfactory tractotomy for control of objectionable urine spraying and urine marking in cats. J. Am. Vet. Med. Assoc. 179:231-234.

Hart, B. L. 1982. Neurosurgery for behavior problems. Vet. Clin. of North Am.: Small Anim. Pract. 12 (4):707-714.

Hart, B. L., and Barrett, R. E. 1973. Effects of castration on fighting, roaming, and urine spraying in adult male cats. J. Am. Vet. Med. Assoc. 163:290-292.

Hart, B. L., and Hart, L. A. 1985. Canine and Feline Behavioral Therapy. Philadelphia, Lea and Febiger, p. 275.

Hart, B. L., and Hart, L. A. 1988. The Perfect Puppy. New York, W.H. Freeman and Company, p. 182.

Hart, B. L., Eckstein, R. A., Powell, K. L., and Dodman, N. H. 1993. Effectiveness of buspirone on urine spraying and inappropriate urination in cats. J. Am. Vet. Med. Assoc. 203 (2):254-258.

Hatch, R. C. 1972. Effect of drugs on catnip (*Nepeta cataria*)-induced pleasure behavior in cats. Am. J. Vet. Res. 33 (1):143-155.

Heffner, H. E., and Heffner, R. S. 1983. The hearing ability of horses. Equine Pract. 5 (3):27-32.

Heffner, R. S., and Heffner, H. E. 1983. Effect of cattle ear mite infestation on hearing in a cow. J. Am. Vet. Med. Assoc. 182:612-614.

Hendricks, J. C., and Morrison, A. R. 1981. Normal and abnormal sleep in mammals. J. Am. Vet. Med. Assoc. 178:121-126.

Heymer, A. 1977. Ethological Dictionary. New York, Garland Publishing, Inc., p. 238.

Hollenbeck, L. 1971. The Dynamics of Canine Gait: A Study of Motion. Erie, PA, A-K-D Printing Company, p. 236.

Houpt, K. A. 1991. Domestic Animal Behavior for Veterinarians and Animal Scientists, 2nd ed. Ames, Iowa State University Press, p. 408.

Hughes, B. O., and Duncan, I. J. H. 1988. The notion of ethological "need," models of motivation and animal welfare. Anim. Behav. 36 (6):1696-1707.

Immelmann, K., and Beer, C. 1989. Dictionary of Ethology. Cambridge, MA, Harvard University Press, p. 336.

Jezierski, T. A., Koziorowski, M., Goszczynski, J., and Sieradzka, I. 1989. Homosexual and social behaviours of young bulls of different geno- and phenotypes and plasma concentrations of some hormones. Appl. Anim. Behav. Sci. 24 (2):101-113.

Ladewig, J., Price, E. O., and Hart, B. L. 1980. Flehmen in male goats: role in sexual behavior. Beh. Neural Biol. 30:312-322.

Lorenz, K. Z. 1981. The Foundation of Ethology. New York, Springer-Verlag.

McFarland, D. 1982. The Oxford Companion to Animal Behavior. New York, Oxford University Press, p. 657.

Mandelker, L. 1990. Uncovering many new psychotherapeutic agents. Veterinary Forum:28.

Manning, A. M., and Rowan, A. N. 1992. Companion animal demographics and sterilization status: results from a survey in four Massachusetts towns. Anthrozoos V (3):192-201.

Marder, A. R., and Voith, V., eds. 1991. Advances in companion animal behavior. Vet. Clin. of North Am.: Small Anim. Pract. 21 (2):203-420.

Miller, R. M. 1991. Imprint Training of the Newborn Foal, Colorado Springs, CO, Western Horseman, p. 144.

Moelk, M. 1944. Vocalizing in the house cat: a phonetic and functional study. Am. J. Psychol. 57:184-205.

Moulton, D. G. 1972. Factors influencing odor sensitivity in the dog: final report for the Air Force Office of Scientific Research, pp. 1-40.

Overall, K. L. 1992. Practical pharmacological approaches to behavior problems. In Purina Specialty Review, Behavioral Problems in Small Animals, St. Louis, Purina, pp. 36-51.

Plumb, D. C. 1991. Veterinary Drug Handbook, Pocket Edition. White Bear Lake, MN, PharmaVet Publishing, p. 688

Price, E. O. 1984. Behavioral aspects of animal domestication. The Quarterly Review of Biology 59 (1):1-31.

Price, E. O., ed. 1987. Farm Animal Behavior. Vet. Clin. of North Am.: Food Anim. Pract. 3 (2):217-481.

Redding, R. W., and Walker, T. L. 1976. Electroconvulsive therapy to control aggression in dogs. Mod. Vet. Pract. 57 (8):595-597.

Remmers, J. E., and Gautier, H. 1972. Neural and mechanical mechanisms of feline purring. Respir. Physio. 16:351-361.

Ruehl, W. W. 1993. Rationale to develop the investigational drug l-deprenyl for use in pet dogs. Newsletter of the Am. Vet. Soc. Anim. Beh. 15 (1):4-6.

Schmidt-Morand, D. 1992. Vision in the animal kingdom. Vet. International 4 (1):3-32.

Scott, J. P., and Fuller, J. L. 1965. Dog Behavior, the Genetic Basis. Chicago, the University of Chicago Press, p. 468.

Shell, L. 1988. Feline ischemic encephalopathy (cerebral infarct). Virg. Vet. Notes 35:3.

Simoni, A., and Sprague, J. M. 1976. Perimetric analysis of binocular and monocular visual fields in Siamese cats. Brain Res. 111:189-196.

Sivak, J. G., and Allen, D. B. 1975. An evaluation of the "ramp" retina of the horse eye. Vision Res. 15:1353-1356.

Syme, G. J., and Syme, L. A. 1979. Social Structure in Farm Animals. New York, Elsevier Scientific Publishing Company, p. 200.

Tan, U., Yaprak, M., and Kutlu, N. 1990. Paw preference in cats: distribution and sex differences. Intern. J. Neurosci. 50:195-208.

Texas A&M University. 1990. Formulary of the Texas A&M University Texas Veterinary Medical Center Veterinary Teaching Hospital. College Station, Texas A&M University, p. 317.

Two Eves for Daisy. Science 264:343, 1994.

Upson, D. W. 1985. Upson's Handbook of Clinical Veterinary Pharmacology, 2nd ed. Lenexa, KS, Veterinary Medicine Publishing Co., p. 660.

Voith, V. L. 1981. Profile of 100 animal behavior cases. Mod. Vet. Pract. 62 (6):483-484.

Voith, V. L. 1989. Behavioral disorders. In Textbook of Veterinary Internal Medicine: Diseases of the Dog and Cat, 3rd ed., S. J. Ettinger, ed. Philadelphia, W.B. Saunders Company, pp. 227-238.

Voith, V. L., and Borchelt, P. L., eds. 1982. Symposium on animal behavior. Vet. Clin. of North Am.: Small Anim. Pract. 12 (4):563-714.

Voith, V. L., and Marder, A. R. 1988. Behavioral disorders. In Handbook of Small Animal Practice, R. V. Morgan, ed. New York, Churchill Livingstone, pp. 1031-1051.

Voith, V. L., and Marder, A. R. 1992. Behavioral disorders: Introduction. In Handbook of Small Animal Practice, R. V. Morgan, ed. New York, Churchill Livingstone, pp. 1245-1247.

Walls, G. L. 1967. The Vertebrate Eye: and Its Adaptive Radiation. New York, Hafner Publishing Company, p. 785.

Waring, G. H. 1983. Horse Behavior: the Behavioral Traits and Adaptations of Domestic and Wild Horses, Including Ponies. Park Ridge, NJ, Noyes Publications, p. 292.

Warren, J. M., Abplanalp, J. M., and Warren, H. B. 1967. The development of handedness in cats and rhesus monkeys. In Early Behavior, Comparative and Developmental Approaches, H. W. Stevenson, E. H. Hess, and H. L. Rheingold, eds. New York, John Wiley and Sons.

West, M. 1974. Social play in the domestic cat. Am. Zool. 14:427-436.

Wever, E. G., Vernon, J. A., Rahm, W. E., and Strother, W. F. 1958. Cochlear potentials in the cat in response to high-frequency sounds. Proc. Natl. Acad. Sci. USA 44:1081-1090.

White, S. D. 1990. Naltrexone for treatment of acral lick dermatitis in dogs. J. Am. Vet. Med. Assoc. 196 (7):1073-1076.

Wilbur, R. H. 1976. Pets, pet ownership and animal control: social and psychological attitudes, 1975. Proc. Natl. Conf. Dog and Cat Control:21-34.

Wilson, E. O. 1975. Sociobiology. Cambridge, MA, The Belknap Press, p. 697.

ISBN 0-8138-2114-2

90000>